MENTAL HEALTH CARE IN THE COLLEGE COMMUNITY

Editors

JERALD KAY
Department of Psychiatry, Boonshoft School of Medicine, Wright State University, Dayton USA

VICTOR SCHWARTZ
Yeshiva University and Albert Einstein College of Medicine New York USA

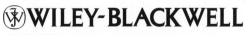

A John Wiley & Sons, Ltd., Publication

This edition first published 2010,
© 2010 John Wiley & Sons Ltd.

Wiley-Blackwell is an imprint of John Wiley & Sons, formed by the merger of Wiley's global Scientific, Technical and Medical business with Blackwell Publishing.

Registered office
John Wiley & Sons Ltd, The Atrium, Southern Gate, Chichester, West Sussex, PO19 8SQ, United Kingdom

Other Editorial Offices:
9600 Garsington Road, Oxford, OX4 2DQ, UK
111 River Street, Hoboken, NJ 07030-5774, USA

For details of our global editorial offices, for customer services and for information about how to apply for permission to reuse the copyright material in this book please see our website at www.wiley.com/wiley-blackwell

The right of the author to be identified as the author of this work has been asserted in accordance with the Copyright, Designs and Patents Act 1988.

All rights reserved. No part of this publication may be reproduced, stored in a retrieval system, or transmitted, in any form or by any means, electronic, mechanical, photocopying, recording or otherwise, except as permitted by the UK Copyright, Designs and Patents Act 1988, without the prior permission of the publisher.

Wiley also publishes its books in a variety of electronic formats. Some content that appears in print may not be available in electronic books.

Designations used by companies to distinguish their products are often claimed as trademarks. All brand names and product names used in this book are trade names, service marks, trademarks or registered trademarks of their respective owners. The publisher is not associated with any product or vendor mentioned in this book. This publication is designed to provide accurate and authoritative information in regard to the subject matter covered. It is sold on the understanding that the publisher is not engaged in rendering professional services. If professional advice or other expert assistance is required, the services of a competent professional should be sought.

The contents of this work are intended to further general scientific research, understanding, and discussion only and are not intended and should not be relied upon as recommending or promoting a specific method, diagnosis, or treatment by physicians for any particular patient. The publisher and the author make no representations or warranties with respect to the accuracy or completeness of the contents of this work and specifically disclaim all warranties, including without limitation any implied warranties of fitness for a particular purpose. In view of ongoing research, equipment modifications, changes in governmental regulations, and the constant flow of information relating to the use of medicines, equipment, and devices, the reader is urged to review and evaluate the information provided in the package insert or instructions for each medicine, equipment, or device for, among other things, any changes in the instructions or indication of usage and for added warnings and precautions. Readers hould consult with a specialist where appropriate. The fact that an organization or Website is referred to in this work as a citation and/or a potential source of further information does not mean that the author or the publisher endorses the information the organization or Website may provide or recommendations it may make. Further, readers should be aware that Internet Websites listed in this work may have changed or disappeared between when this work was written and when it is read. No warranty may be created or extended by any promotional statements for this work. Neither the publisher nor the author shall be liable for any damages arising herefrom.

Library of Congress Cataloguing-in-Publication Data

Textbook of college mental health / edited by Jerald Kay and Victor Schwartz.
        p. ; cm.
  Includes bibliographical references and index.
  ISBN 978-0-470-74618-9 (pbk.)
 1. College students–Mental health–Textbooks. I. Kay, Jerald. II.
Schwartz, Victor, 1955
 [DNLM: 1. Mental Health Services–organization & administration. 2. Student
 Health Services–organization & administration. 3. Students–psychology.
 4. Universities–organization & administration. 5. Young Adult. WA 353 T355 2010
  RC451.4.S7T49 2010
  616.890084'2–dc22

                                                                2009054235

A catalogue record for this book is available from the British Library.

ISBN: 978-0-470-74618-9

Set in 10/12 pt, Times Roman by Thomson Digital, Noida, India
Printed and bound in Singapore by Fabulous Printers Pte Ltd

02 2011

The cover photograph features the campus of Washington University in St. Louis and is reproduced courtesy of Joe Angeles, WUSTL Photo Services

Contents

Preface

Under the rubric of "no good deed goes unpunished", one of us (J.K.) volunteered for the American Psychiatric Association Task Force on College Mental Health, met the other (V.S.), and soon thereafter became the chair of the organization's newly formed Committee on Mental Health on College and University Campuses. Without significant experience in college mental health, this appointment mandated a crash course in all aspects of college mental health. A rapid immersion into the literature and journals in this field revealed few books on the "nuts and bolts" of campus mental health services. The necessary establishment of new collegial relationships with those devoting their professional careers to caring for students in higher education soon followed. Many of these new colleagues in psychiatry, psychology, counseling, social work, medicine, law, and administration, have authored chapters in the *Mental Health Care in the College Community*. They are members of many professional organizations including:

- The American College Counseling Association (ACCA)
- The American College Health Association (ACHA)
- The American College Personnel Association (ACPA)
- The American Psychiatric Association (APA)
- The American Psychological Association (APA)
- The Association for University and College Counseling Center Directors (AUCCCD)
- The Jed Foundation (JED)
- Group for the Advancement of Psychiatry (GAP)
- The Judge David L. Bazelon Center for Mental Health Law
- The National Association of Student Personnel Administrators (NASPA)
- The National Institute on Alcohol Abuse and Alcoholism.

This book then grew out of the recognition of a need for a helpful resource for those currently working in various capacities within and associated with college mental health and for those graduate and professional students fortunate enough to have educational and training experiences in these clinical sites. The former categories include, but are not limited to, health and mental health clinicians, administrators, deans, security personnel, chaplains, and coordinators or directors of professional training programs. Members of the latter category are of keen interest to the editors and authors of this book since we are all committed to the education and training of a new cadre of professionals who will address the ever growing needs of caring for undergraduate and graduate students. (This is of particular importance to the editors' field since there are insufficient numbers of psychiatrists currently working in college mental health.) The subjects of the chapters in this new book, therefore, reflect the scope of roles and functions of many college mental health services. The intent of the editors, is to provide a broad based treatment of the programmatic complexities and challenges facing those responsible for significant aspects of the welfare and wellbeing of today's college and university students.

Although ultimately the readers must judge, we believe there are a number of novel aspects to the *Mental Health Care in the College Community*. First, significant attention has been paid to the attractiveness and contributions of the community mental health and public health models. Given the overwhelming data supporting increased need for many aspects of college mental health, it is prudent to examine the overarching conceptualizations upon which college mental health services have been built. Many of the contributing authors come from very large and prestigious institutions of higher education with enormous responsibilities for the welfare and well being of their students. Some care for populations that exceed the size of many cities and towns in this country and most. Although there is the question of whether increasingly ill students are being treated across the country, there is no disagreement about the heightened concern for student and campus safety that has emerged in the past several years evoked, in part, by the tragedies at Virginia Tech and Northern Illinois University. We are obligated, therefore, to examine the helpfulness of the public health and community mental health experience.

Second, the editors need not convince the readers of this new book about the enduring importance of research. A number of chapters in the book address research challenges and important new research findings. Attention is also devoted to the importance of conducting, and how to conduct, research within the college mental health service. This information should be of interest to those administrators and mental health professionals currently working in campus mental health but also highlights our need to provide research opportunities and mentoring to the graduate and professional students whose clinical training we supervise.

Third, many of the authors of this book are clinician–educators. From reviewing the literature and in speaking with our contributing authors, we perceive there is a need for a book that addresses the clinical and educational experiences of trainees in psychiatry, psychology, counseling, and social work. We have devoted chapters which we hope are accessible and helpful for our students. In these chapters, we have discussed not only issues specific to each discipline, but also important multidisciplinary skills and attitudes required for successful collaboration.

Fourth, although there is the inevitable overlap of edited volumes, we have tried to ensure that each chapter can stand on its own. Many, in fact, augment each other, especially in the areas of public health, service system planning and organization, crisis intervention, research, and of course, clinical education and training. Chapters on innovative programs and approaches have been included as well as a concise overview of the central ethical and legal issues inherent in the provision of clinical services to students. Given the persistent challenges of student alcohol and substance abuse/dependence as well as the less frequent, but no less important, problem of student suicide and violence, we have attempted to include broad coverage of these topics. Throughout the book, we have been careful to provide helpful resources about available programs and foundations supporting college mental health. Because many students elect to study abroad, we invited a chapter on what every student should know, at least regarding UK schools, about mental health resources when they become international students.

We wish to thank Joan Marsh, Associate Publishing Director, and Fiona Woods, our Project Editor, at Wiley-Blackwell. When initially approached with the idea of a book about college mental health, Joan became quite enthusiastic and recognized the need for such a volume.

Above all, readers will undoubtedly appreciate, as we have, the willingness of so many talented contributors who have shared their vast knowledge accumulated over many years at prominent institutions and organizations. We have found the experience of developing this book very rewarding because of the outstanding cooperation and collaboration of the contributors. Since this is the first of what we hope will be many iterations of the *Mental Health Care in the College Community*, we invite readers to inform us about what additional topics would be appropriate for future editions.

JERALD KAY MD
VICTOR SCHWARTZ MD

List of contributors

Paul Barreira MD
Director, Behavioral Health and
Academic Counseling,
Harvard University Health Service,
75 Mt. Auburn Street, Cambridge,
MA 02138, USA

Karen Bower JD
Senior staff Attorney, Judge David L.
Bazelon Center for Mental Health Law,
1101 15th Street, NW, Ste. 1212,
Washington DC 20005, USA

Chris Brownson PhD
Director, Counseling and Mental Health
Center, Clinical Associate Professor,
Department of Educational Psychology,
The University of Texas at Austin,
1 University Station, A3500, Austin,
TX 78712, USA

David A. Davar PhD
Director of Counseling,
Jewish Theological Seminary,
3080 Broadway,
New York, NY 10027, USA

Laurie Davidson MA
Campus Program Manager,
Suicide Prevention Resource Center,
Education Development Center, Inc.,
55 Chapel St., Newton, MA 02458, USA

Gregory T. Eells PhD
Associate Director, Gannett Health
Services, Director, Counseling &
Psychological Services, Gannett Health
Services, Cornell University, Ithaca,
NY 14853-3101, USA

Richard J. Eichler PhD
Director, Counseling and Psychological
Services, 8th Floor, Lerner Hall, 2920
Broadway, Mail Code 2606, Columbia
University, New York NY 10027, USA

Beverly J. Fauman MD
Associate Professor, Department
of Psychiatry, Director, House Officer
Mental Health Program, Director,
Medical Student Mental Health
Program, University of Michigan School
of Medicine, Department of Psychiatry,
1500 East Medical Center Drive,
Ann Arbor, MI 48109, USA

Rachel Lipson Glick MD
Clinical Professor, Associate Chair
for Clinical and Administrative Affairs,
Department of Psychiatry,
University of Michigan Medical School,
1500 E. Medical Center Drive, SPC 5295,
Ann Arbor, MI 48109-5295, USA

Director, Psychiatric Emergency Services,
University of Michigan Health System,
1500 E. Medical Center Drive, SPC 5295,
Ann Arbor, MI 48109-5295, USA

Kristine Girard MD
Associate Chief of Mental Health, MIT
Medical and Clinical Instruction of
Psychiatry, Harvard Medical School,
E23-368, 77 Massachusetts Avenue,
E23-368, Cambridge, MA 02139-4301,
USA

Paul Grayson PhD
Director, Counseling and Psychological
Services, Marymount Manhattan
College, 221 E. 71st St., New York,
NY 10021, USA

Ralph W. Hingson ScD, MPH
Boston University School of Public
Health, 715 Albany St., Boston,
MA 2118, USA

Marta J. Hopkinson MD
Director of Mental Health, Assistant
Director, University Health Center,
University of Maryland, University
Health Center, 2134 Health Center,
College Park, MD 20742, USA

Jerald Kay MD
Professor and Chair, Department of
Psychiatry, Boonshoft School of
Medicine, Wright State University, East
Medical Plaza, 627 S. Edwin Moses Dr,
Dayton, OH 45408, USA

Joanna H. Locke MD, MPH
Program Consultant, The Jed
Foundation, 220 Fifth Avenue, 9th
Floor, New York, NY 10001, USA

Mark Phippen Pg Dip Couns
BACP Senior Accredited Practitioner,
Head of Counselling, Cambridge
University Counselling Service,
2-3 Bene't Place, Lensfield Road,
Cambridge CB2 1EL, UK

Robert A. Rando PhD
Director, Counseling and Wellness
Services, Associate Professor, School of
Professional Psychology, Wright State
University, 053K Student Union, 3640
Colonel Glenn Highway, Dayton,
OH 45435, USA

Victor Schwartz MD
University Dean of Students, Yeshiva
University, Associate Professor of
Clinical Psychiatry and Behavioral
Science, Albert Einstein College of
Medicine, 500 W.185th St., New York,
NY 10033, USA

Lorraine D. Siggins MD
Chief Psychiatrist & Director,
Mental Health and Counseling Center,
Yale University Health Services,
Clinical Professor of Psychiatry, Yale
University School of Medicine, 17
Hillhouse Avenue, PO Box 208237,
New Haven, CT 06520, USA

Morton M. Silverman MD
Senior Advisor, Suicide Prevention
Resource Center, Education Development
Center, Inc., 4858 S. Dorchester Avenue,
Chicago, IL 60615-2012, USA

Malorie Snider
Harvard University Health Service,
75 Mt. Auburn Street, Cambridge,
MA 02138, USA

Aaron White PhD
Assistant Research Professor, Duke
University Medical Center, Department
of Psychiatry, Box 3374, Durham,
NC 27710, USA

1 The Rising Prominence of College and University Mental Health Issues

Jerald Kay

Department of Psychiatry, Boonshoft School of Medicine, Wright State University, Dayton, OH, USA

1.1 Introduction

Throughout parts of the Western World, the increasing visibility of college and university mental health issues has been the result of both unfortunate and fortunate circumstances. In the former category, belong the tragedies of isolated students and the murder-suicides on two particular American campuses. Both of these are rare occurrences within the general population and equally so on the campuses of higher learning. However, within the recent past, a number of student suicides have received broad exposure in the media within the United States. Suicides at prominent universities [1,2] have highlighted the inadequacies of mental health services [3], institutional policies [4], and important ethical and legal concerns [5]. The mass shootings at Virginia Tech on April 16, 2007 [6] followed by the February 14, 2008 incident at Northern Illinois University [7] gripped the attention of the public. Fortunately, clinical and epidemiological research, accompanied by innovative programmatic development, has provided a more comprehensive appreciation of the scope of the issues. Scientific advances in the diagnosis and treatment of mental disorders have undoubtedly permitted some students, who heretofore would not have attended college, to do so. The development of more effective mental health care through advances in psychotherapy and psychopharmacology enables many teenagers to achieve a degree of emotional stability necessary for college and success in their studies and social–emotional development. Increasingly sophisticated college mental health services have ensured continuity of care for these students as well as providing assistance to a growing population of students presenting with new problems after matriculation.

1.2 How Prevalent are Emotional Disturbances and Mental Disorders?

Mental disorders, for the most part, are disorders of young people and many tend to be lifelong. (Figure 1.1 illustrates high-risk periods for psychopathology). More is now known

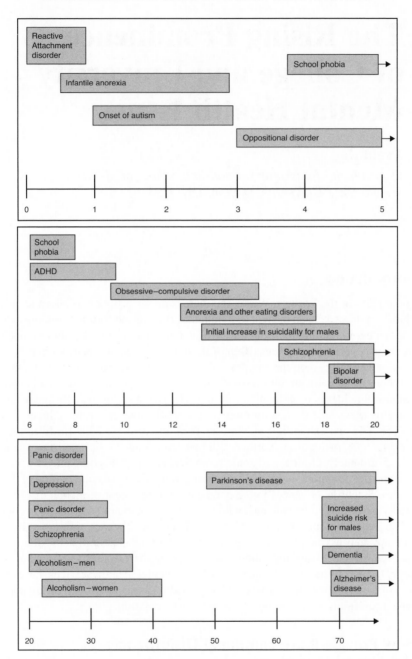

Figure 1.1 *Development of psychopathology. Mrazek DA [9] A psychiatric perspective on human development. In* Psychiatry, *3rd edn (eds A Tasman, J Kay. JA Lieberman, MB First and M Maj). John Wiley & Sons, New York, NY. pp. 97–108, with permission.*

about the vulnerability to and the onset of mood and anxiety disorders, for example, even within grade school children. College mental health clinicians know that the number of matriculating students with a history of mental health treatment and those who enter college on psychotropic medication and/or require ongoing psychotherapy has increased dramatically. One significant pressure on college mental health services therefore, can be attributed to this student population. However, the increased need for mental health services is much broader [8].

1.2.1 Student Surveys

Epidemiological studies of the prevalence of mental health issues among college students are becoming more scientifically rigorous. Some of these will be briefly described shortly. (For an in depth discussion of surveys and research initiatives see Chapter 16.) However, much of the early and continuing indications of increasing college mental health problems have been elucidated by two significant survey mechanisms. The first survey is one conducted annually since 2000 by the American College Health Association (ACHA). Of the approximately18 million students enrolled in the US, the ACHA National College Health Assessment reported on nearly 95 000 student responses during the year 2006 [10]. This survey indicated the percentage of students reporting the following conditions/disorders:

- Anorexia 1.8%

- Anxiety 13.4%

- Bulimia 2.2%

- Depression 18.4%

  - 14.8% of students said they had been diagnosed with depression sometime in their lives

  - 26% of those diagnosed with depression were receiving psychotherapy

  - 36.6% of those diagnosed with depression were taking medication

  - 1.3% made at least one suicide attempt

  - 9.3% considered suicide within the last school year

  - 17.8% experienced depression within the last school year

- Seasonal affective disorder 7.7%

- Substance abuse problems 4.0%.

To place these findings in perspective, only back pain, allergy problems, and sinus infection were reported more frequently than depression. These findings did not change substantially in the spring of 2008 report surveying 80 121 students [11]. This most recent report found that at least once in the past year, 63% of students felt hopeless, 93% felt overwhelmed, 91% felt exhausted (not from physical activity), 79% felt sad, and 45% felt so depressed it was difficult to function.

Figures 1.2–1.5 provide a graphic view of the changes in the numbers of students responding to questions about depression and treatment from 2000 to 2007.

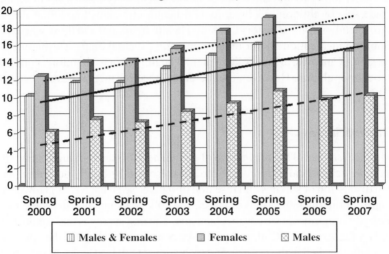

Figure 1.2 *American College Health Association/National Health Assessment, Summarized Mental Health Data and Trends, Spring 2000–Spring 2007.*

The Healthy Minds Study group at the University of Michigan published a number of recent reports utilizing self-report measures such as the Patient Health Questionnaire (PHQ-9), a widely adopted depression screening tool in primary care medicine ([12] illustrated in Figure 1.6). A random sample of approximately 2800 students at a large state university, with demographic characteristics similar to the national student population, completed a web-based survey that found a prevalence of any depressive (major depression/ dysthymia) or anxiety disorder (panic/generalized anxiety disorders) of 15.6% for under- graduates and 13% for graduate students [13]. Students were also queried about mental

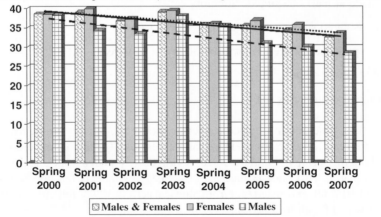

Figure 1.3 *American College Health Association/National Health Assessment, Summarized Mental Health Data and Trends, Spring 2000–Spring 2007.*

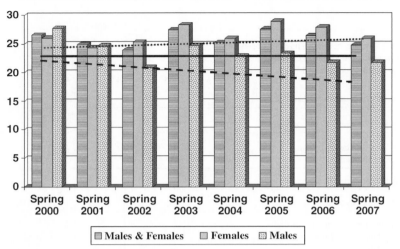

Figure 1.4 *American College Health Association/National Health Assessment, Summarized Mental Health Data and Trends, Spring 2000–Spring 2007.*

health service utilization within the previous year. Fifteen percent of respondents received psychotropic medication or psychotherapy (9% were prescribed medication). However, only 36% of those students with positive screens for major depression sought help. A second report [14] found that over 50% of students suffered from at least one mental health problem at baseline and that this persisted in 60% of this group 2 years later, yet only one half of this second group received mental health services during the 2-year period. Self-injurious

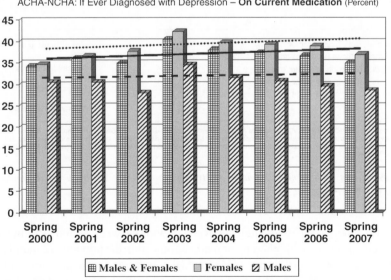

Figure 1.5 *American College Health Association/National Health Assessment, Summarized Mental Health Data and Trends, Spring 2000–Spring 2007.*

PATIENT HEALTH QUESTIONNAIRE (PHQ-9)

NAME: _____   DATE:_____

Over the *last 2 weeks,* how often have you been bothered by any of the following problems? (use "✓" to indicate your answer)	Not at all	Several days	More than half the days	Nearly every day
1. Little interest or pleasure in doing things	0	1	2	3
2. Feeling down, depressed, or hopeless	0	1	2	3
3. Trouble falling or staying asleep, or sleeping too much	0	1	2	3
4. Feeling tired or having little energy	0	1	2	3
5. Poor appetite or overeating	0	1	2	3
6. Feeling bad about yourself – or that you are a failure or have let yourself or your family down	0	1	2	3
7. Trouble concentrating on things, such as reading the newspaper or watching television	0	1	2	3
8. Moving or speaking so slowly that other people could have noticed. Or the opposite – being so fidgety or restless that you have been moving around a lot more than usual	0	1	2	3
9. Thoughts that you would be better off dead, or of hurting yourself in some way	0	1	2	3

add columns: _____ + _____ + _____

TOTAL: _____

10. If you checked off *any* problems, how *difficult* have these problems made it for you to do your work, take care of things at home, or get along with other people?	Not difficult at all _____
	Somewhat difficult _____
	Very difficult _____
	Extremely difficult _____

PHQ-9 is adapted from PRIME MD TODAY, developed by Drs Robert L. Spitzer, Janet B.W. Williams, Kurt Kroenke, and colleagues, with an educational grant from Pfizer Inc. For research information, contact Dr Spitzer at rls8@columbia.edu. Use of the PHQ-9 may only be made in accordance with the Terms of Use available at *http://www.pfizer.com.* Copyright ©1999 Pfizer Inc. All rights reserved. PRIME MD TODAY is a trademark of Pfizer Inc.

Figure 1.6 *Patient Health Questionnaire (PHQ-9). Spitzer RL, Williams JB, Kroenke K et al. Copyright © 1999 Pfizer Inc.*

behavior was reported by 7% of students over a previous 4-week period [15]; but, only one quarter received either psychotherapy or medication within the previous 12 months. Finally, the most recent report from this group [16] found that students with depression characterized by loss of interest and pleasure in activities were twice as likely to drop out of college. Those students with both depression and anxiety were noted as well to have significantly lower grade point average (GPA).

The College Screening Project at Emory University also utilized the PHQ-9 module for depression, accompanied by additional questions on anxiety, suicidal ideation, self-harm behavior, and past suicide attempts [17]. Of 729 respondents, 16.5% acknowledged a previous suicide attempt or self injurious episode, with 11.1% admitting suicidal ideation within the previous 4 weeks. Not surprisingly, those students with higher depression scores on the PHQ-9 reported more suicidal ideation. Of those with moderately severe to severe depression and those experiencing suicidal thoughts, more than 80% were receiving no treatment.

Lastly, 26 000 undergraduate and graduate students from 70 institutions, each with an average enrollment of nearly 18 000, responded to a web-based questionnaire from the National Research Consortium of Counseling Centers in Higher Education. The Survey of College Student Suicidality found 6% percent of undergraduates and 4% of graduate students seriously considered suicide in the previous 12 months [18]. For the majority of these students, suicidal thoughts were fleeting and lasted no longer than one day. However, of those who experienced a recent suicidal crisis, more than 50% sought no help. This study again supports the finding of low mental health utilization by struggling students.

1.2.2 Counseling Director Surveys

The second long-standing survey, The National Survey of Directors, has been conducted annually since 1981 by Dr Robert Gallagher. A limited number of Canadian and American administrative heads of colleges and universities participate in this survey. Some of the relevant findings [19] from the most recent report of 284 participants, representing 3 441 000 students, include:

- 9% of students (310 000) sought counseling in the past year
- 29.6% of students (about 1 million) were seen in other contexts such as workshops, orientations, class presentations
- 60% of campuses have psychiatric services but often with insufficient psychiatric consultation hours
- 16% of center patients are referred for psychiatric evaluation
- 26% of center patients are on psychotropic medication, an increase from 9% in 1994 and 20% in 2003
- 93% of directors reported an increased number of matriculants on medications
- 95% of directors acknowledge greater patient acuity leading to
  - 64% reporting staff burnout
  - 64% reporting shortages during peak times
  - 62% reporting decreased focus on students with normal developmental concerns
  - 33.5% reporting premature termination of treatment
- Directors report nearly 50% of patients have severe psychological problems
  - 7.5% of students have serious impairment that requires leave or continuation only with extensive psychological/psychiatric treatment

- 53% of directors report an increase from the previous year in self injury

- 35.6% of directors noted an increase in students with eating disorders from the previous year

- 25.4% reported an increase in sexual assault cases compared to previous year

- 2075 students hospitalized (average of 8.2 students per school)

- 118 student suicides

• Other stresses reported by directors include

- 67% report increase in crisis counseling

- 66.5% report challenges in finding long-term treatment resources

- 59.5% report growing service demand without increase in resources

- 81% report significant increase of consultation requests from concerned faculty about troubled students.

1.2.3 Toward a More Rigorous Assessment of the Mental Health of College Students

Surveys have played an important role in identifying concerns about the mental health of college students. However, surveys have inherent limitations. In those recent studies relying on screening instruments such as the PHQ-9, symptoms, even when measured with validated instruments, are not equivalent to establishing clinical diagnoses and may not consider contextual issues in the college and university settings [20]. For example, many students become symptomatic secondary to short-lived situational and developmental crises. As well, nearly all of the surveys ascertained only the presence of a limited number of disorders. Cross-sectional studies can provide only associational patterns and not causality. Some surveys may not be representative of the national college mental health picture since study participation by institutions was not random. Moreover, some colleges may join studies because of problems unique to their campuses. Lastly, no studies have included community samples or non-college attending comparison groups. Nevertheless, in reviewing numerous investigations, between 12% and 18% of college students appear to meet diagnostic criteria for mental disorders [21]. How accurate is this finding?

Some findings from a very recent report from the Center for the Study of Collegiate Mental Health [22] are summarized in Table 1.1. The report is a significant contribution since student patients, not the entire student population, provided responses.

Table 1.1	Selected data from the CSCMH Pilot Study

90% of patients had counseling before college, 18% during college and 15% both
10% of patients prescribed medication before college, 14% during and 11% both
5% of patient experienced psychiatric hospitalization before college, 14% during and 1% both
7% of patients admitted to strong fears of losing control acting violently
1% of patients acknowledging binge drinking did so 10 or more times in preceding 2 weeks

Center for the Study of Collegiate Mental Health 2009.

At the end of 2008, an article appeared in the *Archives of General Psychiatry*, which reported on 12-month prevalence rates of psychiatric disorders and mental health utilization rates in college-aged individuals [23]. From the 43 000 participants in the 2001–2002 National Epidemiological Survey on Alcohol and Related Conditions (NESARC), data was abstracted for a subsample of 5092 young adults between the ages of 19 and 25. A group of nearly 2200 college students (studying full-time or part-time within the previous year) was compared to a peer group of approximately 2900 not attending college [24]. What distinguishes this study from previously described ones is:

- Face-to-face interviews administered by trained non-clinicians

- Use of a reliable and valid structured clinical interview based on Diagnostic and Statistical Manual-IV (DSM-IV) criteria

- Assessment for a broad range of psychopathology including:

  - Substance abuse disorders (alcohol and drug abuse or dependence and nicotine dependence)

  - Mood disorders (major depression, dysthymia, and bipolar disorder)

  - Anxiety disorders (panic, social anxiety, generalized anxiety disorders and specific phobia)

  - Lifetime history of conduct and selected personality disorders (paranoid, schizoid, antisocial, histrionic, obsessive-compulsive, dependent, and avoidant disorders)

  - Assessments of stressful life events

  - Specification of sociodemographic characteristics.

Stressful life events were assessed through the 12-item Social Readjustment Rating Scale that examined boyfriend or girlfriend relationship breakup, separation, divorce, and death of a spouse. Mental health service utilization was defined as receiving treatment within the past 12 months for a mood and or anxiety disorder either through hospitalization, emergency department visit, or medication. Substance abuse treatment included being seen by a professional or paraprofessional, inpatient or outpatient treatment (including detoxification, rehabilitation, methadone maintenance, emergency department/crisis center visit, or self-help group). Table 1.2 summarizes some of the psychopathology and treatment findings

Table 1.2	Mental health of college students and their non-college-attending peers	
Disorder	**College**	**Non-college**
Any psychiatric diagnosis	45.79%	47.74%
Any Axis I disorder	39.84%	41.98%
Any mood disorder	10.62%	11.86%
Alcohol use disorder	20.37%	16.98%
Personality disorder	17.68%	21.55%
Avoidant:	2.31%	4.61%
Dependent	0.51%	1.29%
Obsessive Compulsive	8.24%	8.0%
Paranoid	4.86%	8.74%
Schizoid, histrionic, and antisocial	4.7%	8.51%

Modified from Blanco *et al. Archives of General Psychiatry* 65:1429–1437.

from this study employing the National Institute on Alcohol Abuse and Alcoholism Alcohol Use Disorder and Associated Disabilities Interview Schedule [25]. It is important to note that this report did not provide prevalence rates for borderline and narcissistic personality disorders, both of which are challenging treatment conditions in college mental health. However, two recent reports on the Wave 2 National Epidemiologic Survey on Alcohol and Related Conditions, which included 34 653 face-to-face structured interviews of adults using DSM criteria found a 6% lifetime prevalence rate (7.7% men versus 4.8% women) for narcissistic personality disorder with considerable psychosocial disability among men [26]. In addition, there was significant comorbidity in terms of past-year, co-occurrence of substance abuse, major depressive, borderline personality, anxiety, and other personality disorders. The same authors also noted 5.9% prevalence of borderline personality disorder with no gender difference but considerable psychosocial disability among women (Wave 2 National Epidemiologic Survey on Alcohol and Related Conditions) [27].

1.2.4 Alcohol and Substance Use

From a developmental point of view, it is not surprising that alcohol and substance use are so common among college and university students. Late adolescence and early adulthood for many, although not all, is a time for experimentation in this area. However, for some students this evolves into alcohol and substance abuse and dependence. One of the more striking findings in the study by Blanco *et al.* [23] was the higher number of college students, compared to their non-college attending peers, who met criteria for alcohol use disorder. Moreover, college students with drug and alcohol abuse are less likely to receive treatment. One likely reason for this latter finding may be the social acceptance of alcohol and drug use within the campus culture. It is possible students with significant problems are more reluctant to seek treatment for fear of being stigmatized. The National Center on Addiction and Substance Abuse Study (CASA) [28] supported other reports in finding that college students have higher rates of alcohol or drug addiction than the general public: 22.9% of students met the medical definition for alcohol or drug abuse or dependence compared with 8.5% of the general population 12 and older. Despite educational and outreach programs, the percentage of students who reported binge drinking (defined as having five drinks for male students and four drinks for female students during one "drinking occasion" during the previous two weeks) held steady at approximately 40%. The CASA study noted also that in 2003, 83% of all campus arrests involved alcohol. Other findings from this study period of 1993–2005 included:

- Students who abused painkillers (Percocet, Vicodin, OxyContin) during the past month rose from fewer than 1% in 1993 to 3.1% in 2005

- Students reporting smoking marijuana heavily – at least 20 days during the preceding month – more than doubled from 1.9% to 4%

- Students reporting illegal drug use other than marijuana, such as cocaine or heroin, increased from 5.4% to 8.2%.

There is some indication that binge drinking may occur in the context of drinking games and that women appear to have higher blood alcohol levels than their male peers when they

Table 1.3	College alcohol study

Consolidation of 14-year surveys of 120–140 representative 4-year campuses
Binge drinking defined as ≥ 5 drinks for men and ≥ 4 for women on a single occasion in a 2-week period
44% of students reported binge drinking and this was associated with
   Missing class
   Falling behind in school work
   Less studying and lower grades
   More likely when drinking to get in trouble with police
   Engage in unprotected and impulsive sexual activity
Colleges with high levels of binge drinking associated with greater levels of sexual assault
Among students who drive
   13% (2 million students) drove after binge drinking
   23% (3 million students) rode with intoxicated or high driver
60% of binge drinkers met alcohol abuse criteria
20% met criteria for alcohol dependence criteria
Fewer than 25% acknowledged having an alcohol problem
Banning alcohol on campus/dormitories reduced binge drinking risk
Fraternity and sorority membership in freshman increased risk

From Wechsler, H. And Nelson, T.F. (2008) What we have learned from the Harvard school of public health college alcohol study: Focusing attention on college student alcohol consumption and the environmental conditions that promote it. Journal of Studies on Alcohol and Drugs, 69(4):481–490.

attended theme parties [29]. Similarly, it may be that students celebrating their 21st birthday are incorporating more severe alcohol use, as reported at one large southeastern university. Table 1.3 illustrates a recent study [30] that examined binge drinking as detailed in numerous surveys from 120 to 140 representative 4-year campuses utilizing the same criteria as that used in the CASA study.

In short, it is fair to say that, despite significant programmatic efforts, there appear to be few gains in this arena. The Amethyst Initiative, supported initially by approximately 100 college presidents, is an attempt to bring attention to the problem of alcohol on campus through proposing a drop in drinking age from 21 to 18. This group advocates that binge drinking would be decreased with a change in drinking age laws [31].

Increasing stimulant abuse among college students has been the subject of considerable discussion. DeSantis *et al.* [32] reported, that among 1800 students at a large public institution, 34% acknowledged illegal use of stimulants prescribed for the treatment of attention deficit– hyperactivity disorder (ADHD). Many students use these medications to combat fatigue and to study more effectively. Stimulants are readily available on most campuses. Often they are procured from peers with prescriptions for bona fide diagnoses of ADHD. The use of cognitive enhancers is gaining rapid acceptance among students as well as scientists and this practice is the subject of debate by neuroethicists [33].

1.3 Study Limitations

The data from the reviewed studies can, for the most part, present a cross-sectional approach to college student stresses and psychopathology. Nothing can be said of the fate of either after graduation. There are few rigorous, long-term prospective studies, such as that by Vaillant [34], that follow graduates through succeeding phases of life. Indeed, much of what occurs in undergraduate and graduate students must be understood within the context and ethos of the educational experience. This includes issues of alcohol abuse, traumatic experiences, depression and suicidality, to name but a few. (Chapter 5 addresses limitations of self-report measures in greater detail.)

The NESARC study delineates precipitants of emotional difficulties such as a breakup in a dating relationship, marital separation, divorce, or the death of a spouse consistent with significant findings from psychiatric research. Kendler's work in 1995 [35], for example, has demonstrated similar results in adults regarding when individuals are likely to have a major depression as well as what individual genetic characteristics confer greater vulnerability. Individuals with a particular configuration of serotonin genetics require fewer life stresses before developing depression [36]. The NESARC study cannot elucidate the duration of personality disorders diagnosed in surprisingly high numbers of college students. Anecdotally, a number of college mental health clinicians have raised question about the prevalence of obsessive compulsive personality disorder found in this study since most studies support borderline, narcissistic, and antisocial personality disorders as being more prevalent. Could this be a reflection of the academic challenge faced by some students in particularly competitive disciplines? It is clear now, that some personality disorders are not as enduring as once believed [37,38], which invites the question about the time limited contribution of central developmental challenges faced by many college students.

1.4 A Developmental Approach to College Mental Health

1.4.1 Psychosocial Developmental Considerations

Eichler [39] has written about the helpfulness of a developmental approach to college counseling from a psychodynamic perspective. Adolescence is often characterized as the second separation-individuation phase referring to the heightened quest for independence from parents and the establishment of a career trajectory. Although a life-long process, the consolidation of one's self perception is an important developmental task at this age. The ability to initiate and sustain mature, sexual, and loving relationships is yet another aspect of this phase influenced dramatically by earlier interpersonal relationships or the lack of them. Students entering college with few successful relationships are expectedly vulnerable to the challenges of the college years. Such students tend not to be open to new social opportunities, for they are experienced as threatening, which in turn limits social and emotional growth during the years of higher education. Not only may such students be unsuccessful in new relationships; they may not be open to new ideas. Both can limit the college experience significantly.

However, it must be remembered that despite movement away from the nuclear family in one sense, connectedness to one's family must also be maintained. Indeed, most late adolescents enjoy a satisfying relationship with their parents and end up adopting values similar to those held by their parents. This is not to say that some students continue to master these issues in college through inconsistent or charged relationships with professors, administrators, and of course, therapists.

Eichler correctly notes that this ongoing challenge can be seen in the ambivalence which characterizes some therapist-patient relationships. Nearly one fifth of students fail to keep a second appointment at the college mental health service and more than 40% of student treatments were characterized by therapists as having prematurely terminated [40]. Parenthetically, this phenomenon can be especially challenging to student or resident therapists who do not adopt a developmental orientation and who invariably anticipate all college students will be highly intelligent and motivated for treatment.

Indeed, it is often helpful to view therapy for some students as episodic in nature with return to treatment as determined by the student. This is not a novel idea. Many clinicians from differing perspectives emphasize that psychotherapeutic work proceeds during times of hiatus from treatment, often leading to periods of consolidation and integration of gains. Eichler advocates that the central task of therapists is to adopt a developmental view such that interventions, be they brief by default or time limited through planning, promote developmental plasticity at times when students face challenges and stresses. In other words, what can often be most helpful is supporting student strengths during stressful times to promote their mastery of conflict, thereby permitting continued psychological development. Eichler reminds that many students experiencing immobilization from a problem rely on turning the passive into the active. That is, for many students mastery is acquired through action-oriented new initiatives. Some of these may be unhelpful but they can nevertheless be learning experiences if understood within the context of a treatment experience.

This is not to say that interpretive work should not be conducted as appropriate. All therapies reside on a continuum between expressive and supportive orientations depending on the needs of the patient. The college mental health service is a rewarding experience for many therapists who provide, for example, brief dynamic psychotherapies based on a central issue [41], core conflictual relationship theme [42] or cynical maladaptive behaviour [43].

Last, since it has been emphasized that a growing number of students are matriculating with previous psychiatric disorders and treatment experiences, the Jed Foundation and the American Psychiatric Foundation are now addressing the developmental task of transition from high school to college [44]. In addition to the many opportunities for psychosocial and intellectual growth in the college experience, the project reminds that for the vulnerable entering student, the challenges can be overwhelming. However, among students without a previous mental health history, these challenges can precipitate the onset of new disorders. The two organizations are assembling free guides for students and parents to raise awareness around the potential stresses in adapting to college that will encourage the utilization of mental health resources. Concerns about this period in life are also supported, for example, by The High School Youth Risk Survey [45] which has demonstrated the following:

- more than 28% of 13 600 students reported sadness and hopelessness every day for more than 2 weeks

- suicidal ideation is experience by nearly 20%

- specific suicide plans had been made by approximately 15%.

- suicide attempts had been acknowledge by almost 9% of the respondents.

1.4.2 Biological Developmental Considerations

That brain development continues into the third decade of life was unappreciated until recently. Brain structure, it was argued previously, was essentially determined by age three with maturational consolidation completed prior to adolescence. Moreover, 95% of brain cells were considered formed by age 6. It is clear now that the adolescent brain is more precisely a brain in transition and that there are ongoing changes in neuronal circuitry postpubertally. The most significant of these changes are central to the development of higher-order cognition and emotionality and therefore are found in the prefrontal and temporal cortices, the hippocampus and the amygdala. The last structure is considered to be the gateway for emotion, providing affective valence to events that are remembered either within or outside of awareness. It also modulates the storage and strength of memories. The hippocampus is the most central learning and memory structure. Neuronal plasticity is best exemplified in the processes of learning and memory which involve the creation of new genetic material and enhancement of neuronal connectivity. Hippocampal activity changes both brain structure and function through the creation of neurons. In addition, each day approximately 1000 new neurons are created chiefly in the hippocampus and, although their function is not totally clear, it may be that these neurons play an important role in learning through providing temporality to memories. The maturation of the prefrontal cortex is essential in cognitive processing and executive functioning (e.g. abstract reasoning, self awareness, attention). It is clear that maturation, as exemplified by neuronal pruning and growth in myelinization, occurs last in the prefrontal cortex, implying earlier less effective executive functioning. Figure 1.7 illustrates this process.

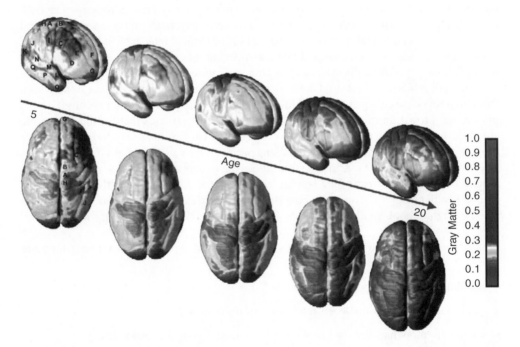

Figure 1.7 *Brain mapping. This is a study of cortical gray matter (GM) development in children and adolescents by using a brain-mapping technique and a prospectively studied sample of 13 healthy children (4–21 years old), who were scanned with magnetic resonance imaging every 2 years for 8–10 years. Because the scans were obtained repeatedly on the same subjects over time, statistical extrapolation of points in between scans enabled construction of an animated time-lapse sequence ("movie") of pediatric brain development. GM development in childhood through early adulthood is non-linear and progresses in a localized, region-specific manner coinciding with the functional maturation. Regions associated with more primary functions (e.g. primary motor cortex) develop earlier compared with the regions that are involved with more complex and integrative tasks (e.g. temporal lobe and prefrontal cortex). Gogtay, N., Giedd, J.N. (2004) Structural magnetic resonance imaging of the adolescent brain.* Annals of the New York Academy of Sciences, **1021**, 77–85.

Last, ADHD, an exceptionally common clinical diagnosis among college students, is characterized by a delay of approximately 3 years in cortical maturation during childhood and adolescence [46]. Even by the ages of 18–20, the thickness of the cortices in those with ADHD is demonstrably less than those without this diagnosis.

There are additional changes to the brain that are worth noting. First, neurotransmitter alterations in dopamine in certain areas are inextricably linked to the modulation of rewarding stimuli. Fluctuations in dopamine, therefore, may be relevant in understanding the frequency of novelty seeking, alcohol and substance abuse, and other high-risk behavior among college students [47]. Greater appreciation of the neurobiology of risk taking has highlighted the health paradox of adolescence. Simply stated, adolescence is the physically healthiest time in the life span, characterized, for example, by increased strength, reasoning capacity, and immune function; yet the overall morbidity and mortality rates increase 200% from childhood to late adolescence [48]. Moreover, the most important contributors to this increase are those related to problems with control of behavior and emotion as manifested in accidents, suicide, violence, mental illness, and risky behavior. Future research must explore the contribution of the immaturity of frontal and temporal lobes to this paradox. Second, it may be that the gradual increase in adolescence of the stress hormone cortisol might explain why some vulnerable students develop emotional or psychiatric difficulties in college [49]. In summary, the relationship between brain development, as observed in structural and functional changes related to learning, and social and emotional development is intriguing.

1.4.3 Toward an Integrative Approach

What is the impact of binge drinking, estimated to be beyond 40% of students in some surveys, on the development of alcohol dependence or personality and brain development? A small study has found white matter abnormalities as demonstrated through functional magnetic resonance imaging and diffusion tensor imaging in teens who binge drink [50]. These findings complement previous work demonstrating teens who binge have less ability to retrieve information (Figure 1.8) [51,52]. In short, although it is true that the human brain

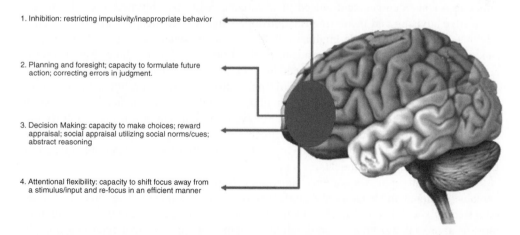

1. Inhibition: restricting impulsivity/inappropriate behavior

2. Planning and foresight; capacity to formulate future action; correcting errors in judgment.

3. Decision Making: capacity to make choices; reward appraisal; social appraisal utilizing social norms/cues; abstract reasoning

4. Attentional flexibility: capacity to shift focus away from a stimulus/input and re-focus in an efficient manner

Figure 1.8 *The role of the prefrontal cortex in executive functions. Based on data from Brown, S., McGue, M., Maggs, J., et al. (2008). Components of executive and sample behaviors. A developmental perspective on alcohol and youths 16 to 20 years of age. Pediatrics, Suppl 4, S290–S230.*

is characterized by its neuroplasticity, it is also true that advances have explicated the sensitivity of the brain to cumulative insults from use of hallucinogens, marijuana, cocaine, and other substances [53–55]. Imaging studies have demonstrated both structural and functional changes in the brain that have significant and enduring effects [56]. It appears, as well, that teens are particularly susceptible to sleep deprivation and that this condition influences not only learning but has significant impact on resiliency. It is likely that insufficient sleep in adolescence may play an important role in aggression, impulsivity, and affect regulation [48].

It is clear that the most accurate model for appreciating human development is based on gene–environment interaction. For example, it is widely accepted that an increasing number of matriculating students enter college with previous treatment experiences. This includes psychotherapy and or psychotropic medications. Yet other students who have suffered childhood maltreatment, but have never received help, bring with them a vulnerability to a number of disorders and often problem situations. The enduring effect of attachment disorders secondary to loss and trauma in their parents' earlier lives is substantial and colors the manner in which such students experience themselves and the world around them. These include the ability to establish intimate and trusting relationships and the constant re-enactment of earlier disappointing relationships. This re-enactment is most frequently characterized by repeated self-defeating behaviors, which may take the form of conflicts about achievement and success in college. In addition, these students are more at risk for mood, anxiety, and eating disorders. Certain ubiquitous behaviors addressed in many of the reviewed surveys will have very different meaning to the student with previous experience of childhood maltreatment and other psychological trauma [57]. In a very different way, the developmental issues facing young adult combat veterans returning to college in increasing numbers will be similar to their non-veteran peers but may also include challenges of integrating previous unfortunate experiences, which may affect learning and socialization.

The same may be said of graduate students, and some professional students, who often experience different stresses by virtue of their age, marital status, family burden, indebtedness, and chosen area of study [58]. The success of those graduate students pursuing science degrees, and indeed their careers, is inextricably tied to establishing a productive advising and mentoring relationship. This often challenging process is generally not one faced by undergraduate students. The persistent pressure of developing successful scientific studies that result in publication as well as teaching responsibilities are other situations often not experienced by undergraduate or medical students unless the latter are enrolled in combined MD–PhD programs. Finally, many medical specialties have noted the unusual developmental challenges faced in 6 year medical schools where students are accepted to medical school directly from high school. Because of curricular time constraints these students take fewer liberal arts courses in the first two years of their equivalent undergraduate phase and have less time for certain social experiences taken for granted by other college students.

In short, neither genetics nor environmental experiences are sufficient in themselves to explain emotional and behavioral disorders among college students. The forces impacting on a student's well being and adjustment to higher education are complex and, therefore, must be appreciated from an overarching developmental approach that addresses both the brain and the mind.

1.5 Ethical and Legal Issues

This chapter began by noting the rising prominence of college mental health issues particularly in the US. Most of this can be attributed to rare, but rather dramatic, large-scale tragedies eventuating in the deaths of many. However, a small number of high profile student suicides also alerted college and university administrators of the need for more clearly articulated policies that respected student needs. As an example, given the frequency of depression on campuses, the practice of suspending all suicidal students has been criticized widely. Because of liability concerns, many institutions insisted on this practice that, in many situations, is short sighted regarding the impact on the student. Chapter 7 will address these issues in detail. In short, accessibility, adequacy and fiduciary responsibility of and for mental health services, health insurance, and confidentiality have been under review.

1.6 Conclusion

This chapter has summarized some of the key issues facing college students and college mental health service providers as indicated in national surveys and epidemiological studies. Only recently has the developmental, clinical, and administrative complexity of these issues been explicated. Higher education is now aware of the need to establish student access to a broad range of services both on campus and off campus, create sophisticated educational programs that address the ubiquity and destigmatization of mental illness and provide accurate and responsible legal and ethical college mental health policies, all within a context of adequate resources. It is clear that much more research is needed in all aspects of college mental health. Moreover, education of mental health professionals from many disciplines will become increasingly critical in ensuring adequate numbers of well-trained clinicians to care for the undergraduate and graduate students in the future.

References

1. Sontag, D. (2002) Who was responsible for Elizabeth Shin? New York Times Magazine.
2. Hegranes, C. (2004) Walking the edge: NYU confronts its suicide problem, Village Voice, September 14, 2004.
3. Voelker, R. (2003) Mounting student depression taxing campus mental health services. *The Journal of the American Medical Association*, **289**, 2055–2056.
4. Appelbaum, P. (2006) Law and Psychiatry: Depressed? Get Out!: Dealing with suicidal students on college campuses. *Psychiatric Services*, **57**(7), 914–916.
5. Lake, P. (2008) Still waiting: The slow evolution of the law in light of the ongoing student suicide crisis. *Journal of College and University Law*, **34**(2).
6. Virginia Tech Review Panel (2007) Mass Shootings at Virginia Tech: Report of the Review Panel, August 2007.
7. Friedman, E. (2008) Who was the Illinois school shooter? http://abcnews.go.com/US/story ?id=429698 &page=3 Accessed March 24, 2008.
8. Benton, S.A., Robertson, J., Tseng, W. *et al.* (2003) Changes in counseling client problems across 13 years. *Professional Psychology: Research and Practice*, **34**(1), 68–72.
9. Mrazek, D.A. (2008) A psychiatric perspective on human development, in *Psychiatry*, 3rd edn (eds A. Tasman, J. Kay, J.A. Lieberman *et al.*), John Wiley & Sons, New York, NY, pp. 97–108.

10. American College Health Association (2007) American College Health Association-National College Health Assessment: Reference Group Executive Summary Fall 2007. Baltimore: American College Health Association: 2008.

11. American College Health Association (2009) College Health Assessment Spring 2008 Reference Group Data Report (Abridged). *Journal of American College Health*, **57**(5), 485.

12. Spitzer, R.K., Williams, J.B.W., Kroeneke, K. *et al.* (1999) Patient Health Questionnaire (PHQ-9). Copyright © 1999 Pfizer Inc. All rights reserved.

13. Eisenberg, D., Gollust, S.E., Golberstein, E. and Hefner, J.L. (2007) Prevalence and correlates of depression, anxiety and suicidality among university students. *American Journal of Orthopsychiatry*, **77**(4), 534–542.

14. Zivin, K. *et al.* (2009) Persistence of mental health problems and needs in a college student population. *Journal of Affective Disorders*, **117**(3), 180–185.

15. Goullust, S.E., Eisenberg, D., and Golberstein, E. (2008) Prevalence and correlates of self-injury among university students. *Journal of American College Health*, **56**(5), 491–498.

16. Eisenberg, D., Golberstein, E., and Hunt, J. (2009) Mental health and academic success in college. *The B.E. Journal of Economic Analysis and Policy*, **9**(1), (Contributions), Article 40.

17. Garlow, S.J., Rosenberg, J., Moore, J.D. *et al.* (2008) Depression, desperation, and suicidal ideation in college students: Results from the American Foundation for Suicide Prevention College Screening Project at Emory University. *Depression Anxiety*, **25**(6), 482–488.

18. Drum, D.J., Brownson, C., Denmark, A.D. and Smith, S.E. (2009) New data on the nature of suicidal crises in college students: Shifting the paradigm. *Professional Psychology: Research and Practice*, **40**(3), 213–222.

19. Gallagher, R.P. (2008) National Survey of Counseling Center Directors. The American College Counseling Association. The International Association of Counseling Services, University of Pittsburg, Series 8Q.

20. Eisenberg, D., Golberstein, E., and Gollust, S.E. (2007) Help-seeking and access to mental health care in a university student population. *Medical Care*, **45**(7), 594–601.

21. Mowbray, C.T., Mandiberg, J.M., Stein, C.H. *et al.* (2006) Campus mental health services: Recommendations for change. *American Journal of Orthopsychiatry*, **76**(2), 226–237.

22. Center for the Study of Collegiate Mental Health (CSCMH) (2009) *CSCMH Pilot Study: Executive Summary*, Pennsylvania State University, PA.

23. Blanco, C., Okuda, M., Hasin, D.S. *et al.* (2008) Mental health of college students and their non-college-attending peers. *Archives of General Psychiatry*, **65**(12), 1429–1437.

24. Grant, B.F., Moore, T.C., and Kaplan, K. (2003) *Source and Accuracy Statement: Wave 1, National Epidemiological Survey on Alcohol and Related Conditions (NESARC)*, National Institute on Alcohol Abuse and Alcoholism, Bethesda, MD.

25. Grant, B.F., Hasin, D.S., Stinson, F.S. *et al.* (2004) Prevalence, correlates, and disability of personality disorders in the United States: Results from the national epidemiologic survey on alcohol and related conditions. *Journal of Clinical Psychiatry*, **65**(7), 948–958.

26. Stinson, F.S., Daswon, D.A., Goldstein, R.B. *et al.* (2008) Prevalence, correlates, disability, and comorbidity of DSM-IV narcissistic personality disorders: Results from the Wave 2 national epidemiologic survey on alcohol and related conditions. *Journal of Clinical Psychiatry*, **69**, 1033–1045.

27. Grant, B.F., Chou, S.P., Goldstein, R.B. *et al.* (2008) Prevalence, correlates, disability, and comorbidity of DSM-IV borderline personality disorder: Results from the Wave 2 National Epidemiologic Survey on Alcohol and Related Conditions. *Journal of Clinical Psychiatry*, **69**(4), 533–545.

28. Casacolumbia.org Website (2008) CASA 2007 Teen Survey Reveals America's Schools Infested with Drugs. National Survey of American Attitudes on Substance Abuse XII: Teens and parents. The National Center on Addiction and Substance Abuse at Columbia University. Retrieved April 27, 2009 from http://www.casacolumbia.org/absolutenm/?a=499.

29. Clapp, J.D., Ketchie, J.M., Reed, M.B. *et al.* (2008) Three exploratory studies of college theme parties. *Drug and Alcohol Review*, **27**(5), 509–518.
30. Wechsler, H. and Nelson, T.F. (2008) What we have learned from the Harvard school of public health college alcohol study: Focusing attention on college student alcohol consumption and the environmental conditions that promote it. *Journal of Studies on Alcohol and Drugs*, **69**(4), 481–490.
31. Wbztv.com Website (2008) 100 College presidents support lower drinking age. Retrieved April 27, 2009 from www.wbztv.com/local/lower.drinking.age.2.798486.html.
32. DeSantis, A.D., Webb, E.M. and Noar, S.M. (2008) Illicit use of prescription ADHD medications on a college campus: A multimethodological approach. *Journal of American College Health*, **57**(3), 315–324.
33. Talbott, M. (2009) Brain gain. The underground world of "neuroenhancing" drugs. New Yorker Magazine April 27, pp. 32–43.
34. Vaillant, G.E. (1977) *Adaptation to Life*, Little, Brown, Boston, MA.
35. Kendler, K.S. (1995) Stressful life events, genetic liability, an onset of an episode of major depression in women. *American Journal of Psychiatry*, **152**, 833–842.
36. Caspi, A., Sugden, K., Moffitt, T.E. *et al.* (2003) Influence of life stress on depression: Moderation by a polymorphism in the 5-HTT gene. *Science*, **301**(5631), 386–389.
37. Zanarini, M.C., Frankenburg, F.R., Hennen, J., and Silk, K.R. (2003) The longitudinal course of borderline psychopathology: 6-year prospective follow-up of the phenomenology of borderline personality disorder. *American Journal of Psychiatry*, **160**, 274–283.
38. Roninnstam, E. (2005) Narcissistic personality disorder: A review, in *Psychiatry-Personality Disorders*, vol. 8, The World Psychiatric Series, Evidence and Experiences (eds M. Maj, H. Askikal, K. Mezzich and A. Okasha), John Wiley & Sons, UK Chichester, New York, pp. 277–327.
39. Eichler, R. (2006) *Developmental Considerations* (eds P. Grayson and P.W. Meilman), College Mental Health Practice, New York: Routledge, pp. 21–41.
40. Hatchett, G.T. and Park, H.L. (2004) Revisiting relationships between sex-related variables and continuation in counseling. *Psychological Reports*, **94**(2), 381.
41. Mann, J. (1973) *Time-Limited Psychotherapy*, Harvard University Press, Cambridge, MA.
42. Luborsky, L. (1984) *Principles of Psychoanalytic Psychotherapy: A Manual for Supportive–Expressive Treatment*, Basic Books, New York.
43. Strupp, H.H. and Binder, J.L. (1984) *Psychotherapy in a New Key: A Guide to Time-Limited Dynamic Psychotherapy*, Basic Books, New York.
44. The Jed Foundation (2009) The Transition Year Project. http://www.jedfoundation.org/programs/transition-year-project ©.
45. Grunbaum, J.A., Kann, L., Kinchen, S.A. *et al.* (2002) Youth risk behavior surveillance – United States.
46. Shaw, P., Eckstrand, K., Sharp, W. *et al.* (2007) Attention-deficit/hyperactivity disorder is characterized by a delay in cortical maturation. *PNAS*, **104**(49), 19649–19654.
47. Spear, L.P. (2002) The adolescent brain and the college drinker: Biological basis of propensity to misuse alcohol. *Journal of Studies on Alcohol*, **63**(2), 571–582.
48. Dahl, R.E. (2008) The neurobiology of risk taking in adolescents: Implications for psychiatric disorders. In The American College of Psychiatrist 2008: Annual Meeting and Pre-Meeting Program Book.
49. Spear, L.P. (2000) Neurobehavioral changes in adolescence. *Current Directions in Psychological Science*, **9**(4), 111–114.
50. McQueeny, T., Schweinsburg, B.C., Schweinsburg, A.D. *et al.* (2009) Altered white matter integrity in adolescent binge drinkers. *Alcoholism, Clinical and Experimental Research*, **33**(7), 1278–1285.
51. Zeigler, D.W., Wang, C.C., Yoast, R.A. *et al.* Council on Scientific Affairs, American Medical Association (2005) The neurocognitive effects of alcohol on adolescents and college students. *Preventive Medicine*, **40**(1), 23–32.

52. Brown, S.A., McGue, M., Maggs, J. *et al.* (2008) A developmental perspective on alcohol and youths 16 to 20 years of age. *Pediatrics*, **121**(Suppl 4), S290–S310.
53. Jacobus, J., Bava, S., Cohen-Zion, M. *et al.* (2009) Functional consequences of marijuana use in adolescents. *Pharmacology, Biochemistry, and Behavior*, **92**(4), 559–565, Epub 2009 Apr 5.
54. Ashtari, M., Cervellione, K., Cottone, J. *et al.* (2009) Diffusion abnormalities in adolescents and young adults with a history of heavy cannabis use. *Journal of Psychiatric Research*, **43**(3), 189–204.
55. Jager, G., de Win, M.M., van der Tweel, I. *et al.* (2008) Assessment of cognitive brain function in ecstasy users and contributions of other drugs of abuse: Results from an FMRI study. *Neuropsychopharmacology*, **33**(2), 247–258, Epub 2007 Apr 25.
56. Schweinsburg, A.D., Nagel, B.J., Schweinsburg, B.C. *et al.* (2008) Abstinent adolescent marijuana users show altered fMRI response during spatial working memory. *Psychiatry Research*, **163**(1), 40–51.
57. Wright, M.O., Crawford, E. and Del Castillo, D. (2009) Childhood emotional maltreatment and later psychological distress among college students: The mediating role of maladaptive schemas. *Child Abuse and Neglect*, **33**, 59–68.
58. Toes, J., Lockyer, J., Dobson, D.S., Simpson, E. *et al.* (1997) Analysis of stress levels among medical students, residents, and graduate students at four Canadian schools of medicine. *Academic Medicine*, **72**(11), 997–1002.
59. American College Health Association, (2007) College Health Assessment Spring 2006 Reference Group Data Report (Abridged). *Journal of American College Health*, **55**(4), 204.
60. Gogtay, N., Giedd, J.N. (2004) Structural magnetic resonance imaging of the adolescent brain. *Annals of the New York Academy of Sciences*, **1021**, 77–85.

2 History of College Counseling and Mental Health Services and Role of the Community Mental Health Model

Paul Barreira and Malorie Snider

Behavioral Health and Academic Counseling, Harvard University Health Service, Cambridge, MA, USA

2.1 Introduction

Colleges are confronted with the challenge to provide comprehensive mental health and counseling services to a growing number of students. By every measure, the number of students seeking counseling and mental health services is increasing. While many explanations are offered to account for this increase in demand, there is no doubt about the consequences: neither the scope nor the structure of traditional services is adequate to meet the level of need. As a result, many counseling and psychological programs feel pressured to abandon or drastically reduce education, prevention, outreach, and more traditional counseling in order to provide clinical care. The dilemma is further complicated by the unique history of the development of college counseling and mental health services. On most campuses counseling evolved from the traditional role of student adviser, both academic and vocational. The function eventually became professionalized through academic training in counseling psychology. Still, the emphasis was on developmental and academic counseling with a clear distinction between clinical counseling or therapy [1]. Clinical or psychiatric services were available through consultation with off campus resources. On a minority of campuses mental health services were established within the student health services following the predominant clinical model of the time. Until recently, on many campuses the two systems existed in parallel, with distinct models of service delivery, budgets, and staff, but overlapping client populations.

In the absence of a conceptual model that helps to explain the need for retaining education, prevention, developmental counseling and psychiatric treatment, it is likely that some services will be provided at the expense of others. It is also likely that the increased pressure to provide services and the absence of a more comprehensive model increases the growing tension between disciplines (counselors versus clinical psychologists and

Mental Health Care in the College Community   Edited by Jerald Kay and Victor Schwartz
© 2010 John Wiley & Sons, Ltd.

psychiatrists), as well as debates about the best models to understand and serve students (developmental versus clinical).

This chapter describes the evolution of campus counseling center and mental health services and presents the case that a community mental health model offers the potential to reconcile the conflict between the two approaches by presenting a coherent model that integrates and validates the strengths of each. The community mental health model embraces developmental, educational, and clinical perspectives to support the well-being of an entire population. We will present the basic principles of the community mental health model and demonstrate its applicability to the college community.

2.2 Early Development of College and University Counseling Centers and Mental Hygiene Programs: Pre-1945

It is difficult to identify the establishment of the first college counseling center, however students in the early 1900s received support from a variety of individuals who called themselves "counselors", "advisors", "student personnel workers", "vocational guidance workers", or "mental hygienists". This eclectic group of individuals described helping students with educational, vocational, financial, moral, and personality problems that interfered with students' academic progress. The earliest example of counseling functions being organized into a separate service occurred in 1932 when the University of Minnesota established the University Testing Bureau. Throughout the 1930s counseling institutions as centers for vocational and academic advising emerged on several Midwestern university campuses. During this period the terms vocational counseling, counseling, and student personnel were often used interchangeably. As quoted in Heppner [2], Brotemarkle wrote in 1936,

> the psychologist, the physician, the psychiatrist, the mental hygienist, the sociologist, for that matter the butcher, the baker and the candlestick maker, each took his turn at claiming. . .that he was the one and only individual to deal with student problems.

In 1939 Williamson recommended the establishment of trained professionals called "clinical counselors". Throughout this period the primary role of counseling centers and counseling psychology was to support the growth and development of students, primarily through vocational counseling. These services were typically located within the academic affairs office of the college, rather than in distinct student health services.

The first recorded appearance of a mental health care service in a college setting was in 1910, with the formation of a small mental hygiene clinic by Dr Stewart Paton at Princeton University. Paton, a psychiatrist and lecturer in neurobiology, became interested in the emotional problems of undergraduates who reportedly flocked to his clinic. As Prescott [3] notes, the growth and development of mental health clinics was in large part a response to the post-war concern that widespread psychological vulnerability amongst college-aged men could weaken the nation's military capabilities; however, these early mental health clinics' mission extended well beyond the production of able-minded soldiers. Dr Paton, who later served in World War I, argued that colleges and universities had not provided students an education that prepared them to withstand the strain and stress of modern life. He hypothesized that other forms of extreme stress, besides war, had the potential to induce a state of psychological disturbance akin to the "shell-shock" observed in traumatized soldiers. In order to address this concern, he emphasized the importance of fostering emotional stability and resilience against many forms of stress in the college's students. In 1920 after two cadets died from suicide, the US Military Academy at West Point hired a psychiatrist, Dr Harry Kerns, to provide clinical care and to study the causes of common maladjustments amongst the cadets. Over the next two decades, a growing number of colleges and universities would follow Princeton's lead by incorporating mental hygiene clinics into their own systems of student health care [3]. These first college and university mental health services were established on the principles of the mental hygiene movement and staffed by psychiatrists and clinical psychologists.

The mental hygiene movement began in 1909 when the National Committee for Mental Hygiene was founded [4]. As described by the Committee's founder, Clifford Beers [5], the primary objective of mental hygiene was to imbed the psychiatric patient within a community-based support system that "would become an unfailing source of information, advice, and comfort" as the individual sought to recover from or to cope with his/her mental health struggles.

In order to create such a system, Beers [5] and his Committee identified six specific goals for the movement. As described in Beers's groundbreaking work *A Mind that Found Itself*, the mission of the movement was to:

1. "work for the protection of the mental health of the public"

2. "help raise the standard of care for those threatened with nervous or mental disorder"

3. "promote the study of mental disorders in all their forms and relations and to disseminate knowledge concerning their causes, treatment and prevention"

4. "obtain from every source, reliable data regarding conditions and methods of dealing with mental disorders"

5. "enlist the aid of the Federal Government"

6. "coordinate the work of existing agencies and to help organize in each state. . .an allied but independent Society for Mental Hygiene".

Within these stated objectives, we can already begin to identify many of the theoretical principles that underlie modern psychiatric practice, particularly within the public sector. Principles including concern for public health, regular monitoring of quality of care, the importance of research and public education, the development of evidence-based treatments, and the responsibility of the government to provide assistance to the disabled and the ill all played substantial roles in defining the theoretical foundations of the Mental Hygiene movement. These principles guided the formation of the first college and university mental hygiene clinics which were located in student health services and would later hold an equally defining position within the theory of community mental health.

2.3 Professionalism and Response to Increase in Student Enrolment

It was not until the mid-1940s, following the nation's experience in World War II, that mental health services truly became a common feature of American colleges and universities.

Millions of returning veterans, who had no signs of previous mental health problems, suffered from serious emotional problems that were understood to stem from the stresses of war. The ability to successfully treat many of these soldiers in the field and the recognition of the need to help soldiers deal more competently with stress encouraged psychiatrists and psychologists to increase mental health services first in the military but also on college campuses. President Truman's Commission on Higher Education concluded that colleges and universities should not only train the intellect, but "make growth in emotional and social adjustment one of its major aims" [6]. In response to the commission report, the newly established Group for the Advancement of Psychiatry (GAP) formed a committee to study college mental hygiene. The first report of the committee, "The Role of Psychiatrists in Colleges and Universities", challenged colleges and universities to "broaden their educational concepts to include the attainment of emotional maturity in addition to the normal goal of intellectual development" [7].

In line with the principles of the Mental Hygiene Movement, college and university counseling centers and mental health services began to emphasize the primary importance of prevention over other forms of intervention. Central to the foundation of these services was the idea that psychological disturbance was produced through a combination of developmental and contextual factors and that this disturbance could be prevented or reduced through manipulation of these factors [7]. The main focus of college mental health thus became developmental rather than clinical. McClusky [8] summarized this ideology in 1949:

> Clinical services to children and youth in schools and colleges will always be important, but in a sense they will always be peripheral because by definition the basic concern of mental hygiene is not remediation but prevention and facilitation.

For this reason, in many universities the task of promoting student mental health became the responsibility of the general "counseling center" rather than student health or psychiatric services. Within 20 years, a significant number of schools had expanded their counseling centers to incorporate "personal adjustment counseling"; though the scope and utilization of these new services remained limited in comparison to vocational counseling [2] Despite these limitations, the expansion of the college counseling center to include services for individuals experiencing social and emotional stress, as well as academic problems, played an important role in defining a new form of mental health service, distinct from the clinical focus of conventional psychiatry.

With the publication of the *Diagnostic and Statistical Manual I* (DSM-I), the official diagnostic manual for psychiatry, in 1952, the line between clinical and counseling models of service delivery became less distinct [9]. The DSM-I emphasized the role of development in determining mental health and emotional problems. All major psychiatric conditions, including depression, anxiety, and personality disorders, were labeled "reactions", suggesting that they developed in response to social and other external forces. While the fundamental distinction between a model that emphasized strength and normal development (hygiology) in contrast to a model that emphasized diagnosis (pathology) persisted, the DSM-I explanatory model for psychiatry offered common ground for responses to individuals in emotional distress. In future decades this common ground would disappear as the diagnostic criteria in successive versions of the DSM become more medical and de-emphasized social and developmental contributions to common psychiatric conditions.

One result was a further polarization of counseling and psychiatric services. With this polarization the value of a community mental health model to guide the organization of counseling and mental health services to college and university students diminished.

2.4 Formalization of Roles and Attention to Developmental Issues and Prevention

A number of organizational and professional developments helped to solidify the identity of the field of counseling psychology and promote the growth of college counseling centers. For example, the American Psychological Association changed the title of Division 17 from Counseling and Guidance to Counseling Psychology in 1952. In 1954 the *Journal of Counseling Psychology* was first published. The American Board of Examiners in Professional Psychology changed the name of its diploma from "Counseling and Guidance" to "Counseling Psychology" [2]. In 1955 Donald Super published a paper that described the transition from vocational guidance to counseling psychology which articulated the distinction between counseling psychology and clinical psychology [10]. In recognition of the increased numbers of counseling centers as well as their expanded roles, the American Board of Counseling Services changed its mission and function and became the International Association of Counseling Services (IACS). IACS is the now the main accreditation body for college counseling centers. With the establishment of IACS as the main accreditation body for college and university counseling centers, the colleges and universities had two accreditation options: IACS for accrediting counseling centers and the Joint Commission on Accreditation of HealthCare Organizations (JACHO) for student health centers which included mental health services. The separate criteria for accreditation of counseling centers and mental health services formalized their distinct identities.

In 1950 a group of mid-western colleges and university counseling directors established the Association of College Counseling Center Directors (AUCCCD) to allow directors to discuss common organizational issues as they developed structured counseling services. The mission of AUCCCD is to assist college/university directors in providing effective leadership and management of their centers, in accordance with the professional principles and standards of Psychology, Counseling, and Higher Education. A second trade organization, American College Counseling Association (ACCA), is an organization for professionals in higher education (including colleges, universities, community and technical settings), whose professional identity is counseling and whose purpose is fostering students' development. While these two organizations helped to establish the identity of counseling centers, a separate trade organization, the American College Health Association (ACHA), was established in 1920 to serve all the health needs of students at colleges and universities, including mental health needs. As one reviews this history, it is clear that counseling centers and mental health services were two systems that developed along parallel tracks to serve broadly the emotional and psychological needs of students, but with different models of how to understand and serve students' developmental, emotional, and psychological needs.

2.5 Community Mental Health Movement

The community mental health movement informed the development of campus mental health services. While the community mental health model of psychiatric care was envisioned to meet the needs of a broader population, its principles are highly relevant to a college community.

The community mental health (CMH) model of psychiatric care developed in response to evolving twentieth century perceptions of both the nature of mental illness and the relationship between the psychiatric patient and society. Building on the ideology of the earlier mental hygiene movement, the CMH model emerged as a truly unified movement in the early 1960s.

In the 50 years following the introduction of the Mental Hygiene movement, mental health care in the United States continued to develop its identity as an increasingly community-based enterprise. Mental hygiene's emphasis on preventive efforts and positive mental health care remained a primary focus of mental health advocacy during this time, and following World War II, these principles began to garner even more widespread support amongst professional psychiatrists. The military's experiences in World War II coping with the apparent epidemic of "combat exhaustion" offered support to the idea that environmental and community factors could not only play a significant role in precipitating cases of mental illness but also in facilitating or impeding recovery [11]. As Lamb has discussed, four key factors were found to positively impact treatment efficacy. These included: proximity of treatment administration to the soldier's home-base; immediacy of treatment following the onset of symptoms; simplicity of treatment and attention to basic physical and social needs; and firm expectancy of future productivity [4]. All four of these principles (community-based treatment centers, early identification and intervention, attention to general well-being, and goal-oriented therapy) would have significant impacts on the developmental trajectory of public psychiatry in the subsequent decades.

In many ways, the earliest supporters of CMH viewed their cause as a direct outgrowth of the prior Mental Hygiene movement, and this influence was particularly pronounced in the CMH model's emphasis on primary prevention. More than a decade before the rise of CMH, the founding director of the NIMH, Robert Felix, identified prevention as one of the institution's primary objectives. "The guiding philosophy which permeates the activities of the National Institute of Mental Health", he wrote, "is that prevention of mental illness, and the production of positive mental health, is an attainable goal" [12]. CMH psychiatry sought to reduce rates of mental illness through the identification and promotion of protective factors and the reduction of exposure to risk-incurring factors. To that end, the CMH model considered preemptive and early-intervention programs as crucial to the fight against mental illness [13]. These programs employed preventive strategies and interventions with targets ranging in scope from the individual to the community and objectives ranging from the development of personal resiliency and individual coping skills, to public education in principles of mental health, to improved accessibility and expansion of supportive social institutions [11].

This last type of program (the development of supportive social infrastructure) can in fact be considered on its own as a hallmark of the CMH model of psychiatric care. From its beginnings, the CMH movement was grounded in the idea that governments and communities have a responsibility to provide for the mental well-being of their citizens and to do so in the most socially inclusive way possible. Inclusion of the non-psychiatrist in prevention and treatment of mental illness therefore developed in response to two lines of reform: social responsibility and patient-centered treatment. Viewed from the perspective of social responsibility, community involvement in these processes may be understood as a response to the emerging idea of a shared burden of care. This notion of shared responsibility found expression in a wide range of social institutions, community-based organizations, and civic professions including primary care, government, the school system, law-enforcement agencies, the media, and religious leadership. Each of these institutions and professions was recognized as having a unique and important role in protecting the mental health of the community members it served. Teachers, for example, were trained in principles of child development and primary prevention, while religious leaders often served a more treatment-oriented role – acting as intermediaries between members of their congregation and mental health professionals (through referrals) and incorporating an understanding of mental health principles into their own counseling practices [14]. Beyond the question of social responsibility, the expansion of mental health services to include professionals outside the realm of psychiatry also served a very pragmatic purpose in promoting effective and inclusive care for the patient. By assigning chronically ill patients to case workers who would oversee both the acute and rehabilitative portions of their treatment, CMH systems sought to increase both continuity and comprehensiveness of care [13]. Within this integrated system, psychiatrists served a three-part role as primary-caregiver, public educator, and consultant to other members of the CMH treatment team [4].

Recalling both the pragmatic lessons of military psychiatry and the theoretical notion of community responsibility, CMH centers were to be located in the heart of the communities they served [4]. They were to provide comprehensive services, ultimately defined as including preventive services (consultation, education, developmental), acute treatment services (outpatient, emergency, short-term inpatient, pre-hospital screenings), and rehabilitative/transitional/maintenance services (elderly care, drug and alcohol programs, post-hospitalization).

2.6 An Example of the Early Application of Community Mental Health at Colleges and Universities: Dana Farnsworth

Even as the bifurcation of psychiatric and counseling services was becoming more and more defined in many areas of the country, some mental health professionals, guided by DSM-I and the community health model, advocated for a more multidisciplinary approach to university mental health care. This view was perhaps most well developed by Dana Farnsworth, MD, director of health services at Harvard and Massachusetts Institute of Technology. In a series of articles published during the 1950s, Dr Farnsworth described his vision for comprehensive university mental health care, emphasizing the critical role that the preservation and promotion of student mental health plays in facilitating the process of education. Describing mental health as a "state of mind that permits full and satisfying participation" in the opportunities one is afforded, Farnsworth argued that proper emotional adjustment serves as "a keystone in the structure of education", enabling the student "to take the greatest possible advantage of the academic, extracurricular, and environmental offerings of the university" [15,16].

For this reason, Farnsworth, like other mental health professionals of his time, emphasized the need for preventative programming – identifying community-based programming, developmental counseling and education, and interdisciplinary intervention, as particularly important components of a comprehensive mental health program. Farnsworth conceptualized the effective college community as one in which the primary focus is on strengthening student mental health in a bottom-up fashion, thereby minimizing the need for top-down efforts to correct mental illness. In this model, a significant portion of the university psychiatrist's efforts are directed toward altering environmental and social factors that contribute to the development of emotional instability and patterns of maladaptive behavior in students, and likewise, toward generating conditions that promote the development of self-esteem, social skills, and positive coping strategies [17].

In order to accomplish this seemingly Herculean task, the psychiatrist was charged with enlisting the support of other members of the college community. Specifically, Farnsworth suggested that the most effective and efficient way to influence the development of students is to incorporate the task of personal counseling into pre-existing systems of interaction, relationships, and advising. Within the college community, the fundamental relationship between professor and student was seen as particularly promising in this regard. In the ideal system of mental health care, Farnsworth argued, "the main portion of student counseling should be an integral part of the total relationship between the teacher and the student, and hence integrated with the intellectual relationships for which a college exists" [16]. For such a model to work, however, all members of the university community would need to be well versed in the principles of positive mental health and developmental counseling.

The psychiatrist thus held two additional responsibilities: public education and professional consultation. As educator, the psychiatrist would both develop a mental-health related curriculum for the edification of the student body and offer instructive programming to members of the faculty and administration in order to increase their knowledge of principles of developmental health and personal counseling and to teach them how to recognize signs of distress in their students. In particularly challenging cases, the psychiatrist would serve as a behind-the-scenes consultant to the educator-counselor, thereby providing the student with individualized professional advice, while still maintaining the counseling relationship. The consultation process would also serve a secondary teaching function, by providing the opportunity to further develop the counselor's skills, perceptiveness, and sensitivity toward his/her students [15]. Farnsworth [16] summarizes:

> The basic goal of a college mental-health service is to organize the knowledge... formulated by the psychological sciences generally and from therapeutic experiences with students specifically, in such a way as to make it useful to the teacher in his enormous responsibility of aiding the optimum development of the student.

In this sense, the psychiatrist functions as a "catalytic agent", educating the community about the importance of mental health, facilitating the formation of beneficial counseling relationships, and offering professional support and advise to administrators and faculty actively engaged in the business of counseling students [15].

In the event that these preventive efforts should prove inadequate or a student's troubles should require more intensive therapeutic intervention, the psychiatrist would assume a final role, as treatment provider and care coordinator. While Farnsworth's writings emphasize the primary importance of developmental counseling in strengthening an individual's mental health, he also stressed the need for college-based psychiatric treatment facilities and personnel to provide care for those students who experience psychiatric illness. Moreover, he suggested that these two types of mental health services should not be considered separate from one another, but rather as part of a single continuum of care. Communication between counselors and psychiatric professionals would be crucial for the referral of distressed students, the assurance of proper follow-up, the provision of appropriate accommodations, and the maintenance of continuity in the counseling relationship [15,18]. In this way, Farnsworth's model exemplified the application of community mental health principles in a university setting.

2.7 Potential Modern Applications of the CMH Model to Educational Settings

Although the current understanding of common psychiatric conditions has dramatically altered diagnosis and treatment, we believe the community mental health model remains relevant to the pressing questions of how to best organize counseling and mental health services on college and university campuses. The key principles of community mental health: community-based services for a defined population, attention to general well-being through education and prevention services, a multidisciplinary team approach, early identification and intervention, and community consultation, address the goals of a counseling psychology model, as well as the goals of a mental health service. Indeed, the basic principles articulated by Dana Farnsworth in the 1950s can easily be translated into our contemporary environment.

The first principle of the community mental health model expects services to be developed locally for a defined population. Obviously, the college/university setting provides such a well-defined population, whether it is a small college with only undergraduates or a large university with graduate and professional students. Moreover, it is quite easy to define the expected educational and developmental tasks of the student population as well as the stresses and risk-incurring factors most likely to be encountered. Finally, the incidence and prevalence of common psychiatric conditions are well-known.

Second, community mental health promotes prevention and positive mental health. The core mission of counseling psychology and many counseling centers includes support of normal development and provision of educational strategies to improve emotional and intellectual growth. In practice, all providers of counseling and mental health services, whatever their professional discipline, should share this mission. In the community mental health model, counseling and mental health services are not set in opposition to one another; rather each uses the methods and tools available to their discipline for the promotion of student well-being. Contrary to some reports, mental health services that operate in the community model do not expect students to recognize their own mental health problems [19]. Indeed, the use of on-campus screenings for alcohol and depression; the use of survey data; the proliferation of peer student groups to provide outreach to students; the use of web sites to allow students to assess their mental health; education programs (Gatekeeper Training) to residential life staff, administration, and faculty, all aim to raise community awareness of mental health issues and help the community recognize common mental health problems and connect students to appropriate services.

The third principle, which builds upon the earlier two, expects the professionals who work within the model to be able to make early identification of significant emotional problems and quickly refer students for treatment. It is implied in the model that working directly together in an integrated or closely coordinated system facilitates both identification and treatment. The more isolated the prevention and education activities are from the treatment activities, the more difficult is referral for services and coordination of care. Moreover, the involvement of clinicians in the education and prevention activities provides an important context for clinicians to understand the problems of students who are referred to them on a spectrum from normal developmental tasks to clear psychiatric conditions. The participation of all types of staff, including faculty, also allows for the earliest identification of students who require a clinical intervention.

Finally, the CMH model expects that clinicians will have expertise in providing the current standard of care for goal-oriented treatment. Staff must be able to deliver documented effective treatments for a variety of conditions including depression, obsessive–compulsive disorder (OCD), alcohol abuse, eating disorder, or trauma. The need for diagnosis specific treatments does not eliminate the potential need for developmental or educational counseling. The current literature suggests a unidirectional model: that is a student receives counseling until the identification of a "serious psychological" problem at which point there is a referral to mental health services with a subtle implication that the student never returns to counseling. The reality for most students is that successful treatment of common conditions; depression, anxiety disorders including OCD, and eating disorders, provides the student the opportunity to function normally in the educational environment which at times may include the need for counseling to deal with normal expected stresses.

The successful implementation of the community mental health model will differ depending on the size of the college or university, as well as on-campus resources. In general, larger colleges and universities have the resources to develop a "counseling and mental health service" that operates within the CMH model. Smaller colleges and universities which don't have the resources may partner with community agencies to supplement the campus programs. The impediments to implementation at the larger schools to a great extent have to do with historical circumstances and the absence of a unifying model. Mergers between counseling centers and mental health services have occurred since the 1970s. As documented by Federman and Emmerling the mergers have resulted in various outcomes: the creation of one unit at the counseling center, or one unit at the mental health center, or a mixed alternative [20]. Whatever the outcome, it isn't clear that the mergers were guided by a comprehensive model for providing the continuum of services from education, prevention to counseling and clinical treatment. Rather, the rationale is often economic; that is, a savings in dollars or administration expenses. Thus most mergers did not present a organizational structure that acknowledges the mutually complementary roles of counseling and clinical services.

2.8 Conclusion

The current pressure to address the growing number of serious problems that students bring to college is forcing counseling centers to choose between helping students with normal developmental problems, providing consultation to students, faculty, and administrators, or delivering more clinical services. This intensifies the divisions between counseling and clinical staff that we have described earlier in this chapter. The CMH model depends on the development of a multidisciplinary team approach where there is mutual participation in support of students and coordination of roles, rather than separate activities. This sense of common effort promotes the understanding that all components of the community mental health system are necessary to accomplish the main goal- the emotional growth and well-being of students. If one component is sacrificed at the expense of the other, everyone loses. Our description of the CMH model emphasizes that it is neither exclusively a clinical model nor an education/prevention model- it expects the presence of both activities.

References

1. Kirk, B.A., Free, J.E., Johnson, A.P. *et al.* (1971) Guidelines for university and college counseling services. *American Psychologist*, **15**, 724–728.
2. Heppner, P. and Neal, G. (1983) Holding up the mirror: research on the roles and functions of counseling centers in higher education. *The Counseling Psychologist*, **11**, 81–98.
3. Prescott, H.M. (2008) College mental health since the early twentieth century. *Harvard Review of Psychiatry*, **16**(4), 258–266.
4. Lamb, H.R. (1999) Public psychiatry and prevention, in *American Psychiatric Association Textbook of Psychiatry*, 3rd edn (eds R.E. Hales, S.C. Yudofsky and J.A. Talbott), American Psychiatric Press, Washington, DC.
5. Beers, C.W. (1908) *A Mind that Found Itself*, Longmans, Green, and Co., New York.
6. (1948) President's Commission on Higher Education, *Higher Education for American Democracy*, Harper & Brothers, New York.
7. Group for the Advancement of Psychiatry (1951) Committee on Academic Education. The role of psychiatrists in colleges and universities [GAP Report No. 17]. New York: GAP.
8. McClusky, H.Y. (1949) Mental health in schools and colleges. *American Educational Research Association*, 405–412.
9. (1952) *Diagnostic and Statistical Manual: Mental Disorders*, American Psychiatric Association, Washington, D.C.
10. Super, D.E. (1955) Transition: From vocational guidance to counseling psychology. *Journal of Counseling Psychology*, **2**, 3–9.
11. Grob, G. (1991) From hospital to community: Mental health policy in modern america. *Psychiatric Quarterly*, **62**(3), 187–212.
12. Felix, R. (1949) Mental disorders as a public health problem. *The American Journal of Psychiatry*, **106**, 401–406.
13. Caplan, G. (1964) *Principles of Preventive Psychiatry*, Basic Books Inc., New York.
14. Ridenour, N. (1961) *Mental Health in the United States: A Fifty-Year History*, Harvard University Press, Cambridge.
15. Farnsworth, D. (1953) Mental health-keystone of education. *The Journal of School Health*, 289–301.
16. Farnsworth, D. (1952) What is mental health in a university? *Mental Hygiene*, 34–48.
17. Farnsworth, D. (1955) Success and failure as viewed by the college psychiatrist. *New England Association Review*, 2–10.
18. Farnsworth, D. (1954) Potential problems areas of mutual interest to the dean and the psychiatrist. *Mental Hygiene*, 209–218.
19. Mowbray, C.T., Megivern, D., Mandiberg, J.M. *et al.* (2006) Campus mental health services: Recommendations for change. *American Journal of Orthopsychiatry*, **76**(2), 226–237.
20. Federman, R. and Emmerling, D. (1997) An outcome survey of mergers between university student counseling centers and student health mental health services. *Journal of College Student Psychotherapy*, **12**(1), 15–27.

3 The Reporting Structure and Relationship of Mental Health Services with Health Services

Gregory T. Eells[1] and Victor Schwartz[2]

[1]*Counseling & Psychological Services Gannett Health Services, Cornell University, Ithaca, NY, USA*
[2]*Yeshiva University Albert Einstein College of Medicine, NY, USA*

3.1 Introduction

There are a variety of reporting and administrative structures in college counseling and mental health services and they reflect the history and priorities of the Institutions of Higher Education (IHE) they serve. The structures are sometimes a byproduct of historical circumstances and at other times reflect carefully considered assessments of need. In a recent survey of 391 counseling center directors, 95% indicated that their mental health service reported within a student affairs division. This structure promotes important connections with other IHE staff who work to support students. Forty-eight percent of those directors reported to a vice president or an associate/assistant vice president of student affairs. An additional 34% reported to a dean of students or an associate/assistant dean of students. Nine percent reported to a health services director and most of the remaining respondents reported within an academic division such as psychology or counseling [1].

Reporting structures raise essential questions about the relationship of a counseling or mental health service to the university health service. The first is whether the counseling service is administratively and clinically integrated with the university health service or functions as an independent administratively parallel office. In the same survey of directors, 66.5% of counseling services fall into the latter independent category while an additional 31.4% report varying degrees of integration ranging from fully integrated (sharing the same building and administrative structures) to being partially integrated and sharing either administrative structures or space [1].

Among integrated counseling and health services there is also a variety of administrative structures. In a recent white paper that surveyed 77 health and counseling services that described themselves as integrated, four types of administrative structures were described and all of them reported within a student affairs division:

- a counseling services director reporting to a health services director (31%),

- a counseling and health service director independently reporting to student affairs while being integrated (31%)

- a health and counseling director reporting to a chief health officer (27%)

- a health services director reporting to a counseling services director who in turn reported to a senior administrator (10%) [2].

The integration of counseling and health services is an issue of considerable complexity that raises questions about the optimal ways to develop relationships between these services.

The potential advantages to developing closer working relationships and/or administratively integrating counseling and health services include providing the most comprehensive care to students, identifying campus societal and cultural shifts, aligning resources, enhancing relationships amongst clinicians that are providing care to the same students, and positioning both services well for taking leadership on campus for health and mental health issues. This chapter will review relevant literature on the integration of these services, explore a variety of administrative and clinical issues related to integrating or enhancing working relationships, and conclude with recommendations on how to improve these essential relationships.

3.2 Review of Literature

The integration and/or increased cooperation of physical and mental health services at IHEs undercuts the persistently unhelpful mind-body dualism by acknowledging the biological components of many mental health concerns, and behavioral, psychological and emotional components of most "physical" concerns. A truly biopsychosocial approach to student health and wellbeing, and indeed the entire US health care system, supports a tightly coordinated, integrated care model, which increases cost-effectiveness and reduces morbidity and mortality [3]. The majority of patient visits in primary care have some behavioral health component but not a specifically identified mental health disorders [4]. Reports from The Institute of Medicine (5,6) targeted issues of integrated care as pervasive problems within the US healthcare system. One overarching recommendation made by the IOM [6] was:

> Healthcare for general, mental and substance-use problems and illnesses must be delivered with an understanding of the inherent interaction between the mind/brain and the rest of the body (p. 9).

Despite the attractiveness of integrated care, strong empirical support for the superiority of this type of system is lacking. A meta-analysis reviewing these issues found that although integrated care sites report positive treatment outcomes (such as symptom severity, treatment response and remission), none of the studies demonstrated better clinical outcomes for integrated services when compared to non-integrated care models [7]. Walker and Collins [8] also acknowledge that the financial and organizational barriers to integrating care (such as professional identity issues, history of different systems and perspectives on confidentiality) are often serious barriers to a widespread implementation of a more integrated care model.

There are a limited number of studies examining the integration of counseling and health services in an IHE setting. More than 25 years ago, Foster [9] described the process of merging a counseling center with a comprehensive student mental health unit at a health center and highlighted the importance of the existing relationships between participating agencies, the awareness of partial interdependence amongst agencies, the resource asymmetry between the involved units, and the types of tasks to be coordinated, as keys to successful integration. Foster advocated the use of "supplemental integrating devices", such as interdisciplinary teams, clinical seminars and coordinators for research, training, and developmental services as vehicles to bring about greater integration.

Federman and Emmerling [10] conducted an outcome survey of organizational mergers between university student counseling centers and student mental health services. Statistically significant positive outcome ratings were noted in quality of clinical services, ability to meet the needs of students, and administrative structure. Most goals for change and improvement were achieved post-merger. The authors concluded that though there were some positive benefits, no specific organizational configuration was found to be more effective or desirable than any other.

An article examining the integration of physical health and mental health services at the University of Rochester, Cornell University, and Northeastern University concluded that collaboration between medical and mental heath services is essential, especially, around informed consent for referrals between services, resolving ambivalence from mental health staff, and establishing strong ties to the larger administrative structure supporting integrated care [11].

3.3 Administrative Integration Issues

3.3.1 Staff Professional Identity

Moves toward clinical and administrative integration or increased cooperation frequently raise issues of differing professional philosophy and identity which may become significant challenges. Differing models are characterized by assumptions that sometimes seem antithetical,. For example, commonly a more developmental model may appear to have values that conflict with a traditional medical model. Although, those trained in the medical and in mental health professions have similar purposes, there are subtle, unrealized differences in viewpoints that can lead to misunderstandings. Kingsbury [12], in relating his experiences as a physician and a psychologist, discussed differences in these training approaches with respect to science, case conceptualization, interdisciplinary relations, and hierarchy. He concludes that good well-meaning individuals trained from these different perspectives inevitably experience difficulty in communicating with each other and often question each other's competence and training.

One common dynamic that arises in the process of integration is the different approach to clinical services. Traditional health services often focus on obtaining a diagnosis as quickly as possible through asking specific symptom focused questions. Once accomplished, treatment often is self-evident in uncomplicated medical complaints. In mental health services, arriving at a diagnostic conclusion through unstructured interviewing may be less important initially and provides less clarity in how to respond to the student since establishing an in depth therapeutic alliance is essential.

One potential consequence of this dynamic is that counseling staff may feel devalued given the abstract nature of mental health work. This is particularly ironic given the potential for higher morbidity and mortality related to mental health issues in IHE students. There is a risk that counseling staff feel like an ancillary service such as laboratory or pharmacy rather than an essential service that is integrated into the fabric of an overall system of care. The key to successful discussions about integrating services or cooperating more closely is ensuring that professionals from each service acknowledge and value the unique perspectives and skills brought by their colleagues from different fields.

3.3.2 Mission and Vision

For services to think more deliberately about integration first requires a very intentional discussion about the vision and mission of what health and mental health services do at a particular IHE. An ACHA [2] white paper found that 43% of merged services had a shared mission statement and that the majority of the other centers in the study indicated a separate mission statements for each functional area. If counseling and health services each view themselves as devoted to being a single cooperating entity then specific practical administrative decisions flow from that shared sense of purpose. We will now turn to some of those decisions.

3.3.3 Accreditation

The extent of service integration may determine accreditation routes. If services are more separate in their mission and vision, then the counseling service is more likely to be accredited by the International Association of Counseling Services (IACS) and the health service is more likely to be accredited by either the Accreditation Association for Ambulatory Health Care (AAAHC) or by the Joint Commission on Accreditation of Health Care Organizations (JCHAO). In a survey of accredited counseling services integrated with health services, the highest percentage (33%) were accredited under AAAHC, with 15% accredited by IACS, and 12% by the JCHAO. AAAHC appears to be the most popular and most applicable accreditation for more integrated services [2].

3.3.4 Scheduling and Electronic Health Records

Decisions about software packages and electronic health records also flow from discussions about vision and mission. Service integration permits the use of a single scheduling/records software package. If the services decide to operate in a more parallel fashion, then counseling and health services will likely choose separate software packages that operate on separate servers.

3.3.5 Confidentiality

Decisions about selecting software packages for record keeping inevitably lead to concerns about confidentiality and what information counseling and medical clinicians can access in each others' records. Privacy is uppermost in the minds of students seeking counseling services (see Chapter 7). If students perceive that information from the counseling service is too easily shared with the health service, they may not be comforted by the assurance that these are administratively fused offices and have the right to share clinical information. Access to each others' records may erode student confidence in the privacy of counseling service visits

However, the reality is that these same students are sharing very private information with their medical providers and often the same or similar legal privacy protections govern the disclosure of both health and mental health information. Also, a more integrated approach can reduce the stigma that is historically associated with mental health services. Broad-based discussion about information sharing between counseling and medical staff is critical to the provision of the best possible care That information is shared between services and the nature and limits of the communication should be clearly communicated to students when this occurs.

3.3.6 Financial Support

One of the often cited benefits of integration of services is cost savings through fiscal efficiencies. Integrated services may allow for the elimination of redundancies in administrative, IT support and support staffing for both services. Contracts for electronic health records and the ordering of other supplies may be more economical when done cooperatively for both health and mental health services. Influence with the central university administration may grow as a larger integrated service speaking with one voice and being the primary advocate for health and mental health matters on campus will likely garner greater financial support. A physician executive director advocating for more social workers or psychologists for counseling services or a psychologist executive director advocating for more nursing support can be very compelling. This dynamic can reduce competition between health and mental health services in which each director is meeting with a non-clinician university administrator and advocating for the needs of their respective services.

This financial support can also play a role in the construction of a shared facility. There are many services that have constructed shared facilities across that US. Having an integrated facility can provide a single location that can work to address both individual and public health needs and can highlight that health is a core value of the IHE community.

3.4 Clinical Issues

3.4.1 Multidisciplinary Teams

A benefit of integrated services is the bringing together of medical, mental health and health promotion staff to respond to areas of common interest and concern. This section will examine the usefulness of multidisciplinary teams in addressing eating disorders, sexual health, and alcohol and other drugs.

The challenging treatment of eating disordered students requires an integrated approach. Multidisciplinary teams that meet weekly with representatives from nursing, nutrition, medicine, psychiatry, psychology and social work can coordinate care more effectively and provide a higher quality of clinical care. These teams can address family involvement in treatment, need for hospitalization, and arranging health leaves of absence.

Responding to students with sexual health issues offers another way to facilitate integrated care. Sexual health teams allow counseling staff, health promotion staff, and medical staff to take a collaborative approach in providing clinical services, student education materials, coordinated outreach, special needs, and sexual health awareness and promotion. This can take the form of information about counselling and treatment for sexual dysfunction, availability and proper use of condoms and other birth control approaches, and integrated strategies on prevention of sexually transmitted infections. Materials about sexual health and safety can be better informed by clinicians who respond to these issues and can allow for feedback to health promotion staff on areas that may need more targeted public health or educational approaches.

Clinical integration of services through multidisciplinary teams is especially helpful in addressing alcohol and other drug (AOD) issues. This approach facilitates decision making around important clinical and public health issues such as the use of programmatic efforts like the Brief Alcohol Screening and Intervention for College Students (BASICS), building and maintaining individual counseling and community referrals, and the development of recovery groups. The team approach is an effective mechanism to implement campus wide educational policy and programs; programs like AlcoholWise, an on-line substance use educational tool, and medical amnesty programs. A medical amnesty program is one that encourages students to seek appropriate help by substituting an institutional clinical response for a judicial response. For example when a student is in need of emergency transport to a hospital for substance-related issues they can request medical amnesty and receive some type of evaluation and counseling after the hospitalization rather than face some form of judicial sanction. These types of policies can be implemented with the advocacy of a well-integrated team.

3.4.2 Mental health Screening in Primary Care

Integrating counseling and health services offers an excellent pathway to reach students in distress through primary care. New York University (NYU) Health Services, which is integrated with counseling services, participates in the Breakthrough Collaborative to conduct depression screening in primary care. NYU has also involved a variety of other schools in the US to participate in this project. Inspired by recommendations of the US Preventive Services Task Force [13] that addressed under detection and inadequate treatment of depression, NYU has also involved a variety of other schools in the United States to participate in this project.

Yearly depression screening in primary care encourages medical, nursing, counseling, and health promotion staff members to collaborate and offer intervention by either primary care providers and/or care managers, provide self-help materials and identify campus resources, and conduct evaluations with referral to mental health services where appropriate.

Screening for depression in primary care also encourages implementation of other primary care screening programs in substance abuse and anxiety disorders for example. The risk of morbidity and mortality is significantly higher for students with mental health issues. The two leading causes of death in college students, accidents (often related to substance use) and suicide (www.afsp.org/files/college_film/factsheets.pdf) makes it incumbent on any IHE to provide as many opportunities to get students with mental health needs to care. As Schwartz [14] noted, approximately 80% of the completed suicides never receive counseling services and if they do receive counseling, they are six times less likely to kill themselves. If the integration of counseling and health services can help students get the care they need it can save lives.

3.4.3 *Reporting of Psychiatry Services*

Another key question is the location and availability of prescribers of psychotropic medications. In the most recent AUCCCD survey (2008) [1], psychiatry services are available only in 39% and 15% of counseling services and health services respectively. An additional 6% report the presence of psychiatry in both mental health and health services. Unfortunately, 31% of responding centers reported no access to psychiatry at all on their campuses.

Working within an integrated service, psychiatrists can have access to the essential medical workups to prescribe medication while developing a relationship and sharing information with counseling center psychotherapists. This is vital in college mental health settings where rapid assessment and treatment decisions are required. No matter where psychiatry resides administratively, a structure must be in place to facilitate interaction about shared patients with the clinicians at the counseling center.

Psychotropic medication in uncomplicated clinical situations also may be prescribed by general practitioners, nurse practitioners or supervised physician assistants located at the health service and this is the solution at many IHEs without psychiatry. Non-psychiatric clinicians can provide psychotropic medication management including refills for stabilized students. Ideally this is only done if there is capacity for consultation with a psychiatrist either on or off campus. Again, it is less important where the various clinicians reside than that there be a strong cooperative relationship between the various clinicians on campus [15].

3.5 Recommendations

1. Any discussion of the value of integrating counseling and health services should be grounded primarily in the desire to provide better care to students.

2. Any discussion about integrating services should emphasize the importance and value of the different perspectives brought to the discussion by various counseling and health professionals.

3. Discussions about integrating services should begin with discussions of shared mission and vision.

4. Issues of accreditation, scheduling and record keeping software, financial support and other administrative decisions should flow from the discussions about shared mission and vision.

5. Though there are potential benefits to the integration of health and counseling services there are also benefits and costs to these services being independent parallel services.

6. Administrative integration does not necessarily imply clinical or functional integration; nor, does integration necessarily result in cooperation.

7. No matter what model is in place, a balance must be struck between the need to share clinical information as necessary and the essential need to protect the privacy of patients and their perception of that privacy.

8. Efficiencies and cost saving opportunities do not necessarily require administrative restructuring and an integration of services will not necessarily result in these savings-

sometimes enhanced and strategic cooperation amongst departments is all that is required.

9. If changes in administrative structure are to be made, the focus should be ground up with clinicians in both counseling and health services providing a clear outline of potential benefits and concerns and a transparent discussion of whether or not the administrative change is the best way to resolve these issues.

10. Ultimately, the success or failure of any of these administrative structures has more to do with the cooperative spirit, professional collegial respect and thoughtful leadership in the various stakeholders than with the actual administrative designs.

3.6 Conclusion

This chapter has reviewed the literature on administrative and clinical issues that arise when considering integration, or enhancing relationships between these services.

As dramatic changes in the US healthcare system emerge, IHEs will be pressed to examine the potential value of these services developing closer working relationships. More IHEs are recognizing that both the physical and mental health of their students are essential to their overall mission as educational institutions and will look to counseling and health services to assume leadership on campus for health and mental health issues.

References

1. Association of University and College Counseling Center Directors (2008) Survey of Counseling Center Directors.
2. American College Health Association (2009) Integration of Counseling and Health Services on College and University Campuses. Unpublished white paper.
3. Blount, A., Schoenbaum, M., Kathol, R. *et al.* (2007) The economics of behavioral health services in medical settings: A summary of evidence. *Professional Psychology Research and Practice*, **38** (3), 290–297.
4. Kroenke, K. and Mangelsdorff, A.D. (1989) Common symptoms in ambulatory care: Incidence, evaluation, therapy and outcome. *American Journal of Medicine*, **86**, 262–266.
5. Institute of Medicine (2001) *Crossing the Quality Chasm: A New Health System for the 21st Century*, National Academies Press, Washington DC.
6. Institute of Medicine (2006) Improving the quality of health care for mental and substance use conditions, in *Committee on Crossing the Quality Chasm: Adaptation to Mental Health and Addictive Disorders*, National Academies Press, Washington DC.
7. Butler, M., Kane, R., McAlpine, D. *et al.* (2008) Integration of Mental Health/Substance Abuse and Primary Care. No. 173 (Prepared by the Minnesota Evidence-based Practice Center under Contract No. 290-02-0009.) AHRQ Publication No. 09-E003. Rockville, MD. Agency for Healthcare Research and Quality.
8. Walker, B. and Collins, C. (2009) Developing an integrated primary care practice: strategies, techniques, and a case illustration. *Journal of Clinical Psychology*, **65**(3), 268–281.
9. Foster, T. (1982) Merger 1980: The organizational integration of college mental health services. *Journal of American College Health Association*, **30**(4), 171–174.
10. Federman, R. and Emmerling, D. (1997) An outcome survey of mergers between university student counseling centers and student health mental health. *Journal of College Student Psychotherapy*, **12**(1), 15–27.

11. Manderscheid, R., Masi, D., Rossignol, C., and Masi, D. (2007) The integration of physical health and behavioral health services: Three university case examples. *Archives of Psychiatric Nursing*, **21**(3), 141–149.

12. Kingsbury, S.K. (1987) Cognitive differences between clinical psychologists and psychiatrists. *American Psychologist*, **42**, 152–156.

13. US Preventive Services Task Force (2008) The Guide to Clinical Preventive Services, AHRQ Publication No. 08-05122.

14. Schwartz, A. (2006) College student suicide in the United States: 1990–1991 through 2003. *Journal of American College Health*, **54** (6), 341–352.

15. Schwartz, V. (2006) Medications, in *College Mental Health Practice* (eds P. Grayson and P. Meilman), Routledge, NY.

4 Components of an Effective College Mental Health Service

Gregory T. Eells[1] and Robert A. Rando[2]

[1]*Counseling & Psychological Services Gannett Health Services, Cornell University, Ithaca, NY, USA*
[2]*Counseling & Wellness Services, School of Professional Psychology, Wright State University, Dayton, OH, USA*

4.1 Introduction

Institutions of Higher Education (IHEs) are recognizing with greater clarity that they cannot educate the minds of their students without attending to the health of those same minds. As this shift unfolds, mental health services are increasingly being seen as serving an essential function in the mission of IHEs. This raises questions about how mental health and counseling services operate. There is a considerable diversity of structures and practices within these mental health and counseling service operations. When working to understand the operations of any one individual counseling service, the context within which the center operates as well as the range and breadth of services provided are critical factors for consideration. All centers generally provide some form of individual counseling or psychotherapy. Beyond this, centers vary tremendously, with some providing only individual work and others providing other forms of treatment such as couples, group and family counseling, alcohol and drug treatment, eating disorders treatment, psychological assessment, psychotropic medication, and career counseling.

This chapter will outline effective practice examples in the structuring of services while also outlining the importance of service director's developing a sound leadership philosophy that values the attention to relationships with and amongst staff and staff morale. Key administrative issues such as the location and layout of the clinic, scheduling and recordkeeping, funding, and providing threat assessment for the campus at large will then be addressed. Issues related to clinical services such as the value of triage/phone screening, case management and disposition, the coordination of counseling and psychiatry, various challenging clinical presentations, and confidentiality will be examined in the next section. Finally the importance of working with mental health resources outside of the university community will be addressed. Policies and procedures for psychiatric hospitalizations will be reviewed along with procedures for referring students to community providers.

Mental Health Care in the College Community   Edited by Jerald Kay and Victor Schwartz
© 2010 John Wiley & Sons, Ltd.

4.2 Leadership Philosophy and Staff Morale

The ability of a counseling service director to build good relationships in the counseling service is essential and flows from solid management principles. The first of these principles is to manage by influence rather than by the imposition of will. When persons in power operate by trying to impose their will, the best they ever elicit from others around them is an appearance of compliance with no real buy-in or enthusiasm. Truly living by the "managing by influence" principle increases the likelihood that staff become proactive problem solvers and effective employees. Inclusion and involvement promote ownership and accountability by all members of an agency. The second principle of good management is having a well-defined mission and clearly defined staff roles. The third principle is that form follows function. Thoughtful directors recognize and accept that change will occur and ask questions about the change process with a final form in mind. The fourth principle is minimizing distorted communication. Distorted communication is often a function of high competition and low collaboration within an agency and decreases the likelihood of organizational viability and success. The fifth principle asserts that directors must manage people while ensuring that necessary tasks are also accomplished. Administrators who are very good at accomplishing tasks frequently lose sight of the people who complete the tasks. The fine balance that directors must maintain is pursuing the achievement of organizational goals in concert with the satisfaction of staff members' needs. The final principle is to establish a work climate in which the intrinsic needs of staff can be satisfied. Directors must understand what motivates their employees, celebrate the diversity amongst them, and discern ways to maintain their own positive energy and model self care for the entire organization [1]. All of these principles highlight the developmental framework and foundation on which many counseling services rest. A framework that acknowledges the importance of relationships, transparency and balance as we work to meet the mental health needs of our students.

4.3 Administrative Issues

4.3.1 Clinic Location

These principles also provide a foundation for decisions about the more tangible aspects of a mental health service. One of these aspects is clinic location. This issue like many issues with counseling services is highly dependant on the unique history and culture of the supporting IHE. The majority of centers (66.5%) [2] are independent services operating within a student affairs division and can be located in a private setting on campus or are sometimes integrated into a more visible "one stop shop" student services building.

Some counseling services (15.6%) are completely integrated within the IHEs health service. This arrangement offers considerable opportunity for providing holistic care to students and also creates some administrative challenges in terms of operations and blending the different cultures of counseling and health services. An additional 15.8% [2] of counseling services are partially integrated with the health services either sharing the same building or sharing some administrative functions. All of these factors influence location in ways that are unique to the hosting IHE. A larger tension with location is balancing the privacy concerns of students with accessibility. Institutions have responded to this tension by developing satellite clinics or by placing counseling staff in specific colleges, residence halls or student support programs.

4.3.2 Clinic Layout

The layout of many counseling services is often determined by the office space allocated and available to the service at the time decisions about location were being made. With the increased recognition that health and mental health services are critical to student success, many IHEs are designing and building new facilities and/or remodelling current structures. Willis [3] highlighted two primary areas of concern in the design or mental health service facilities. Counseling center design must balance the needs of staff and administration with consideration for the comfort of the client. Carr [4] noted that facilities must promote staff efficiency, allow for supervision of clients and staff and provide a therapeutic environment that is clean, with sufficient lighting (preferably natural lighting), acoustic privacy, and the use of frosting and other techniques to provide privacy in waiting areas. The second issue noted by Willis involves the focus on uniqueness and architectural design at the cost of service and program operations. Counseling center design should include a private reception area that both provides a welcoming environment (music, video, print materials and accessibility) and an unambiguous message to clients as to the procedures that they should follow upon arrival and at subsequent visits [3]. Therapist offices should include comfortable furniture for client seating, be able to accommodate clients with mobility issues, and provide a work area for the therapist that is separate from the treatment area. Some counseling centers integrate the training of graduate level clinicians. This will often result in the addition of video cameras and/or two-way mirrors that allow for the viewing and recording of session content. Many counseling centers use technology to record clinical notes as well as view recorded sessions. It is important to consider the placement of computer monitors in all areas of the counseling center to secure the privacy of any information that may appear on a computer screen. Security is a final consideration in the design and layout of counseling centers. Security features including reception desks with security glass, panic buttons connected directly to campus or local security departments, and the use of multiply locked cabinets and rooms for client data as well as secure network servers are all integral considerations in the counseling center design.

4.3.3 Scheduling and Record Keeping

The vast majority of counseling services are moving to some type of electronic scheduling and record keeping system. Changing demands in counseling practice and the need for data to justify continued financial support for the service makes this essential. In a recent survey of counseling center directors, 81% reported using electronic systems for scheduling and 68% reported using electronic systems for clinical notes [5]. The most frequently used software amongst counseling services not integrated with the IHE health service is Titanium Schedule, which is best described as a counseling center management software system (www.titaniumschedule.com). Their web site lists over 400 customers internationally and their system is well reviewed by directors balancing factors such as cost and effectiveness. The developers of Titanium Schedule are also collaborating with Pennsylvania State University to support the Center for the Study of Collegiate Mental Health (CSCMH). The goal of CSCMH is to "create a collaborative and technology-powered national infrastructure for the purpose of gathering, sharing, and reporting on the real time trends in college student mental health".

Other software systems used by counseling services for scheduling and record keeping tend to be larger and more multifunctional and are often used by counseling services integrated within a larger health service. These systems include Point and Click, Medicat, PyraMed and eClinical Works. These systems are considerably more expensive than Titanium Schedule but offer a much broader range of functionality including billing and medical documentation.

Critical to all scheduling and record keeping is the maintenance of client confidentiality and record security. State and Federal law regulates those procedures necessary for the maintenance of client data in both paper and electronic formats. Collaboration with IHE information technology department is vital in the development and implementation of security systems for counseling center client records.

4.3.4 Funding

The issue of funding for centers also highlights the incredible diversity that exists in the management of counseling services. In reviewing Figure 4.1, [5] 55% of centers do not charge a mandatory fee and are funded by an allocation from the operating budget of the IHE. An additional 17% receive less than half of their funding from some type of mandatory fee receiving the rest of their funding from an IHE allocation. An additional 12% of services receive between 50–99% of their funding from a mandatory fee and 16% of services are completely funded through charging students a mandatory fee.

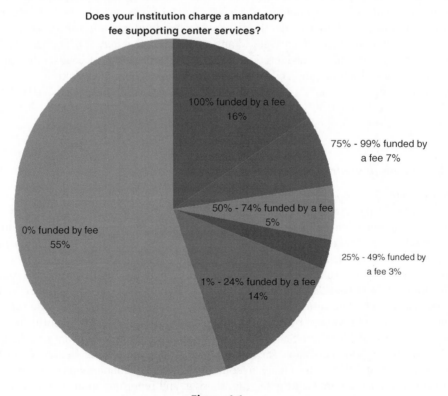

Does your Institution charge a mandatory fee supporting center services?

100% funded by a fee 16%

75% - 99% funded by a fee 7%

50% - 74% funded by a fee 5%

0% funded by fee 55%

25% - 49% funded by a fee 3%

1% - 24% funded by a fee 14%

Figure 4.1

Counseling services also have additional ways of raising revenue. Of 391 respondents to the AUCCCD survey [5] 11 reported collecting third party payments with annual revenues ranging from $2000 to $200 000. An additional 86 services reported receiving some funding from grants and contracts. The mean income from these grants and contracts was $35 450 with a minimum income of $300 and a maximum of $320 000.

In the 2008 fiscal year 38% of counseling services reported budget increase ranging from 1 to 7%, 50% reported that their budget stayed the same and 10% reported a decrease in their budget [5]. This data indicates considerable support for counseling services.

4.3.5 Campus Consultation/Threat Assessment

The role of the counseling service and the service director in consulting with campus partners and providing some type of risk or threat assessment to the campus is one that has received considerable attention in IHE circles especially in the aftermath of high profile campus tragedies. Data suggests that at least 3% of counseling center clients report fear that they may lose control and act in a violent manner [6]. Many IHEs have developed some type of student of concern committee comprised of various IHE staff that deal with student life issues. However, many IHEs had these committees prior to the more recent campus tragedies. In states where there have been high profile campus tragedies like Illinois and Virginia, the reports by the governors and legislators have recommended the presence of these teams.

Functionally student of concern teams collect information and intervene early, providing a safety net for students experiencing difficulties. The teams provide early coordination of communication, a direction for information gathering, necessary case management, structure for identifying, training and supporting campus partners such as academic units who report concerns to the team, and a vehicle to identify various policy issues. There is also a growing consensus on how these teams operate. These team generally function better if they have a designated leader who takes a consensus approach while weighing more heavily some members' area of expertise. The team dynamic also develops in a way that is more effective if the team meets weekly. The team also needs someone dedicated to documenting team discussion and outcomes of decisions. It is important to involve legal counsel at the IHE to agree on documentation standards. When counseling service staff or the director are members of this team they generally serve as a consultant and are still obligated to maintain the legal standards of confidentiality that are required of them as mental health professionals.

Another issue for these teams is their role in conducting some type of risk or threat assessment process when there is some concern about targeted violence. Threat assessment committees are multidisciplinary teams involving key campus representatives who meet to discuss IHE community members who are evidencing risk for harm to self, others, or the institution, are disruptive to IHE operations, and/or disruptive to the learning process [7]. Each IHE and mental health service must negotiate the involvement of their counseling services staff based on their resources and local need. However, it is essential that IHE staff have a basic understanding of some facts about targeted violence and what a threat assessment process is designed to accomplish. Important facts about targeted violence include the fact that perpetrators do not "just snap", though there are triggers. Also it important for all IHE staff to realize that there is no useful profile in predicting targeted violence in terms of gender, SES or ethnic background, though it is often common for others in the community to be concerned about the person's behavior. Most individuals who engage in targeted violence are suicidal with no escape plan. For an IHE to respond effectively staff must act quickly to determine if the person is on a pathway to violence. This is accomplished by having a process that is designed to identify persons of concern, investigate persons and situations that have come to attention of staff, assess the information gathered and if necessary, manage persons and situations to reduce the posed threat [7].

4.4 Clinical Services

4.4.1 Triage/Screening

Increasingly, the primary mission of counseling services is to provide much more immediate access to clinical care especially in response to higher acuity levels in students. Oftentimes the system services have in place to allocate care is no longer meeting the demands of the students or other campus constituents. Counseling services have brief "windows of opportunity" when students are willing to access care and if services are not available, students may not return. Brown, Parker and Godding [8] discuss the frequent use of waiting lists in outpatient mental health services as a function of demand outstripping capacity. They highlight the costs of waiting lists including increased emotional distress, potential danger to self or others, a poor image of the service, loss of revenue and a missed opportunity for treatment. They conclude that a triage system is an alternative to a waiting list system, with multiple benefits.

Triage systems have been developed and implemented at approximately 13% of counseling services [5]. Originally used during World War I, the concept of triage has been widely adopted in disaster response and hospital emergency rooms. The use of triage systems in outpatient mental health settings services have been linked to increased recognition of acuity, increased accuracy of screening, enhanced clinical care, more timely response, high patient and staff satisfaction and a more efficient utilization of limited resources [9–11].

Implementing a triage system at an IHE counseling service first requires providing an effective rationale for the need for this service and then building a foundation of significant support amongst the clinical and office staff at the counseling service. The next step is to construct a system that is a good fit within existing structures that allows for 15–30 minute triage appointments immediately available for students. Once this is accomplished, it is then essential to educate the community about what this new service is and how it does not replace the existing more thorough assessment/intake process. Triage serves as an entry point into the system allowing for rapid access and matching with the appropriate level of care [12].

Components of a successful system include outlining what a student will be told when they want to access the service. When a student phones, it is explained to them that they will speak with a senior clinician in a confidential appointment who will gather some basic information that will allow for a rapid matching of services, based upon their individual needs. Same-day appointments are set up at the front desk. If the student self-identifies at that point as being in an emergency, they are immediately referred to the daily on-call clinician, bypassing the standard triage system [12].

During the actual triage appointment, most efficiently conducted by phone, students are told that the counselor will be "gathering some basic information that will allow us to best match our services with your individual situation". The conversation can be conceptualized as having four key components: basic demographic information; an inquiry into what led the student to call; specific questions about past and current treatment (suicidality, violence risk, history of hospitalization, substance abuse, eating concerns, medical concerns and current medications); and disposition where the clinician is assigning the student to an emergency (seen immediately by on-call clinician), urgent (appointment within 48–72 hours) or routine level of care. An example of a triage form used at Cornell University to document a triage encounter can be found in Appendix A.

One common concern with a triage system is that with increased access to services comes increased client flow through the mental health service. This can lead to increased stress on the system as well as the clinicians that provide the services. For some staff managing the shifting demands of triage are difficult-while others embrace the change. Those who find it challenging may require support during the transition.

Another concern expressed from some students has been that the triage system adds another layer of assessment and that they have to tell their "story" to a triage clinician and conduct an intake/assessment before treatment commences. This is a very valid concern and ultimately is inherent in the triage system. In most systems the benefits previously outlined far outweigh the concerns.

A final concern of telephone triage systems focuses on risk management issues [13]. Overall, triage systems offer significant reductions in risk-management concerns by capturing acute situations more quickly thus potentially avoiding adverse outcomes such as harm to self or others, or avoidable hospitalizations.

4.4.2 Case Management and Case Disposition

Once students are triaged, assessed and in the counseling system one key question is how the case is actually managed. Generally most services rely on the professional judgment of their clinicians to determine how the student is treated. However, some services do rely on a session limit to meet the demand for services. Of surveyed centers, 17.4% reported having a fixed session limit for students, another 30.7% report having a session limit but they make it flexible based on the students clinical presentation, 51.4% do not have any type of session limit [14]. There are costs and benefits to each approach. The benefits to fixed session limits are the service knows available resources and can plan accordingly. The primary cost is that some students care is disrupted when they may still be experiencing severe symptoms. The benefits of a session limit that is flexible is that the service gets the benefits of a session limits and has a response for the primary concern by giving some students additional care based on clinical need. The cost to this approach is an administrative structure must be put in place to determine which students get an exception to the session limit. This is often done by a group of clinicians who are now using their time to make disposition decisions rather than providing clinical care.

The modal response for services is to not have a session limit. The benefit of this approach is that clinicians can focus on providing the needed clinical care. The cost is that it is more difficult to plan for case management as demand for services increase. One response of some services that do not have session limits is to expect all clinicians to see a predetermined number of new clients every week. This allows for the overall management of clinic flow and places the decision of which clients get extended care in the hands of the people best able to make the decisions, the clinician providing the care.

4.4.3 Coordination of Counseling and Psychiatry

Many mental health services at IHEs provide both counseling and psychotropic medication management. In a recent survey 39.7% of counseling services reported that psychiatric services were available on campus only at the counseling service, 16% reported that they were only available at the student health service and 6.6% reported that they were available at both the counseling and health service. Additionally, 30.9% of mental health services reported that psychiatric services were available through contracting out or a referral to the community [2]. Many of the most common mental health disorders are treated with a combination of both counseling and medication and an IHE setting is uniquely complex both clinically and administratively regarding providing effective treatment. Clinically, clients and patients are culturally diverse, generally good therapy candidates and are sensitive and responsive to medications. Administratively, treatment providers are in the role of coordinating the interface between the student and the university.

One of the primary challenges in providing treatment in IHE settings is that providers are often in different buildings and different administrative units sometimes making communication difficult. However, one primary benefit is they are more often in the mental health service where communication between counselor and prescriber has the potential to be very effective. One of the key issues is for both counselor and prescriber to see their relationship as foundational for each of their individual relationships with the student. If this foundation is in place there is considerable opportunity for improved treatment outcomes. From various theories we know that these triadic relationships can be laden with competition, envy, jealousy, alliances and enemies. However, family systems theory informs us that triangular relationships are often the most stable structures for containing conflict and anxiety. The triangular relationship of student, prescriber, and counselor can lends itself to coalitions, splitting, and side-taking. The prescriber and the counselor must be attuned to this potential and build their relationship with each other focusing on each others' strength and potential contribution [2]. Psychiatry, brings the expertise with medications and the management of sever psychopathology. Counseling can help identify and modify maladaptive thinking and behavior of clients to more effectively handle interpersonal conflict. Counselors can use their relationships to bolster trust in psychiatry. Psychiatry can emphasize the value of psychotherapy. Both parties can work together to address the all too common problem of medication non-compliance. Many patients never fill their prescriptions or stop taking their medication. Compliance rates vary across psychotropic medications but are between 65–85% for antidepressants, 55% for antipsychotics, and 60% for lithium [15].

4.4.4 Challenging Clinical Issues

There is growing data that more students are arriving on the campuses of IHEs presenting with increasingly complex psychological, emotional and behavioral challenges. The Executive Summary of the Center for the Study of Collegiate Mental Health [6] reported that, for a sample of clients from college and university counseling centers (approximately 28 000 students), 9% had reported being hospitalized for a mental health concern, 8% reported a prior suicide attempt, 35% reported taking psychotropic medication, and 9% endorsing symptoms of post-traumatic stress disorder. They continue to note that clients reporting traumatic experiences were significantly more likely to also have problems with substance use, self-harming behavior, suicidal thoughts, suicide attempts, thoughts of harming others, generalized anxiety, depression, hostility, and academic distress. Some mental health issues have result in more complex intervention strategies. For example, students diagnosed with developmental and learning disorders (e.g. attention-deficit hyperactivity disorders (AHDH), learning disorders (LD), Asperger's disorder, etc.) may require a multidisciplinary approach to treatment. The National College Health Assessment Fall 2008 Executive Summary [16] reported that 23.6% of surveyed college students reported having some form of disability. The impact of disability was highlighted by 4.3% of students diagnosed with AHDH and 2.9% diagnosed with LD reporting that these conditions had a significant impact on their academic success. Another group of students presenting with issues that may require more complex and multidisciplinary interventions are those with substance abuse and dependence. The CSCMH Executive Summary [6] reported that 5% of clients noted prior treatment for drug and alcohol use. Sixteen percent of students surveyed in the ACHA/NCHA survey (2009) reported drinking seven or more drinks at one time with 3.5% reported having engaged in driving behavior after consuming at least five alcoholic beverages. Fourteen percent of students reported taking prescription drugs that were not prescribed for them. The impact of substance use is highlighted when 1.8% drug using students and 4% of alcohol using students reported that their substance use had a significant impact on their academic functioning. CSCMH [6] reported that binge drinking had a negative relationship with student's academic performance measured by both grade point average and scores on an academic distress scale.

4.4.5 Confidentiality

The increase in the complexity of issues students are presenting with at mental health services have increased the pressures on services to alert student affairs colleagues and parents if there is any concern regarding risk of harm. However, the students seen in these services are legally adults and are entitled to the same confidentiality protection afforded all adults who seek counseling. This confidentiality provides the foundation for treatment and does save lives. There has been some confusion in IHE circles about what laws apply to the records of students receiving mental health services. The federal law known as the Family Educational Rights and Privacy Act (FERPA) is often cited but has an exemption for mental health records, though these records can be covered under FERPA if used for health leaves or other academic decisions. The Health Insurance Portability and Accountability Act is another legal protection often cited but does not apply to most counseling centers because they do not bill for third party reimbursement. The primary source protecting confidentiality at a mental health service in an IHE are state laws protecting this information and the various licensing laws governing the practice of various mental health professionals.

4.5 Working with Outside Community Mental Health Resources

4.5.1 Psychiatric Hospitalizations

On average each mental health service at an IHE will be involved in 8.6 psychiatric hospitalizations per school, and 66% of services will be involved in at least one hospitalization in a year [17]. Table 4.1 breaks down the average rate of student hospitalization based on IHE size. Hospitalizations generally work best for all parties involved when there is close collaboration between the inpatient hospital and the counseling service at the IHE. When this happens there is an increased likelihood of successful reintegration of the student back into the college environment.

To accomplish this the counseling service needs to view this relationship development as their responsibility by reaching out to the local hospitals and arranging meetings with

Table 4.1	Number of students who were hospitalized for psychological reasons
Institution size	**Mean**
under 1500	4.04
1501–2500	5.06
2501–5000	5.66
5001–7500	6.68
7501–10 000	7.46
10 001–15 000	11.40
15 001–20 000	11.40
20 001–25 000	18.50
25 001–30 000	23.88
30 001–35 000	43.50
35 001 and over	24.00

critical personnel. A first step in this relationship development is counseling staff becoming familiar with the major managed care companies represented within the IHE student body. The counseling service can take a leadership role in determining if these companies have contracts with local hospitals. This can facilitate a rapid and effective inpatient referral. If a large number of students are on a student health insurance plan offered by the college or university, the counseling center director can serve as an advocate to ensure that these policies include parity around benefits for psychiatric hospitalization. At the very least the local hospital(s) can be placed on the preferred provider list for the insurance plan.

When a hospitalization does occur the best way for the service to feel prepared is to have well articulated protocols. The first question that needs to be asked in these protocols when considering hospitalization is "Does the student meet the criteria for an inpatient level of care?" These criteria vary from state to state but common criteria include acute danger to self or others, acute need for medication stabilization that cannot be done on an outpatient basis, acute need for medically supervised detoxification, as well as having ruled out the safe use of a less intensive level of care such as a crisis stabilization bed, respite bed, partial hospitalization, or intensive outpatient treatment.

Another key question is whether or not the hospitalization should be done on a voluntary or involuntary basis. When a student appears to meet the criteria for hospitalization and is deemed to be stable enough to get to the hospital a voluntary hospitalization is appropriate. If there is any reluctance on the part of the student to go to the hospital with imminent risk factors then an involuntary hospitalization should be conducted. All mental health service staff should be very familiar with the statutes and procedures for involuntary hospitaliza-tions in their state. A key component of making the process successful is to discuss in a transparent way the recommendation of hospitalization with the patient. This should be in a manner that is clear, calm, respectful, and yet firm in position. Once the decision to hospitalize, in the presence of imminent risk, it should be made clear to the patient that not going to the hospital is not up for negotiation.

All counseling services staff should have a basic understanding of protocols for transporting students to the hospital especially in cases of an involuntary hospitalization. One way of approaching these situations is to have all staff be aware of their specific roles. Clinical staff ideally will have the license and state designation to legally request the transport of the student to the hospital. Emergency commitment paperwork should be readily available and staff should be fully familiar with laws and procedures around hospitalization. Transport ideally will occur through cooperation with campus safety and local ambulance services. The counselor responsible for the hospitalization should continue to be clear and firm and can inform the student that "You are going to be evaluated further for safety. These officers and ambulance staff are now going to escort you to the ambulance." After the student has been transported the counselor can call the hospital to convey any additional facts of the case that are needed to help facilitate admission or treatment. More specific issues around psychiatric hospitalizations are outlined in Rockland-Miller and Eells [18].

4.5.2 Referrals to Community Providers

Often counseling services see students whose presenting concerns are outside of the service's stated scope of practice and a referral to a community provider is needed. Practices around referrals again vary considerably based on the location of the service's IHE. IHEs located in urban environments generally have a wider range of available local resources whereas more rural environments are often more limited. However there are several general procedures for cultivating strong community referral networks. First, it is important to cultivate relationships with community clinics that provide both counseling and psychotropic medications and to develop other networks with private therapists that also will take responsibility for any medication management. Second, it is useful to work out relationships and procedures so adequate referral follow-up can be conducted.

4.6 Conclusion

By reviewing the ways in which mental health services at IHEs interact with other community resources and local hospitals, understanding the challenging clinical issues presenting to these services and the ways in which these services respond, and reviewing the various practices around administrative structures in how these services operate the goal is that there will be a better understanding of what makes an effective mental health service. When a service considers all of these issues within a well articulated leadership philosophy it will be better able to serve the health of the minds of the students its institution is educating.

Appendix A: Triage Form (Adapted from Cornell University)

Counseling & Psychological Services

Service Date	

Student Information:

Name:	ID #:
Local Address:	
Phones:	

Male	Female	Age

Year in school: __ Fr __ So __ Jr __ Sr **X** Grad __ Other	College/Major:
Who is requesting service: __ Self __ Peer __ Fac/Staff __ Parent __ Other (specify below)	

Reason for Calling:

History & Relevant Information:

No	Yes		
		Currently receiving MH treatment?	Where & for what?
		Prior treatment, including inpatient or brief hospitalization?	When & for what?
		Current medical concerns or problems?	Details: Had bad car accident and brain surgery
		All current medications?	Med, dosage, prescribed by whom & for what?
		Concerns about food, weight, dieting, or exercise?	Details: Feels a little out of shape. Is exercising
		Alcohol use?	Details: 1-2 drinks on weekends. Drunk once a week. Smokes pot socially. A lot last week because friend was in town
		On a scale from 0 to 10, with 0 being never and 10 being every time you use, when you consume alcohol, how often do each of the following occur?	Score Blackouts - (unable to remember what happened the next day) Get into physical fight. Hurt or injure yourself. Unwanted sexual experience or consequence.
		Have you ever gone to the hospital because of alcohol or other drug use?	Details:
		Other substance use?	Details:
		Have you ever attempted to hurt yourself?	Details: .In H.S. thoughts of killing himself. No recent thoughts last 2 days or 3-4 mos. No SIB.
		Are you currently having thoughts of harming yourself or anyone else?	Details:

Always inform caller: "If you start feeling worse before your next appointment, please call (Emergency number)

Rationale for appointment at CAPS - Check all that apply

__ Unstable Situation
__ International &/or minority student
__ No resources to pay for care in Ithaca dissatisfied
__ Likely not to follow through off campus
__ Discharge from hospital
__ Concern from other campus resources
__ Need for coordination between multiple Gannett providers &/or campus resources
Comments:

__ Freshman
__ New to counseling services
__ Student tried other options and is

__ Substance use
__ MLOA
__ Concern by parent or others

Level of Service Response Needed   **Current GAF -**

	Emergency	"E"	Schedule client within **24 hours**...GAF 50 & below Serious symptoms, serious impairment in functioning, critical incidents, unstable
	Urgent	"2"	Schedule client within **72 hours**...GAF 51-60 Moderate symptoms, moderate difficulty in functioning
	Routine	"C"	Schedule client within 10 days.....GAF 61 or higher Mild symptoms, may have some mild difficulty in functioning

Case Disposition (Please indicate additional information for * items)

	(REF) Direct Referral – To Community Provider

	Provider	Phone	Scope	# Visits
	Local Resource		Diagnostic Evaluation	5
	Local resource		Medication Management	15
			Psychological Services	40
	Other:			

	In House Referral
	AOD – must consult before scheduling client
	CHEP – must consult before scheduling client
	E – Emergency
	2 – Urgent
	C & A – Routine

	Psychiatry Alerted Immediately, Because:
	Sig. Suicidal or Homicidal
	Probable Need to Hospitalize
	Agitated Psychosis
	Emergent + Panic

	*Clinician	
	*Date	
	*Time	*(Tell student to arrive 15 minutes early for paperwork)*

Other On-Campus Resource/Referrals Provided	
Health Services	Phone #s
Disability Services	
Career Services	
Other:	

*Client to call back with treatment decision by following date:

*Counselor will arrange for client to be called back with a CAPS appointment by time/date:

(TRM) Terminated – Phone Consult Only

Staff Name	Date of dictation or signature:
Staff Signature:	

References

1. Eells, G.T., Seals, T., Rockett, J. and Hayes, D. (2005) Enjoying the roller coaster ride: Directors' perspectives on fostering staff morale in university counseling centers. *Journal of College Student Psychotherapy*, **20**(2), 17–28.
2. Association of University and College Counseling Center Directors (2008) *Survey of Counseling Center Directors*.
3. Willis, VJ. (1980) Design considerations for mental health facilities. *Hospital and Community Psychiatry*, **31**(7), 483–490.
4. Carr, R.F. (2008) *Psychiatric Facility*, NIKA Technologies, Inc., For VA office of construction and Facility Management (CFM) 1–4.
5. Association of University and College Counseling Center Directors (2009) *Survey of Counseling Center Directors*.
6. Center for the Study of Collegiate Mental Health (CSCMH) (2009) *2009 Pilot Study Executive Summary*, State College, Pennsylvania State University.
7. Deisinger, G., Randazzo, M., O'Neill, D. and Savage, J. (2008) *The Handbook for Campus Threat Assessment & Management Teams*, Applied Risk Management, LLC, Boston.
8. Brown, S.A., Parker, J.D. and Godding, P.R. (2002) Administrative, clinical, and ethical issues surrounding the use of waiting lists in the delivery of mental health services. *Journal of Behavioral Health Services Research*, **29**(2), 217–228.
9. Broadbent, M., Jarman, H. and Berk, M. (2002) Improving competence in emergency mental health triage. *Accident & Emergency Nursing*, **10**(3), 155–162.
10. Kevin, J. (2002) An examination of telephone triage in a mental health context. *Issues in Mental Health Nursing*, **23**(8), 757–769.
11. Smart, D., Pollard, C. and Walpole, B. (1999) Mental health triage in emergency medicine. *Australian and New Zealand Journal of Psychiatry*, **33**(1), 57–66.
12. Rockland-Miller, H. and Eells, G.T. (2006) The implementation of mental health clinical triage systems in university health services. *Journal of College Student Psychotherapy*, **20**(4), 39–52.
13. Erdman, C. (2001) The medical/legal dangers of telephone triage in mental health care. *Journal of Legal Medicine*, **22**(4), 553–579.
14. Riba, M.B. and Tasman, A. (2006) Psychodynamic perspective on combining therapies. *Psychiatric Annals*, **36**(5).
15. Cramer, J.A. and Rosenheck, R. (1998) Compliance with medication regimens for psychiatric and medical disorders. *Psychiatric Services*, **49**, 196–210.

16. American College Health Association (2009) *American College Health Association-National College Health Assessment II Executive Summary Fall 2008*, American College Health Association, Baltimore.
17. Association of University and College Counseling Center Directors (2006) *Survey of Counseling Center Directors*.
18. Rockland-Miller, H. and Eells, G.T. (2008) Strategies for effective psychiatric hospitalizations of college and university students. *Journal of College Student Psychotherapy*, **22**(3), 3–12.

5 Essential Services in College Counseling

Richard J. Eichler[1] and Victor Schwartz[2]

[1]*Counseling and Psychological Services, Columbia University, New York, NY, USA*
[2]*Yeshiva University, Albert Einstein College of Medicine, New York, NY, USA*

5.1 Introduction

College counseling centers have undergone a dramatic expansion and role redefinition in the last several decades. While the earliest roots of many services may be found in academic and career advisement programs, often provided by faculty members [1], vocational and educational guidance has lost its primacy in the field of college counseling–and indeed is no longer even a counseling center function at many institutions, where it is provided, instead, by specialized career counseling offices. The Counseling and Psychological Services (as they are frequently called) of today, either by design or of necessity, tend to be principally defined by the tasks of personal counseling, often with a distinct psychiatric focus, and by their role in community outreach, consultation, prevention and postvention.[1]

The current emphasis in college counseling is reflected in the standards that have been adopted by national organizations in their efforts to define the essentials of service provision on college campuses. For example, the International Association of Counseling Services (IACS), a body which accredits many university and college counseling centers, requires for accreditation that a center provide the following services [2]:

- Individual and group counseling/psychotherapy, including the use of psychological tests and other assessment techniques "as needed"

- Crisis intervention

- Emergency coverage either directly or through cooperative arrangements with outside facilities

- Psychiatric care, either on campus, or through arrangements with community providers

---

[1] For a discussion of models of care in college mental health see Chapter 2 in this volume.

Mental Health Care in the College Community   Edited by Jerald Kay and Victor Schwartz
© 2010 John Wiley & Sons, Ltd.

- Outreach programming including both preventive and developmental interventions

- Consultation to members of the university community and, optionally to parents, spouses and other collaterals

- Referral resources

In addition, centers are required to conduct continuous program evaluations and accountability research and provide ongoing professional development and continuing education for staff and trainees.

Consultative functions are addressed in Chapter 8 of this volume; crisis intervention is discussed in Chapter 9; training in Chapters 11 and 12; and research in Chapter 16. In this chapter, we provide an over-view of all other essential services, including afterhours and emergency coverage; individual and group therapy; psychiatric evaluation and medication management; psychological testing; and community outreach.

5.2 Access to Care

College counseling personnel differ markedly in how they conceptualize their work, debating, for example, the relative merits of the developmental model that dominated the early years of the field, when counselors primarily aimed to facilitate normative transitions from adolescence to adulthood, compared to today's increasingly widespread "medical" model, which emphasizes the diagnosis and treatment of psychiatric disorders [1]. However, no matter how centers envision their mission, nearly all must contend with a shared reality: large numbers of students, often with acute psychiatric problems, presenting for care.

According to national survey data, during a 12-month period ending in the spring semester of 2008, 43% of college students report having at least once felt too depressed to function; 9% say they seriously considered suicide, and 1.2% say they actually made a suicide attempt; and of those who drink alcohol, over 18% say they physically injured themselves, and almost 4% say they physically injured someone else as a consequence of alcohol consumption [3]. In addition, 17% report at least one occasion in their lives when they intentionally injured themselves [4]. In view of the high levels of distress, breakdowns in functioning and potentially life-threatening behaviors in the student population, it is critical that every counseling center have some mechanism by which to identify students who require immediate treatment.

Urgent care or walk-in hours are perhaps the most common means of guaranteeing that students in crisis are seen in a timely fashion. However, there are potential shortcomings to this arrangement especially when clinical resources are limited. Because students, rather than clinicians, make the initial determination as to who requires immediate assistance, walk-in hours typically attract a mix of truly at-risk students, along with students experiencing painful, but highly transitory affective storms, students who are too impatient, impulsive or entitled to schedule appointments, and so forth. Clinical time best spent managing emergencies may, on busy days, instead be devoted to *ad hoc* triage, detracting from the care of the neediest students, while leaving students with less urgent problems feeling neglected if it becomes necessary to cut their visits short to accommodate emergencies.

Increasingly, schools are adopting variants of a telephone triage system [5] to prioritize the care of students in advance of scheduling face-to-face clinical encounters. Of course, when phone triage suggests an acute emergency, an immediate face-to-face appointment is arranged. National survey data finds that 13.5% of schools now have some such system in place [6]. Preliminary data suggests that telephone triage systems are effective at identifying students at risk for life-threatening behaviors, while simultaneously promoting early positive connections to the counseling center (R.J. Eichler and C. Chin, presentation at the American College Health Association Annual Meeting, 6 June 2008).

Psychiatric crises are, of course, not limited to business hours. Therefore counseling centers must have 24 hour coverage in place. A recent national survey finds that about 26% of schools provide the general student body with direct access to mental health professionals on-call; the more common arrangement, by far, makes counselors available to key campus personnel, such as Public Safety, residence life advisors and student affairs administrators for after hours consultation, and, as needed, for direct intervention with students [7]. The former arrangement is generally more appealing to students and provides those who are distressed, but not in crisis, with late night assistance, but it is resource intensive and often impractical at institutions with large student bodies (and therefore large numbers of prospective late-night callers). The latter arrangement insures that only true emergencies reach mental health clinicians and therefore provides a more cost effective, if less encompassing, safety net. An increasingly widespread third alternative is to outsource twenty-four hour hotlines to agencies specializing in emergency care. When this option is elected, it is strongly recommended that the counseling center also place a staff member on-call as a resource both to the hotline staff and to student affairs personnel and other campus stakeholders. There is no substitute for a clinician who understands the campus culture, local resources and the like. In addition, in the event of a tragedy requiring immediate postvention, it is critical that there is timely access to counseling center staff who can arrange support for the community.

A dwindling number of health services maintain infirmaries or urgent care clinics where after hours psychiatric care is also provided. While infirmaries may spare some students the often unpleasant experience of a visit to the local psychiatric emergency room, they are very costly, cannot provide the same level of safety as a hospital, nor offer the same range of medical and diagnostic care. All of these limitations also raise significant liability concerns.

5.3 Clinical Consultation, Treatment Planning and Referral

5.3.1 The Initial Interviews

Ideally, treatment begins with an explicitly defined consultation period, typically consisting of two to three visits. The consultation may be introduced with words to the effect that the therapist would like to take a few sessions to get to know the student, to understand what she or he hopes to derive from treatment, and to work together to develop the best practical plan for meeting the student's goals, be it at the counseling center, or elsewhere. Emphasizing the value of a consultation in determining the kind of treatment from which the student is most likely to benefit may seem obvious enough, but in practice some clinicians take for granted that students will understand the necessity and intrinsic worth of treatment planning. Other therapists, anxious to protect their time, or guilty about the limitations on the care their center provides, may be inclined to initiate treatment by underscoring what they *cannot* do (with statements like "we *only* offer brief therapy") and in the process implicitly diminish the value of what they *can* do. Emphasizing the negative invites students to do the same, and may compromise the therapeutic relationship before it gets off the ground. For an excellent discussion of countertransferential impediments to conducting short-term treatment, see [8].

A well demarcated consultation provides a context for the conversations to follow. As students begin telling their story, they often naturally assume, even if treatment is publicized as short-term, that they will receive all their care on campus. Defining the first visits as a discrete assessment period to determine, among other things, where the remainder of treatment will occur, reduces the likelihood that students will experience a subsequent recommendation for off-campus treatment as an abrupt empathic rupture, a personal rejection, or a betrayal of the trust implied by sharing intimate details of one's life. An explicit consultation period also begins to convey the participatory, collaborative nature of the therapeutic enterprise to students, many of whom have little prior understanding of the activity required of them in psychotherapy. The degree to which students are or are not able to reflect on their experience and behavior, tolerate anxiety, and exhibit capacities for resiliency, trust and for self-regulation during the consultation are all important barometers of the kinds of treatment suited to their current level of functioning. The consultation, in other words, is an opportunity to uncover not only vulnerabilities but strengths, and to plan treatment accordingly.

In extending a consultation over several sessions, clinicians have an opportunity to assess patients at different points in time. This can aid in discriminating between the transitory affective storms or bouts of anxiety not uncommon during the college years and more enduring problems. It provides an opportunity, as well, to evaluate whether a patient appears to be progressively deteriorating which, in turn, can be helpful in monitoring whether symptoms such as social withdrawal or unusual behaviors are reactive to specific and possibly transient life stressors or prodromal to more insidious developments.

The consultation period will, of course, ordinarily include a somewhat systematic review of:

- family, academic, developmental and social history

- current and past life stressors and trauma

- current and past levels of functioning

- social supports

- medical problems

- past psychiatric history

- a mental status exam

While all of this information is valuable – and some of it, such as suicidal intent, is vital to assess – all of it is also rendered essentially useless if patients drop out of treatment. Therefore, the task of gathering information needs to be balanced with the work of engaging students. To the extent possible, it is helpful to relate questions that might otherwise seem gratuitous or intrusive back to the complaints in the forefront of students' minds. Asking about, say, disturbances in sleep or appetite may seem superfluous or irrelevant to a student distraught over a romantic break-up. By contrast, the same questions may be perceived as empathic and caring if framed in the context of the student's concerns: "You say you are devastated over this break-up. That could mean a lot of things; I want to be sure I understand what you are going through, so I can be of help. So tell me, when some people are really upset they have trouble falling asleep or staying asleep – is that happening to you?" And so forth.

There is, in short, a critical distinction between doggedly pursuing a mental checklist of symptomatic behaviors, with few words of explanation or with little regard for students' subjective state, as opposed to carefully monitoring, and working to mitigate, students' anxiety, embarrassment, or agitation. This is not to suggest that inquiry should be abandoned at the first sign of discomfort, but therapists should bear in mind that students who experience their first sessions as overwhelming are obviously less likely to return for more of the same. These first critical encounters need to convey some experience of benefit or hope, be it in the form of a new insight or perspective or of a promising new interpersonal connection. As Harry Stack Sullivan wrote years ago [9]:

> The *quid pro quo* which keeps people going in this necessarily disturbing business of trying to be foresquare and straightforward about one's most lamentable failures and one's most chagrining mistakes is that one is learning something that promises to be useful. (1970, p. 16).

In this spirit, it is often helpful to summarize, however tentatively, initial impressions and thoughts about treatment, so students do not leave "empty-handed". That said, patients differ greatly in what they find helpful: For one patient, a tentative interpretation may dilute anxiety; for another, interpretation may be experienced as criticism, or may increase an uncomfortable sense of transparency. For some students, the catharsis of sharing long concealed fears or secrets with a therapist who is at once authoritative, kind, and non-judgmental may suffice to convey a sense of therapeutic possibility and optimism; for others, emotional release rapidly gives way to a flood of disorganizing feeling, and empathic reassurance is what is needed.

Fluctuations in patients' affect, relatedness, motor behavior and the like are, of course, every bit as vital a source of information as are the answers patients supply to questions. Indeed patients' descriptions of their lives are subject to a variety of distortions, intentional or otherwise, whereas patients' behavior is directly observable. It need be remembered, however, that conduct is influenced by the interpersonal context in which it unfolds, and there is no situation completely analogous to that of a psychiatric interview. Constructing a reasonably complete and accurate picture of a student's behavior outside the consulting room is a daunting undertaking, and the clinician should take care "having discovered a few of the patient's handicaps [not to] use a lively imagination to provide us with something like a comprehensive picture of him as a person" ([9], p. 54). For example, a student may appear restless and agitated in the consulting room; before concluding that he or she is chronically on edge, the clinician is well advised to consider whether the patient's behavior is situational: Is the patient from a culture in which it is shameful to see a mental health professional, and if so, could this result in anxious agitation? Is the patient discussing a particularly embarrassing subject, like sexual dysfunction? Are the restlessness and agitation indeed indicative of anxiety – or might the student be impatient with the therapist's line of questioning? For detailed discussion of the initial interview the reader is directed to MacKinnon *et al.* [10].

5.3.2 Diagnostic and Extradiagnostic Factors in Treatment Planning

Treatment in college counseling centers is generally very brief [6,11]. In part, the brevity of counseling in campus mental health settings is dictated by the sheer weight of numbers. Demand for services has risen steadily, often without a commensurate increase in counseling resources [12,13].

A common solution when demand outstrips resources is the imposition of *session limits*, a practice which has been adopted in some form by about 52% of colleges nationwide [6]. Advocates of session limits contend that brief, circumscribed treatment is cost effective; equitable; alleviates many symptoms; improves overall psychological functioning; and reduces or eliminates waiting lists, and by extension reduces the number of students lost to treatment. Critics of session limits variously challenge the efficacy of short-term treatment; question whether session limits effectively control utilization of services;[2] suggest that an *a priori* limit on treatment may drive off fragile students; contend that session limits privilege symptom relief at the expense of promoting more enduring life skills; and argue that dictating the length of treatment is contrary to supporting students' developmental strivings toward greater personal autonomy. The debate over session limits is cogently summarized by Ghetie [14].

An alternative to straightforward session limits is an individualized approach in which centers establish an overarching philosophy of services provided, and each student seeking treatment is assessed to determine whether her or his needs can realistically be met within these broad service parameters.[3] The literature on psychotherapy outcomes may usefully inform this approach by suggesting which complaints can and cannot typically be addressed through the relatively circumscribed interventions most college counseling centers have time to provide. For example, studies have repeatedly demonstrated that acute subjective distress as well as certain more chronic symptoms, such as dysphoria, self-consciousness, and guilt can be significantly reduced for many patients in brief treatment and that many interpersonal problems – other than those associated with severe personality disorders – can be usefully addressed within somewhat longer, but still reasonably limited, time constraints [15–17]. When the amelioration of these sorts of complaints is mutually agreed upon as a goal, and students appear to have the inner resources prerequisite to brief therapy, a trial course of treatment at the counseling center may be appropriate. Fundamentally healthy students seeking assistance for problems with academics, acculturation, bereavement issues and the like are also obvious candidates for in-house treatment. It should be emphasized that the fact that a given student is likely to benefit from brief therapy does not negate that he or she might profit further from longer courses of treatment. In fact, beneficial courses of brief therapy during the college years may motivate some students, later in life, to undertake more intensive treatments.

---

[2] The little available research data indicate that centers with session limits do not meaningfully differ from those without such limits in the percentage of students they serve nor in the average duration of the treatments they offer; however, centers with session limits actually have substantially longer waiting lists [101].

[3] The ensuing discussion pertains exclusively to counseling/brief psychotherapy, not to medication management, which is taken up later in this chapter; some centers may choose to adopt different policies governing limits on counseling, on the one hand, and pharmacotherapy, on the other. This discussion also presumes the availability of a reasonably robust network of affordable off-campus treatment options. Cultivating such a network, to the extent that local resources permit, should be high on the list of a counseling center's priorities.

To the surprise of perhaps few practicing clinicians, research finds that short term treatment is generally insufficient to treat the symptoms of significant personality disorders, such as hostility, social detachment and paranoia [17], nor is it sufficient for many patients with multiple or chronic mental disorders (see also [18]),[4] though many of these patients will benefit from longer-term therapy [19]. Therefore, at all but the most well-staffed counseling centers, students with these complex, entrenched psychiatric conditions are strong candidates for referral to longer term treatment facilities.

This is not to imply that individual clinical decisions should be predicated solely on research data. On the contrary, outcome research speaks only to how groups of people, on average, respond to different interventions, whereas treatment plans are formulated for individuals who may differ greatly from one another and from group norms [20]. It is precisely for this reason that treatment guidelines founded on psychotherapy research are best applied flexibly in light of individualized clinical judgments, in keeping with an emerging consensus in the field that psychotherapy planning should synthesize empirical findings and clinical reasoning [20]. Psychiatric diagnosis, which after all is essentially a means of grouping patients together on the basis of shared symptoms and behaviors, need be qualified by the attributes that distinguish patients within a given diagnostic category from one another, with particular attention to those factors in a patient's psychological make-up and life circumstances most likely to affect the acceptance, use, and absorption of a given treatment modality. An assessment of the consequences or sources of a student's troubles may also suggest the need for any of a variety of ancillary services. Table 5.1 provides an illustrative summary of some extra-diagnostic considerations that may usefully contribute to a comprehensive treatment plan.

5.3.3 Implications of Phase of Life Issues for Treatment Planning

That the treatment of college students tends to be brief is not simply a product of budgetary constraints. When no limits are imposed on duration of treatment, many students will opt out on their own, often quite quickly (e.g. [22]). The social stigma associated with mental health services, anxiety aroused by the prospect of treatment, the disappointment at not achieving a rapid cure and a host of other factors may dissuade people of all ages from ongoing treatment. In addition, normative developmental factors may fuel college students' ambivalence [23]. A central feature of the transition to adulthood, at least in much of American culture, is a lessening of dependence on adults in the service of achieving a greater sense of self-reliance, competence, and individuality [24]. Thus, college students may have an ambivalent attitude toward adult authority figures, such as therapists, at once desiring support and connection, but at the same time regarding such desires as somewhat regressive and childish. This helps account for the fact that many students seek treatment, only to beat a hasty retreat from deepening involvement with their counselors.

---

[4] The preponderance of clinical opinion is aligned with research on this point. The patient selection criteria for most formal systems of short term therapy rules out psychotic and borderline levels of ego organization, and favors patients with some insight into their problems, depressed patients, and patients in crisis. For a fuller discussion, see Groves [18].

Table 5.1	Illustrative extradiagnostic considerations in treatment planning

Context of the problem: Are problems circumscribed or trans-situational? Acute or chronic? To what extent is functioning impaired? What are the consequences of continuing to function at this level in the near future? Are protective measures needed? Should family or social supports be mobilized? Is the student disruptive to others in class or in residence halls? Are academic accommodations or medical leave of absence warranted to mitigate the adverse consequences of functional impairment?

Subjective distress: Is the patient's level of distress a motivating factor for talk therapy? Is the student's distress overwhelming, and if so, is a medication consultation indicated to provide immediate relief?

Level of cooperation: Is the student self-reflective, open to new points of view, trusting? Excessively rigid, resistant or oppositional to accepting treatment advice? Superficially compliant, but passive? Overly deferential and therefore disinclined to report treatment failures? Does the patient romanticize symptoms? Do the symptoms confer significant secondary gains (e.g. attention from friends and family; relief from psychic pain by self-cutting, etc.) that might act as a deterrent to making good use of treatment? Are motivational enhancement techniques appropriate as a prelude to therapy or referral?

Patient expectations:[1] Is the patient hopeful with regard to treatment or especially skeptical? Has the patient had positive or negative experiences with a particular form of treatment or with medication in the past? Have family members? What forms of help-giving/advice are most consistent with the patient's temperament and cultural expectations? Is the patient comfortable with discussing feelings? More inclined toward practical advice and problem-solving techniques?

Familial factors: Are parents, friends, spouse or partner supportive of treatment? Discouraging? Actively opposed? Are family members insistent on treatment to the extent that it is experienced by the student as a punishment or as something undertaken for the benefit of others? Would the student's recovery disrupt a family system in which he or she inhabits the "sick role?" Would involving family members in treatment planning improve outcomes?

Need for other services: Is the student in an abusive relationship that merits enlisting Public Safety, or other campus resources? Is the student experiencing conflicts with faculty or administrators that warrant the intervention of a Dean, Faculty Chair or the Ombud's Office? Does the student have a disability that might require academic accommodations or other assistance from the campus Disability Office? Is the student religious, and, if so, might some concerns best be addressed by campus clergy? Is the student practicing safe sex? Is testing for HIV or an STD indicated? Does the student have other potential medical issues warranting referral to Primary Care?

[1]Patient expectations have a modest, but significant, impact on treatment outcomes [21].

Age-expectable pre-occupations with identity may further contribute to ambivalence about psychotherapy (and medication) during the college years. A developmental imperative during late adolescence is the refinement and reorganization of the self-representations of childhood into a more adult identity [25,26]. The process of establishing one's identity in the adult world is a very public one; it is insufficient to lay claim to a particular social niche – one's qualifications for that niche must be ratified, as it were, by the larger community. Ongoing participation in psychotherapy is experienced by some students as a liability in asserting a positive identity, for they associate it with weakness, helplessness, neediness or mental illness – in short with qualities they very much wish to exclude from both their inner self-representation and their public presentation [23]. The syllogism, faulty though it is, goes something like this: "I go to therapy, ergo I am dysfunctional; I don't want to be dysfunctional; ergo I will quit therapy."

To reflexively treat student ambivalence about therapy as "resistance" to be surmounted is therefore often a clinical error. For the reasons outlined above, many students are unready to commit to regular weekly appointments for even a limited duration of time. In these situations, unless personal safety is at issue, it is usually unwise to insist on an explicit appointment schedule as part of a treatment plan. It is much more tolerable for highly ambivalent students to be asked weekly if they would like to return for another session than to be "offered" up front eight or ten consecutive appointments. For other students, weekly treatment, whether pre-arranged or organized "on the fly" still requires too much commitment; these students may need to modulate the emergence of strong dependent, transferential feelings and/or minimize the sense of becoming a "patient" by attending treatment on an intermittent basis [23]. Individualized treatment planning should allow for this possibility.

5.3.4 The Referral Process

When it becomes clear in consultation that a student will be best served in another treatment setting, it is generally advisable to refer as quickly as practical. It rarely makes sense to delay the initiation of the treatment from which it is believed a student is most likely to benefit. Along with exhausting the precious resource of time, attempting to treat pathology that cannot be managed in the counseling center may demoralize staff and thereby indirectly detract from the overall quality of care rendered [27]. Unnecessarily prolonging treatment in the counseling center may also, in some cases, reduce the likelihood of a successful transition to off-campus resources. To offer one obvious example, for students who form rapid, overly-intense, if shallow, attachments, and for whom separations are likely to be experienced as abandonment or rejection, putting off a referral may succeed only in deepening attachment to the counselor, magnify the sense of loss at separation, and thereby harden resistance to accepting treatment off campus. Of course, some students, particularly those with borderline levels of ego organization, may have pronounced negative reactions to the recommendation of an off-campus referral no matter when it is raised, underscoring again the importance of clarifying limitations on treatment from the outset, so as to have a reference point by which to challenge students' interpretation of referral as a personal rejection.

Perhaps the most problematic cases are those in which students attempt, consciously or otherwise, to coerce ongoing treatment at the center by injuring themselves, threatening or attempting suicide, or otherwise recklessly acting out at the point of referral. Terminating with, or transferring the care of, a student at significant risk has obvious ethical and legal ramifications and should only be undertaken in consultation with a senior colleague or clinic administrator, and legal counsel and with careful consideration to applicable institutional policies and state law. Legal issues are addressed in greater depth later in this volume, but it is worth stating here that while there is potential liability in referring a student off-campus, there is also liability in undertaking to treat a student in a setting that lacks the personnel or other resources sufficient to meet a student's needs.

In some instances, it is possible to strike a middle ground and refer students for the more intensive treatment they require off-campus, while the Counseling Center retains a case management role, continuing to assist, as needed, with academic, residence-life and related issues and serving as a liaison between administration and family. Maintaining a case management relationship after referral is not, of course without risks: It may inadvertently promote splitting, or may dilute or otherwise interfere with the therapeutic relationship, and therefore this arrangement should be undertaken cautiously on a case-by-case basis.

In other instances, the referral of students who initially refuse to consider a higher level of care may be facilitated by setting aside a small, predetermined number of visits in which to process the referral recommendation. The purpose and duration of these sessions should be very clearly defined as an opportunity to better articulate the proposed treatment plan, and explore the student's reservations. Arranging sessions along these lines is not to be confused with agreeing to an inappropriate long-term treatment plan out of "concern" for the student's welfare, which in truth is sometimes coded language for a desire to avoid student anger or acting out in response to referral. Ideally, a cluster of four or five well defined preparatory sessions affords students an opportunity to achieve some elementary recognition that the rage and anxiety prompted by the prospect of separation invariably have a long and complicated pedigree – that is, that they are feelings rooted in the past, rather than a reasonable response to separating from a counselor they have only just met. These sessions also provide an occasion to establish a basic safety plan and to introduce students to the experience of managing, rather than acting out, painful affects, an experience, which may, in turn, be leveraged to promote interest in dialectical-behavior therapy (DBT) or similar longer-term treatments. The preparatory period may also be used, as needed, to assist students in weighing such options as medical leaves of absence or academic accommodations, and to enlist, as appropriate, the support of family, friends, advisors or deans – tasks for which college counselors are better equipped than therapists working at a remove from campus culture. Finally, the preparatory period almost invariably involves setting limits, which is not to be confused with establishing rigid, unenforceable rules for the therapeutic relationship. Rather, by setting limits we mean articulating the limits of what the counseling center can and will do for the patient, and establishing that the patient must share in the responsibility for getting well [23]. Once a student at significantly elevated risk is referred, the referring clinician should, of course, make a concerted effort to insure that the student follows up [28].

Among the other more challenging referral situations are those in which students are in denial as to the severity of their problems, a state of affairs that is not uncommon in work with eating disorders, substance abuse and dependence, and bipolar disorder, among other conditions. To prolong on-campus treatment with such students often amounts to colluding with their denial insofar as their condition cannot be effectively treated within the counseling center. At the same time, insisting upon an expedited referral may effectively constitute abandonment: patients who reject the notion that they have significant problems have no incentive to pursue treatment off campus, but do have multiple disincentives, including the unconscious desire to remain in denial.

Dilemmas such as these again underscore that referral is not the simple act of providing information about available outside resources, but rather a process-oriented psychoeducational intervention that often requires considerable therapeutic skill. The techniques of motivational interviewing [29] are illustrative of a collaborative approach to stimulating a desire for change that may be usefully adapted to many referral situations. Motivational interviewing, treated in greater depth later in this volume, seeks to enhance patients' belief in their own efficacy and to increase awareness of the disparity between their goals, on the one hand, and their behaviors, on the other. The socially awkward student who significantly abuses alcohol as a social lubricant may, for example, be helped to recognize that his or her drinking has not, in fact, engendered social or romantic success, but on the contrary, has resulted in numerous quarrels and embarrassing social displays, and has, if anything, been a detriment to a fulfilling social life. Realizations of this kind may serve as an incentive for change, and thereby smooth the path for referral for substance abuse counseling. Note that in this example the student is motivated to seek substance abuse counseling not because the denial of alcohol abuse is necessarily overcome or because he or she "learns" that excessive drinking is unhealthy – something known to virtually all college students, without the benefit of a lecture – but because the value of moderating drinking is brought into alignment with the student's aspirations for an improved social life.

Of course, no matter how skilled the clinician, there can be no guarantee that a referral will take hold or even that a student will remain in treatment long enough to raise the subject of referral. Therefore, particularly when working with students at elevated risk for self-harm, counselors are well advised to treat each session as if it might be the last, and to engage students in safety planning and similar targeted active interventions at every opportunity. These interventions are not incompatible with the overall treatment goal of referral to a higher level of care; in fact, to the extent that they demonstrate the potential efficacy of treatment, they may serve as an inducement to pursue referral recommendations.

5.4 Personal Counseling and Brief Psychotherapy

In the broadest of strokes, college counseling is most likely to prove beneficial when it is understood as a distinct specialty with guiding principles that transcend practitioners' theoretical orientation. Effective college mental health professionals adapt their approach – be it cognitive–behavioral, interpersonal, psychodynamic, or otherwise – to account for the developmental opportunities and vulnerabilities of their late adolescent and young adult patients, and to account, as well, for the realities of the college setting, among them, the fast-paced, often unforgiving academic calendar; the local campus culture; and the constraints on services that can be provided in the university counseling center. Successful treatment, as already noted, begins with thoughtful patient selection and collaborative treatment planning. Beyond this, it is focused, but flexible, active and activating, solution-oriented, culturally sensitive, and attuned to the transformative possibilities intrinsic to therapeutic relationships. Finally, like all good clinicians, college counselors are attentive to countertransferential barriers to delivering quality care.

5.4.1 Solution-Oriented, Focused Treatment

Common to almost all forms of short-term therapy is an effort to establish a therapeutic focus early on, and to maintain that focus going forward. In the ideal, the focus of treatment embodies goals that "can be stated in positive language, assessed as observable behavior, that are dear to the patient, that are congruent with the patient's culture, and that are – *possible*" ([18], p. 98). The treatment focus defines a scope of work to be undertaken, and provides a coherent organizing principle for the treatment to come, but is neither monolithic nor immutable. The therapist strives to "be flexible, yet focused; to use different perspectives and interventions, as necessary; yet to bring them together into a unified, integrative treatment" ([30], pp. 132–133). Insofar as a treatment focus emerges from a dialogue between student and counselor, in the ideal it encourages curiosity, thoughtfulness, self-reflection, an orientation toward reality, and problem-solving in the student. In the language of psychoanalysis, it is in and of itself an ego building activity.

In short, brief psychotherapy is defined by a time-limited treatment plan, not by default, as when students simply drop out of treatment or exhaust their allocation of visits. The content and form of the treatment focus will vary across theoretical orientations, but is typically stated in terms of an overarching symptom, a defining intrapsychic conflict, a developmental impasse, a recurrent interpersonal quandary, a persistent pattern of maladaptive behavior, or a life theme, such as separation-individuation [31]. By way of illustration, Mann [32] describes a highly anxious patient with a long history of loss who presents with baseless fears of being discharged from his job. Mann suggests to this patient that all his life he has been excessively nervous and has expected the worst because of the many sudden, unanticipated and painful events in his past. In other words, he conceptualizes the patient's presenting problem in terms of the "central conflict" of loss which then becomes the focus of treatment. The early articulation of a dynamic treatment focus, as it is usually understood, is somewhat incompatible with the increasingly influential constructivist/relational perspective from which therapists are viewed as much participants as observers in treatment, who therefore cannot divorce themselves from interpersonal involvement with patients sufficiently to articulate a reasonably objective formulation of patients' problems. That said, even from this relational perspective, there is an appreciation that short term treatment requires a focus; within this model, however, a process focus may replace a content focus. That is, the stated focus of treatment may be on developing generalizable capacities for self-observation and awareness of how one's inner processes unfold in interaction with others [33].

The point of departure for establishing a therapeutic focus is, then, the patient's presenting complaints and expectations, but the patient's initial understanding of the source and nature of these complaints and of available avenues for addressing them may undergo varying degrees of transformation as the student and counselor devise a preliminary course of action. While some students have a fairly good understanding of what ails them, others may benefit from psychoeducational intervention in reformulating their problems and developing a better appreciation of realistic means of addressing them. A somewhat oversimplified illustration is that of the first year student with a history of mild learning disability who complains of being "too stupid to manage" after receiving grades of B + , as compared to A's earned in high school, and is now contemplating transfer to another, less demanding university. Here, in the course of elaborating a treatment focus, it may be useful, first, to draw a sharp distinction between difficulties secondary to intellectual capacity and difficulties attendant upon a learning disability; second, to educate the student about the normative adjustment period between high school and college; and third to challenge the accuracy of the student's negative appraisal of his or her grades. Should the student prove receptive to these sorts of interventions, the focus of treatment may seamlessly shift from the question "Shall I transfer?" to "What academic supports and accommodations do I require, and how shall I arrange for them?"

An initial psychoeducational approach, even when ineffective, may usefully help surface underlying psychodynamics and/or personality traits, and suggest a productive focus of treatment. For instance, in the case of our hypothetical learning disorder student an acceptance of the reality of the learning problem but a refusal to seek needed academic accommodations and support services might segue into work on intrapsychic conflicts about autonomy and dependence and/or about perfectionism and narcissistic vulnerability.

Brief therapy necessitates a more explicit and narrower focus than longer term treatments, and, even more than this, demands more of the therapist in actively maintaining a focus. "Focus", as Groves [18] observed, is not just a noun, but a verb as well; it is the counselor's task to refocus students on issues that can reasonably be addressed in treatment. This is not to suggest a rigid or mechanical adherence to a treatment plan; obviously the emergence of new facts, or a change in a student's life circumstances, such as an unexpected loss or trauma, may require a shift in direction. College counselors also do well to remember that their adolescent and young adult patients are in a phase of life noteworthy for waves of intense, even overwhelming feelings that may dissipate almost as suddenly as they surface, and should be prepared to discard treatment plans that, seemingly overnight, are rendered obsolete by a marked change in young patients' mood and outlook.

In general, however, therapists are charged with maintaining fidelity to a mutually ratified treatment focus, which, after all, embodies, and is intended to ameliorate, students' principle complaints. Refocusing students often also provides an opportunity to comment on maladaptive strategies for managing anxiety. By way once more of a much over-simplified example, consider the situation of a student on academic probation, who is not progressing with her schoolwork, because, she says, there are just too many competing demands on her time. In counseling, she quickly turns the conversation to a trivial quarrel with her boyfriend, even as a critical academic deadline looms near. It is neither terribly helpful nor empathic to protest that the student is not here to discuss her romantic life. By contrast, it might have therapeutic utility to suggest that the student is made so anxious by her work that she, understandably, wishes to direct her attention elsewhere, and to wonder aloud if she is replicating in therapy the same mechanism for managing anxiety – avoidance – as undermines her scholastic endeavors. Such a statement capitalizes on observations in the here and now to offer a hypothesis about the source of the student's problem (anxiety), about the maladaptive means of contending with the problem (avoidance) and about an approach to solving the problem (developing better strategies for managing anxiety).

Maintaining a therapeutic focus emphatically introduces into treatment the critical dimension of *time*, which very often is perceived or managed unrealistically by students. The ticking clock in the background of brief treatment can be used to therapeutic advantage.[5] After all, the clock is not merely ticking in the therapist's office; it is ticking away the minutes of the patient's life. Students, in particular, are often on the clock. Those who are struggling academically do not have a year or two to unravel the depression, anxiety, psychodynamic conflicts or character traits that impede their progress – by then they are likely to be on academic suspension or worse. Students who are socially inhibited cannot reclaim the unique opportunities for interpersonal growth college affords if they only emerge from self-imposed isolation after graduation. And so on.

At a deeper level, "The link between time and reality is insoluble. We can divorce ourselves from time only by undoing reality or from reality only by undoing the sense of time". ([32], p. 66). If treatment does not explicitly incorporate reference to the insistent passage of time, it may unintentionally collude with the desire, present to some degree in virtually every patient, to avoid change, to cling to self-defeating, fundamentally unful-filling ways of life, if only because there is a certain comfort and feeling of safety in the familiar, no matter how maladaptive [34].

Patients are not alone in wishing to negate the passage of time, which, after all, is intimately entwined with the bitter fact of mortality. Thus, therapists too may shrink from realistic engagement with time. However, the brevity of short-term work introduces time into the treatment in ways that are much harder for patient – or therapist – to ignore. In the ideal, treatment can capitalize on this: much as transference affords a medium for demonstrating and reworking maladaptive relational patterns, students' response or lack of response to the time constraints of treatment is potentially a useful window into, and opportunity to address, their relationship to the progress – or lack of progress – in their lives outside the consulting room.

---

[5] Provocative in this respect is the work of Michael Brakham and his colleagues [15] who have found a quicker rate of improvement in patients randomly assigned to 8-session treatments than to those assigned to 16-session treatments, raising the possibility that change occurs more rapidly when tighter time limits are imposed.

A distortion in the sense of time is an especially relevant phenomenon in working with late adolescents, for whom it is developmentally normative to feel at once an excessive sense of urgency, even as they behave as if the future stretches infinitely before them. Adolescents typically entertain "a decided disbelief in the possibility that time may bring change, and yet also of a violent fear that it might" ([35], p. 169). Their disbelief is understandable enough: they are painfully aware of their immaturities which they often exaggerate in comparison to their peers, and which leads them to question their ability to take their place in adult society. Their fear of changing – of maturing – is rooted in a dread of adult levels of commitment and responsibility, in the loss of the gratifications and seemingly unlimited potential of childhood, and in the recognition that to grow up is to discover and confront "the finiteness of life, as well as the finiteness of personal abilities and choices" ([23], p. 36).

5.4.2 The Counseling Relationship

Psychotherapy research has repeatedly demonstrated that the quality of the patient-therapist alliance is an important, if modest,[6] predictor of therapeutic outcomes across all modalities of treatment, including pharmacotherapy [21,36–39]. Research is less instructive in specifying the therapist characteristics and behaviors that contribute to a strong alliance, although there is evidence linking a positive working relationship to an empathic, collaborative approach and to shared treatment goals [36,40] and to techniques that specifically convey engagement, support, understanding and affirmation of successes; that help patients increase their understanding of their problems; and that focus on patients' subjective experience during sessions [41]. Techniques at the extremes – for example, excessive structuring of sessions, or conversely, a failure to proceed in any coherent, organized manner (i.e. a failure to develop and maintain a therapeutic focus) – appear to compromise the formation of a strong working alliance [41].

Of course, psychotherapeutic technique is rarely clear-cut. While it is intuitive to suppose that empathy, attentiveness, reliability and similar qualities could only further treatment, clinical experience demonstrates that this is not always the case [42]. For example, active listening may be received by some students as passive or depriving. A non-judgmental stance may be experienced as infuriatingly nondirective and unhelpful. Cultural factors may figure prominently in how a counselor's interpersonal style is received. For example, therapists who adhere to a process-oriented approach may alienate or confuse students whose cultural expectations and preferences are for authoritative advice and concrete problem-solving strategies. At the same time, therapists are well advised to exercise caution in responding to students based on cultural "sensitivities" that might unwittingly sacrifice an appreciation of their individuality, and in this respect end up just another form of stereotyping [43,44]. A student's cultural identification should not be assumed a priori; students may identify with racial or ethnic affiliations very different from those an outside

---

[6] Averaging the findings of hundreds of psychotherapy outcome studies and many meta-analyses, Norcross and Lambert [36] estimated that the therapist-patient relationship accounts for 10% of the variance in psychotherapy outcomes. While this figure may seem low, contrast the impact of the relationship to that of specific treatment methods which account for only 5–8% of the outcome variance. In fact, patient variables (expectations of help; diagnosis; readiness for change, etc.) is the only factor which has been shown to contribute more to the success of treatment than the therapeutic relationship does.

observer might assign them, and may also differ dramatically from others within their ethnic/racial group in their degree of acculturation and in their stage of racial identity development [45].

In tailoring therapeutic style to students from a variety of backgrounds, it behoves college counselors to develop as broad as possible an understanding of different value systems, and to avoid using the mores of the counselor's own culture as a frame of reference for "normality". For example, counseling practices often place a premium on promoting individuality, independence, and personal responsibility – values prevalent in the Caucasian majority culture but contrary to those of many traditional Asian–American and Hispanic families, in which the culturally accepted norm is to place the welfare of the family unit above the pursuit of individual success [46,47].

Beyond cultural considerations, in the context of college health mental practice, attunement to the vicissitudes of late adolescent and young adult development may usefully inform a counselor's therapeutic stance. An appreciation of developmentally expectable strivings, fears, and conflicts and of the age-specific coping strategies of late adolescence can help in managing a wide range of relational challenges in treatment, such as mistrust, ambivalence, acting out, and the externalization of conflicts, as detailed elsewhere by Eichler [23]. Beyond this, a developmental orientation can foster greater creativity in using the relationship as a central instrument of growth. Years ago, Mahler and her collaborators observed that toddlers more readily step out into the world, both literally and figuratively, if they are certain of a secure "home base" to which to return for "emotional refueling" [48]. Almost all parents are familiar with the phenomenon Mahler described: their toddlers, intoxicated with the newly acquired ability to walk, race across the playground, only to be momentarily overcome by panic at finding themselves alone and unsupported in what feels like a forbiddingly large and unfamiliar world. Upon searching frantically for their parent, and reconnecting through gaze or touch, toddlers are reassured and happily resume exploring. In much the same way, college students more readily experiment with the rich psychosocial possibilities of college life, and better meet the challenges of transitioning to adulthood when fortified by secure attachments [49,50].

For students whose attachment figures have proven less than reliable, or who, at 18 or 19 are simply still young and somewhat at a loss when geography or circumstances deprives them of close familial contact, college counseling centers may assume, to some extent, the function of secure "home bases". The awareness of ongoing access to care, albeit if only for very brief episodes of counseling, affords some students a sense of support and connection that emboldens them to meet developmental challenges. This is, however, once again only possible when centers are flexible in their administrative arrangements, and counselors are flexible in their therapeutic stance.

None of this is to contradict our earlier assertion that students with significant personality disorders or severe or multiple psychiatric diagnoses are best referred as soon as practical. Intermittent therapy is not long-term therapy. It is, in essence, a flexible distribution of a handful of sessions over an extended period of time, and in that sense, it is actually best classified as brief treatment. For more severely disturbed students, prolonged but intermittent treatment is unlikely to provide a platform for developmental expansion; at best, it may succeed in temporarily restablizing chronically unstable students. While perhaps at times unavoidable, intermittent treatment for more seriously disturbed students "may be akin to the enabling behavior that partners of alcoholics engage in, which allows the condition to continue and, over the long haul, worsen" ([51], p. 697).

5.5 Medication Services

The use of medications has increased dramatically in college mental health practice over the last decade or two. In 1994, counseling center directors reported that only 9% of students treated at their centers were prescribed medication on campus; by 2007, that figure had risen to 26% [12]. Currently, 60% of college counseling services report offering some form of psychiatric coverage and most directors say that they would prefer increased professional resources for medication management on campus [12].

Some prominent clinicians within the college mental health community voice serious reservations about prescribing psychiatric medications to students [52], and, certainly, given the vicissitudes of adolescent and young adult psychological development, caution is warranted in prescribing, especially for less severe symptoms. However, there is growing consensus that under many clinical circumstances, medication (and medication combined with psychotherapy) is quite beneficial [53]. Moreover, since many students arrive on campus already on a regimen of medication [54] and many others expect or want access to medication management, it is preferable to provide these services as an integrated element of counseling center treatment.

5.5.1 Models of Care

As noted in Chapters 2 and 3 there are varying models of care within college mental health systems. These derive in part from historical tradition, in part from issues of turf and professional identity, and in part from funding and administrative concerns that differ among campuses. As a result, a variety of relationships exist between medicating clinician and therapist. Psychotropic medication may be prescribed by a non-psychiatrist physician at the college health service or by a psychiatrist, physician's assistant or nurse practitioner each of whom may be housed at either the health center or at the counseling center. On some campuses, counseling center psychiatrists combine psychotherapy with medication, while on other campuses psychiatric practice is typically limited to pharmacotherapy while psychotherapy is provided by non-medical clinicians. And at the 40% of colleges in which there is no capacity to prescribe psychiatric medication on site, prescribing may be done through any number of off-campus settings.

When medication services and psychotherapy are delivered by different practitioners, careful consideration need be given to *coordination and communication* between therapist and prescribing clinician. Inadequate communication is by far the most frequent source of difficulty in split treatments, particularly as patients may present very different information to each practitioner, and the usual transference–countertransference challenges may be amplified in a therapeutic triad, as opposed to the more common therapeutic dyad [55].

Coordination of care in split treatments is obviously simplest when the prescribing clinician is housed at the college mental health service. If this is not the case, when a referral for medication evaluation is made, permission should routinely be requested (and, if appropriate, a release signed) for the treating clinicians to confer, as necessary. Students who self refer for medication assessment or treatment should be asked whether they are also being seen for psychotherapy, and again arrangements should be made for communication between prescriber and therapist. If a student is not participating in talk therapy, it is generally wise to explore whether counseling should be incorporated into the treatment plan. For further discussion of combining psychotherapy and medication see Hollon and Fawcett [56].

5.6 Referring Students for Consultation

Referral for psychiatric assessment should generally be considered for students who present with:

- psychosis

- significant or persistent anxiety or depression

- significant mood swings

- significant attention or concentration problems that have not responded to behavioral or environmental interventions

- panic attacks

- significant sleep problems

- symptoms of post-traumatic stress disorder

- significant symptoms of obsessive–compulsive disorder or other impulse problems

- repeated self-injurious behaviors

- eating disorders

It is also usually advisable for students already taking medication when they first present at the counseling center to be seen for a re-evaluation, unless they are stable and have a viable, ongoing treatment arrangement with a clinician "back home". Even when there is a home-based prescriber, if clinical resources permit, it is often prudent for students to develop a backup relationship with a college area psychiatrist[7] in case problems emerge that require a face to face assessment. This is particularly true when the student's primary treating clinician is situated at a great distance from the university.

In the case of students manifesting psychosis, severe depression and/or severe anxiety (especially when accompanied by suicidal ideation or impulses), psychiatric assessment should be arranged as soon as feasible, since hospitalization may be a required in addition to the urgent initiation of medication. Furthermore, timely treatment with a benzodiazepine may forestall the need for ongoing medication for students experiencing acute or frequent panic symptoms [57,58].

In less urgent circumstances, it is often makes sense to see students for a few psychotherapeutic visits before making a referral for medication assessment. This can be beneficial since many young adults have significant variation in mood, thought and functioning and often, seemingly serious problems can resolve with a bit of supportive care and watchful waiting. Starting medication prematurely can obscure the reasons for any improvements noted (i.e. is improvement due to changing circumstances or to medication?) and this could, in turn, result in students taking medicine needlessly. It may also precipitate unnecessary anxiety about relapse when the decision is made to discontinue medication [57]. In addition, taking time to develop trusting relationships with patients facilitates referral for a

---

[7] For the sake of convenience, we use "psychiatrist" in the text to denote the prescribing clinician, even though the medicating clinician may not, in fact, be a psychiatrist.

medication evaluation by, among other things, reassuring patients that the decision to recommend such a consultation has not been taken lightly.

When the issue of psychiatric assessment is raised, therapists should explain the reasons for referral in fairly specific terms. Since psychiatric medications are not diagnosis specific [59], it is vital to explain the symptoms that are the target of treatment. Therapists should explain that an assessment is a conversation, and will not necessarily result in the prescription of medication. Again, it is important to discuss the value of ongoing communication between the treating therapist and psychiatrist and to emphasize the value of a treatment combining talk therapy and medicine when this is indicated. It is also imperative to explore the patient's expectations, fantasies and concerns about medicine. It is particularly important to dispel the notion that response to medicine implies either a long-term need for medicine or a specific "illness". It should also be made clear that medicine will likely not be a panacea but is often effective in lessening symptoms to some extent.

5.6.1 Medication Consultation

As noted above, colleges have varying structures for managing medication consultation. As circumstances allow, consultation is best performed by someone with the greatest degree of psychiatric specialization and the greatest degree of proximity (or at least communication) with the treating therapist. In any case, the reason for the consultation should be conveyed by the primary therapist to the psychiatrist in advance of the medication evaluation. This allows the psychiatrist to focus clinical attention and to explore differences in clinical presentation that may emerge in the consultation visit.

Even when extensive information is conveyed by the treating therapist, the college psychiatrist should always conduct an independent, thorough assessment of the patient. It is imperative that the psychiatrist have a firm grounding, not only in psychopharmacology, but also in the developmental issues relevant to college students. The college psychiatrist must also be cognizant of, and sensitive to, the ebb and flow of university life (More about this later).

The assessment should include a careful evaluation of the intensity, duration and persistence of current symptoms; and a review of family history and medical history (including possibility of pregnancy). Careful attention should be paid to subtle signs of thought disorder, as the college age is frequently the age of first presentation of psychiatric illness. Past treatment experiences should be assessed both for potential indicators of pre-existing diagnoses or problems, and for what they might reveal of patients' feelings toward treatment. It is essential to probe past and current substance use with recognition that substance abuse is often under-reported in this setting [60]. It is also important to assess environmental factors such as sleep and eating patterns or their disturbances, not only because they may be symptoms of depression or anxiety, but because they can also cause these problems [57]. Some clinicians find rating scales a helpful adjunct to assessment but, as discussed more fully below, rating scales are not a substitute for a thorough clinical assessment.

5.6.2 To Medicate, or not to Medicate

The decision to prescribe medication should not be predicated on symptom severity and diagnostic impression alone, but should also take account of the patient's desire or hesitation about taking medication, as well as, for most undergraduates, their parents' attitudes and concerns about psychiatric medication. Matters of timing are of major concern when prescribing for students. For example, starting a selective serotonin reuptake inhibitor (SSRI) that takes several weeks to impart clinical benefit, but which may have rapid onset of troubling side effects, may be ill advised shortly before a period of exams for a student who does not currently exhibit marked functional impairment. While side effects tend to be of short duration, even relatively minor levels of fatigue, jitteriness or sleeplessness over a week or 10 days can significantly compromise the efforts of students struggling to study for finals or to catch up on papers, particularly when they are already grappling with anxiety or depression.

It is sensible to explore whether environmental manipulation, talk therapy, reduction in substance use, or behavioral interventions such as aerobic exercise may be adequate to address mild to moderate symptoms of anxiety or depression. However, in cases of psychosis or severe depression or anxiety, it is best not to delay initiating medication treatment unless there is a specific contraindication. In general, one should consider whether acute, intermittent or short-term medications might suffice to stabilize a situation. This is especially important since many young people are less than fully compliant and consistent in taking regularly prescribed medicine. While it may not be practical (or necessary) to perform a full medical evaluation for every patient for whom medicine may be prescribed, clinicians should carefully re-examine medical history, other medications currently taken, and recent medical care and should be alert to possible indications of an organic cause for symptoms. For example, a student with unexplained and abrupt surges of anxiety may be suffering from thyroid disease; a student with fatigue and depression inconsistent with past history or present circumstances may be suffering from mononucleosis. A student who has had no recent physical exam or who has indication of possible physical illness should be referred for a physical assessment. Students who are candidates for treatment with stimulant medication and mood stabilizers like lithium carbonate should also be screened for any evidence of underlying cardiac disease [61].

5.6.3 Talking to Students About Medication

Students' attitudes toward medication range from those who might well benefit from, but nevertheless resist, a medication trial for any of a variety of irrational reasons to those who lack clear indications for medication treatment, but nevertheless seek it. Some students experience taking medication as a sign of weakness or fear that responding to medicine implies a specific illness or lifelong need for psychopharmacological treatment and therefore are reluctant to entertain pharmacological intervention. At the other end of the spectrum, some students have come to see any troubling mood or thought as an illness based deformity that ought to be addressed through medication [62]. Prescribers need be attuned to the ways in which students process recommendations concerning medication even when their overt responses seem measured and rational. Among the many negative transference reactions that may arise from the prescription of psychotropic medication are a fear of being controlled; a belief that the psychiatrist is uninterested in, or overwhelmed by, the student's feelings or experience and wishes to blunt the student's affect; or a conviction that the psychiatrist lacks the skill to assist the student through psychotherapy [55]. When psychiatrists decline to prescribe an inappropriate medication, students may experience them as withholding; and when medications, even when efficacious, disappoint inflated expectations, psychiatrists may be devalued along with the pills they dispense.

The prescribing psychiatrist must convey a balanced explanation of the value and limits of medication treatment. As already noted, psychiatric medications do not treat specific illnesses (with the possible exception of psychostimulants for the treatment of attention deficit hyperactivity disorder) and response to medicine does not necessarily imply a particular diagnosis or clinical course. Even young people who have a severe episode of depression have a significant likelihood of not re-experiencing another severe episode. While a full blown psychotic episode outside the context of intoxication, substance abuse or medical illness may be more prognostically worrisome, it is still no guarantee of lifelong psychiatric disturbance [63].

It is important for the psychiatrist to be both modest in claims about medicine, but at the same time hopeful about treatment. Medicine should be presented as one component of a comprehensive treatment plan. Patients should be informed of the importance of taking medication as prescribed, following up with visits, not taking any other medicines without first checking with the psychiatrist and not abusing substances while on medication. It is best for the psychiatrist to review the possible risks of mixing medication and substances, but these risks should not be overstated. If the dangers of mixing medication and substances are exaggerated, a student who drinks while on medication without untoward effect may develop a cavalier attitude toward potentially volatile combinations going forward. Please see Table 5.2 for more "helpful hints for prescribers".

Since certain psychiatric medications, such as anti-anxiety agents and psychostimulants, have potential for abuse, psychiatrists need remain alert to patients who may be seeking medication for recreational or non-clinical purposes. Presentations that seem too perfect (as if they are being read out of the *Diagnostic and Statistical Manual*), patients who are too insistent or demanding, have frequent need for early refills (especially of controlled substances) or who have histories of substance abuse, should be evaluated and managed

Table 5.2	Helpful hints for prescribers

Start low and go slow: In general, students who are new to medication can be fairly sensitive to side effects, especially when they are trying to continue to function actively at school. It is usually preferable to start medications at approximately half the recommended dose and increase slowly. Students are more likely to comply when they are not overwhelmed with side effects.

Side effects typically precede benefits: Most psychiatric medications, but especially the SSRIs, are likely to cause side effects before they help. It is important to make sure patients are aware of this. At least in the case of SSRIs, typically mild side effects can predict a robust response

Don't forget to discuss weight gain: Many psychiatric medications can cause weight gain and this will often result in non-compliance. Make sure to discuss weight gain ahead of time. For more information see Fava [64].

Discuss sexual side effects: Many patients are hesitant to discuss the adverse sexual side effects of medications. These side effects can often result in non-compliance if not managed properly. There are several approaches to minimizing sexual side effects; it also helpful to inform students that depression and anxiety can diminish sexual interest and to the extent that it diminishes symptoms, medication can also have a positive effect on libido. The reader is referred for a more detailed discussion to Hirschfeld [65].

Don't stop medicine abruptly: Remind patients that many medicines need to be tapered. Students should not stop medicine without discussing this with their psychiatrist and without supervision. Management of medication and plans for refilling medicine over breaks and summer need to be discussed carefully and well in advance of the break.

SSRI, selective serotonin reuptake inhibitor.

especially carefully and every attempt should be made to obtain confirmatory or corroborating evidence for diagnosis and treatment.

5.7 Group Therapy in College Mental Health Services

While recent academic literature on group therapy in college mental health is somewhat spare, group programs are in fact quite widespread and robust. A random review of 20 college counseling center web sites performed by one of the authors (Schwartz) in March 2009 demonstrated that group counseling has become a routine offering in college mental health services. This should come as no surprise since groups afford a number of valuable therapeutic and strategic benefits. Whitaker [66] has noted that groups may offer advantages for students struggling with relationship problems, and Sheehy and Commerford [67] have suggested groups may be more effective than individual therapy for some students with eating disorders. For late adolescents and young adults concerned with how to relate to others or how to retain a sense of autonomy while remaining connected to family and community, group counseling provides a natural setting in which to examine these and similar concerns.

Groups provide an appealing alternative for many services that struggle with limited clinical resources since perhaps five to ten patients can be treated in a single session. However the time savings conferred by group treatment may be somewhat illusory. In a survey of group programs in college counseling centers, Golden and colleagues [68] found that typically 20% or fewer of patients were seen in a group modality and that 90% of them had been referred by individual therapists within the service. This finding suggests that many, if not most, students treated in groups are also seen for individual therapy (although it is likely that some students are seen several times for assessment sessions and then referred for group treatment exclusively). Initiating groups is a fairly labor and time intensive process. Publicizing, prescreening, and preparing members for participation are all important components to successful group programs, and all take time. In short then, counseling centers appear to offer group programs primarily because of their perceived therapeutic value rather than to stretch limited resources. And indeed, in Golden's survey, 83% of respondents (counseling center directors) rated their group programs as either successful or very successful.

5.7.1 Types of Groups

The great variety of groups offered at counseling centers may be categorized along several lines. The most frequent offerings are traditional *"process" groups*. These are groups that primarily focus on interpersonal relationships and social interaction. They may be ongoing (which presents several logistical challenges for a college population), but are more commonly relatively brief in duration, and are usually informed by one of several psychodynamic models (described more fully in [69,70]). Participation in these groups may be open to all members of the student community or may be limited to specific populations (such as groups for men or students of color or graduate students). They are sometimes focused on particular symptoms or problems (e.g. students who have experienced loss, or abuse, or are children of alcoholics).

In recent years, there has been growth in the popularity of therapy groups based on either cognitive behavioral therapy (CBT) or dialectical-behavior therapy (DBT) approaches. The reader is referred to White and Freeman [71] and to Dimeff *et al.* [72], respectively, for more detailed descriptions. These groups are typically focused on particular symptoms such as anxiety or depression management, or on particular diagnoses such as eating disorders, or, in the case of DBT, on borderline spectrum problems.

Universities also offer a range of psychoeducational groups, which are typically short term and have a specific focus, such as teaching techniques to cope with anxiety (e.g. Harvard's, "The worrier's guide to the universe" and Duke's "meditation and mindfulness" groups[8]), or to improve time management or study skills. Support groups addressing developmental issues relevant to particular groups of students are also common. For example, many universities run support groups for doctoral students working on dissertations, for international students acculturating to the American educational system, and increasingly, for combat veterans transitioning back to civilian life after tours of duty in Iraq or Afghanistan. Psychoeducation groups are less exploratory and more supportive in nature and are not intended to promote an examination of group process. They are usually open to any student who may wish to attend. Many times these groups can also be run as single session workshop programs.

Finally, there are groups for special populations, special circumstances, and innovative group designs. Many campuses have Alcoholics Anonymous programs, although these are often not run directly through the counseling service. The University of Iowa has begun a group for students on the Asperger's spectrum called "Making a connection". Special circumstances groups are exemplified by a group at Brigham Young University that has met with success focusing on self defeating perfectionism in a devout Mormon student group [73]. California State University at Sacramento has several groups for survivors of sexual assault or domestic violence that combine yoga and traditional talk therapy. Both report high ratings for participant satisfaction. Group treatment can also be quite helpful for students for whom interpersonal conflicts impede academic progress in programs that place a significant emphasis on collaborative work. An example is a focused group for MBA students who have had interpersonal difficulty in group projects. (M. Bailey, former director of group program, NYU, personal communication).

5.7.2 Considerations in Setting Up a Group Program

There are several significant challenges to establishing a group program on college campuses. Since universities function largely as self contained communities, there are often greater issues than in other less cloistered settings related to both privacy and to managing the relationships students may develop with one another outside the group. On smaller campuses, in particular, this can be a formidable challenge. Also, college students' schedules frequently change and students often take for granted that attendance is optional for the many activities in which they are engaged. This can create problems with commitment to regular attendance at group sessions [74].

With these considerations in mind, it is important to prepare the group program with adequate forethought and planning. When feasible, it is helpful to designate one staff member to coordinate and oversee the program. Thought should be given to the nature of the campus community and to which groups have been successful and well received by students in prior years. Scheduling of groups should allow for the greatest likelihood of student attendance. Early evening hours often work well for many students at residential universities, whereas mid-day/lunchtime groups are more suitable for colleges with larger commuter populations.

---

[8] Except where otherwise indicated, all reports of specific group programs are from an informal request for group information posted to the AUCCCD listserv in late February 2009.

As noted above, most group referrals come from clinicians within the counseling service so these clinicians should be kept well informed about the group program and provided details about specific groups: whether they are therapy or psychoeducational, time limited or ongoing, and so on. Inclusion and exclusion criteria should be shared.

Prescreening students for therapy groups is highly recommended. When groups are organized around treating specific symptoms, establishing a diagnosis is, of course, a critical inclusionary (or exclusionary) criterion for participation. While there is little empirical research to define a precise approach to screening for groups that are not diagnosis-specific, common sense is often a sufficient guide. It seems reasonable, for instance, to suppose that students appropriate for therapy/interpersonal groups are those who have some difficulty with social interaction but are not struggling with either intense social anxiety or severe anger problems. Prescreening allows group leaders to identify students who might find certain types of groups problematic. For example, some people with history of panic attacks find meditation based groups extremely anxiety provoking.

Motivation to participate in group treatment is another significant consideration in the screening process. As part of this screening process, information needs to be shared about scheduling, length of the time the group will be meeting, and policies around absences. This allows the group leaders to make certain that group members are adequately committed to group attendance. It is important to be clear from the outset about group boundaries and ground rules, as well about the degree to which there will or will not be communication with therapists treating group members in individual psychotherapy. This may help to alleviate some concerns about privacy and confidentiality.

Policies around privacy and around group participants forming relationships outside the group should be made explicit, along with other boundary issues. It is not necessarily indicated, nor is it practical, to prohibit outside-the-group contact, and in some supportive groups (such as those for bereavement), extra-group contact may actually be helpful to group members. The essential issue is that therapists make rules explicit, give group members an opportunity for input into these rules, and monitor the group for problems or concerns around these issues. (M. Bailey, personal communication)

Many colleges use co-leaders for groups. This affords continuity if one leader is unable to attend, allows for better monitoring of group process and affords an excellent training opportunity when a senior clinician is paired with a trainee. It obviously makes sense to note which groups run successfully in order to make plans and husband resources for upcoming semesters and school years. It is also useful to think strategically about scheduling of workshop-style groups. For example, time management and study skills are logically offered during the early part of school year before students lacking these skills have dug too deep a hole for themselves. It may also be useful to partner with offices that provide academic support or disabilities services to help them address student needs.

5.8 Psychological Testing and Assessment

Psychological assessment may, in the context of college counseling serve a variety of ends, including:

- Screening for psychiatric illness
- Estimating current level of cognitive functioning or severity of psychiatric disturbance

- Assisting in differential diagnosis of psychological and cognitive disorders
- Evaluating the success of treatment interventions over time
- Providing a source of data for continuous quality improvement programs
- Assisting in educational and vocational planning.

Formal assessment instruments confer certain advantages. They help insure that critical areas of functioning are not overlooked; help control for (but do not entirely eliminate) problems arising from poor or biased reporting of symptoms by patients; allow for more systematic and standardized comparisons of patients' behaviors to those of relevant peer cohorts; and have established levels of reliability and validity that enable clinicians to realistically assess the strengths–and limitations–of findings. The validity of psychological measures (that is, the likelihood they actually measure what they purport to measure) is generally comparable to that of medical tests [75].

5.8.1 Types of Measures

Psychological assessment instruments can crudely be divided into two categories: (1) psychological tests that *directly* examine aspects of *observable* behaviors, and (2) self-report questionnaires, symptom inventories and other similar behavior rating scales that essentially ask respondents to *describe* their behavior or that of persons well known to them. Psychological tests sample behaviors through the presentation of a consistent set of tasks (e. g. factual questions to be answered, reading passages to be analyzed, numbers to be memorized, puzzles to be solved, inkblots to be described), whereas rating scales present observers (e.g. family members, clinicians, teachers) or patients themselves with a list of attributes on which to rate the patient in some consistent fashion. For example, an ADHD rating scale might ask the observer to indicate, among other things, whether the patient forgets important work or school assignments "never", "once in a while", "sometimes" or "often". The advantage of posing questions in relation to behavioral anchors of this type is that it allows responses to more readily be compared to group norms; comparing findings to normative data is fundamental to tests of all kinds.

Tables 5.3 and 5.4 provide a small sample of commonly used tests and rating scales, respectively, selected from among the vast array of such instruments available.

5.8.2 When to Use Tests and Other Measures

In college counseling centers, it is generally more practical to employ rating scales than psychological tests. Administering tests typically requires extensive training and proficiency. In addition, many take hours to administer and interpret, and most presenting questions can only be adequately answered by administering a battery of several such tests. Self-report inventories, on the other hand, are easily administered, scored and analyzed with a minimum of professional input, and for this reason often serve as excellent screening instruments, with certain caveats, which are discussed below. Self-report questionnaires minimize interviewer bias, and also typically include means of measuring the consistency with which patients respond to items, and hence the validity of their responses. That is to say, if patients provide radically different responses to items with similar content, the clinician is alerted to the

Table 5.3	Commonly used psychological tests	
Category of test	**General purposes within college counseling context**	**Examples of widely used tests**
Intelligence	Measure general intellectual endowment and assess specific strengths and weaknesses in various domains (e.g. verbal comprehension, working memory, processing speed) Essential part of any comprehensive psychological, psychoeducational or neuropsychological assessment	Wechsler Adult Intelligence Scale (WAIS-R) Stanford-Binet Intelligence Scales
Achievement	Measure competence in one or more academic areas (e.g. phonetic decoding of words, reading comprehension, reading rate, spelling, arithmetic); assist in educational planning In conjunction with a general intelligence test, and often neuropsychological tests, used to diagnose learning disabilities	Woodcock–Johnson-III Tests of Achievement (WJ-III-ACH) Wide Range Achievement Test Nelson Denny Test of Silent Reading
Neuropsychological	Identify strengths and weaknesses in specific neurological functions (e.g. attention, executive functions, memory, language processing) that contribute to learning Assist in diagnosing learning disabilities and in confirming the diagnosis of attention deficit disorder Measure cognitive impairment secondary to neurological insult	*Measures of attention, vigilance* (for example, Continuous Performance Test) *Measures of executive functions* (for example, Delis–Kaplan Executive Function System) *Measures of memory, learning* (for example, Rey Auditory–Verbal Learning Test) *Measures of perceptual organization & planning* (for example, Complex figure Test)
Projective	Controversy as to whether projective tests should be considered methods of generating hypotheses or tests As tests, purport to measure psychopathology, coping skills As methods of generating information, provide data about personality functioning subject to clinical interpretation [77]	Rorschach Inkblot Test Thematic Apperception Test (TAT)
Sources: [76–79,102].		

possibility that the test has not been completed thoughtfully or honestly, and that findings may be invalid.

For all their attributes, rating scales also have marked limitations, notably the inflexibility of their format which does not allow for follow-up and qualification of responses [81].

There is no simple way to summarize the conditions under which extensive testing, in contrast to brief screening, is appropriate. In fact, rigid protocols, such as those mandating repeated testing of patients on a fixed schedule, are "highly suspect" ([75], p. 129). Rather, testing decisions are best governed by individual clinical circumstances, weighing, among other factors, potential costs and benefits. For example, referring every underachieving student for a comprehensive battery of educational, intelligence and neuropsychological

Table 5.4	Commonly used behavioral rating and self-report scales	
Category	**Common uses in college health settings**	**Examples of widely used measures**
General Symptom Inventories	Screen for overall level of psychiatric distress and symptom severity	SCL-90-R
	Screen for symptomatology in 9 broad domains (e.g. phobic anxiety, interpersonal sensitivity, paranoia, etc.) Measure progress in treatment	Brief Symptom Inventory (BSI)
Personality inventories	Aid in the assessment of mental disorders, degree of emotional upset, identification of specific problem areas and strengths, and in treatment planning Generate hypotheses about psychodynamic functioning and prognosis	Minnesota Multiphasic Personality Inventory (Two versions currently in use: The MMPI-2 and MMPI-2-RF)[1]
	Screen for clinical patterns more easily related to DSM-IV syndromes than findings from the MMPI	Millon Clinical Multiaxial Inventory (MCMI-III)
	Generate personality patterns along dimensions derived from Jungian theory Most often used to assist in career choice	Myers-Brigg Personality Inventory
Depression scales	Screen for depression in general populations	PHQ-9
	Assess severity of depression	Beck Depression Inventory
	Monitor therapeutic outcomes	Revised Hamilton Rating Scale for Depression (*semi-structured interview*)
ADHD scales	Screen for ADHD Screen broad domains of impairment (e.g. inattention, hyperactivity, impulsivity)	Conners' Adult ADHD Rating Scale (CAARS)
Alcohol abuse/ questionnaires	Screen for abuse as well as hazardous/harmful drinking	Alcohol Use Disorders Identification Test (AUDIT)
Interest inventories	Assist in career and educational planning by identifying personality types (e.g. "Artistic", "Social", "Enterprising") and/or interests thought to correlate with occupational preferences	Strong Interest Inventories
		Kuder Occupational Interest Inventory, Kuder Career Search with Person Match
	Predictive of job satisfaction, but not of success–these are measures of preference, not of aptitude	Self-Directed Search (SDS-R)

Sources: [76,77,79–85].
[1]Controversy about the soundest ways of interpreting the MMPI is reflected in the publication of alternative versions of clinical scales. See Butcher and Williams [80] for a detailed discussion.

tests to rule out a learning disability is clearly unwarranted, whereas it often makes sense to refer for evaluation of nonverbal learning disabilities those students who have trouble setting priorities, developing outlines, organizing papers, distinguishing main ideas from details, understanding mathematical concepts, and negotiating social relationships – a constellation of complaints often associated with this disorder.

5.8.3 Interpreting Test Results

While an overview of psychometric considerations in testing is well beyond the scope of this chapter, by way of introduction to the subject we highlight below four broad areas of caution for the college mental health professional:

Testing is not the same as assessment

Diagnosis and treatment planning requires *comprehensive assessment*; over-reliance on the findings of psychological instruments considered in relative isolation can yield very wrong impressions. Consider, by way of a simple example, a college student who is found, on a standardized reading comprehension test, to score at the ninth grade level. This single finding may simply reflect overall intellectual endowment; or it could be indicative of a learning disability, or of a lack of adequate past instruction, or of a poor command of English if English is a second language; or it may reflect a highly idiosyncratic interpretation of reality consistent with serious mental illness; or problems in concentration, which, in turn may be secondary to trauma, depression, substance abuse, or a primary attention deficit. To properly interpret this single score, one might, then, require any or all of the following: a thorough developmental and family history; clinical interview and observation; the results of intelligence tests and of a variety of tests of language processing and other neuropsychological functions; interviews with collaterals; and a review of academic and/or psychiatric records. In short, testing is a subset of psychological assessment, which is a complex idiographic process of interpreting data gleaned from multiple sources [75].

Screening is not the same as diagnosing

To be useful in diagnosis and prognosis, scales must be sensitive – that is, effective in identifying those people who have a particular syndrome or trait of interest (so-called "true positives"). They must also be specific – that is, effective in ruling out those people who do not possess the attribute of interest. *Specificity* and *sensitivity* are generally reported as proportions. For example, a depression inventory that correctly identifies 85% of the true depressives in the population assessed is said to have a sensitivity of 0.85. An inventory that screens out 95% of those people who are not depressed ("true negatives") is said to have a specificity of 0.95. Specificity and sensitivity of 0.90 are considered "quite respectable for a psychological test" ([86], p. 412)

Although it may not at first be obvious, the diagnostic or predictive value of a scale is situational. A scale may possess excellent sensitivity and specificity and still be of limited practical use to the clinician if the *base rate*, or prevalence, of the behavior of interest is low in the population assessed [87]; under these circumstances such an instrument may well assign the diagnosis of interest to far more people who *don't* actually have the disorder than to those who do!. The mathematically adventurous reader is referred to Appendix A for a more detailed illustration of how this can occur.

This is not to suggest that rating scales are worthless in evaluating students for relatively rare disorders or behaviors. When prevalence is low, behavioral rating scales, if applied judiciously, may usefully serve as *screening* instruments to identify a group of people who merit further clinical evaluation.[9] Problems arise, however, when the findings of a screening are treated as definitive diagnoses, rather than as a first step in a more comprehensive diagnostic process, or when counseling centers lack the resources or administrative capacity to follow up with the very large number of students who may be identified as potentially at risk through screening protocols.

---

[9] This process is described in greater detail in Appendix A.

Measures may function differently in different settings
As noted above, the predictive value of scales depends, in part, on the prevalence of the behaviors or disorders they measure. Since prevalence may vary from one setting to the next, the utility of these tools may also vary from setting to setting. For example, screening every student on campus with a suicide inventory is likely to turn up a substantial proportion of false positives – that is, students who identified as suicidal who will not actually make suicide attempts. Using the same tool to screen students who present at the counseling center with a history of at least one past major depressive episode is likely to generate a significantly lower rate of false positives, since suicidal risk is likely to be much more prevalent in this group than in the general campus population.

Improvement on a rating scale is not necessarily meaningful progress
Improvement may be noted on a scale over time, but the fact that scores improve does not necessarily imply that treatment is working. Clinicians are cautioned against confusing statistical significance with clinical significance. Consider for example, a student in treatment for depression whose progress is monitored by monthly administration of a depression inventory on which her or his score declines a seemingly dramatic 20% before leveling off. While at first blush treatment may appear to be impressively beneficial, the student may well still meet the criteria for a major depressive episode, in which case there is little reason to be content with the outcome of therapy. The point is that even statistically significant progress on any scale of health is not a particularly consequential metric; what matters is whether improvement makes a meaningful difference in a patient's life [88]. In this vein, broad outcome measures have certain advantages. While it may seem natural enough to measure the progress of a patient in treatment for depression with a depression rating scale, such a scale may not register, for example, a marked increase in anxiety that results in continued compromise in quality of life even as dysphoria abates. Given the high incidence of depression and anxiety over the lifespan, at minimum it is recommended that both dimensions be incorporated into an instrument used as a global index of therapeutic progress, with serious consideration also given, if possible, to the quality of social relationships [89]. For a more thorough discussion of the use of measures to assess therapeutic outcomes, the reader is referred to Maruish [90]. In addition, it is important to bear in mind that improvement on a rating scale may be transitory; for example, depression is often a chronic, episodic illness and many patients will experience at least one recurrence of major depression, with the risk of recurrence rising if there have been multiple episodes [91]. Therefore, it is not generally wise to discontinue medication or other treatments based solely on symptom remission; the full clinical picture, including risk factors for recurrence, need be taken into account.

5.9 Community Outreach

A single finding from a recent national survey of 284 college counseling center directors calls into relief the importance of community outreach: 86.4% of students who died by suicide in 2007 at the colleges surveyed never sought psychological services on campus [12]. Clearly, then, there is a group of deeply distressed students – small in numbers, perhaps, but enormous in importance – that counseling centers must strive to reach. In addition, many international students and American-born minority students come from backgrounds in which there is significant shame associated with seeking mental health services, or in which it is considered disloyal to family members to discuss personal problems outside the home, or in which there are other significant cultural barriers to care [44,92]. It may be necessary for counselors to move out of their offices into the "home turf" of these students to demonstrate their commitment and relevance, and to dispel the many myths and misconceptions (as well as reality-based concerns) these students may have about mental health services [44,46].

However, there are significant challenges to mounting effective outreach efforts. Outreach often takes the form of programs intended to raise student awareness and overcome inaccurate and stigmatizing information about mental health problems and their treatment. The hope is that such programs will encourage students to reach out to friends in need or, even more optimistically, will inspire students who themselves are troubled to alter problematic behaviors or to seek help. Educational programs are, for example, the most common interventions employed by colleges to reduce alcohol abuse [103]. Yet, there is little reason to suppose that students who are suspicious of counseling or in denial about their own psychiatric or substance abuse problems will voluntarily attend these programs. Even if students do participate, knowledge or attitudinal change does not necessarily promote behavior change. For example, in thorough reviews of the salient literature, Larimer and Cronce [93] found little evidence to support the efficacy of educational or awareness programs in directly reducing problematic alcohol consumption, and similarly, Gould and Kramer [94] found contradictory evidence that educational programs, designed to stimulate self-disclosure or to promote the identification of peers at-risk, are effective in reducing youth suicide. In addition, if not well designed and well managed, educational programs have the potential to backfire. For example, programs designed to heighten awareness of eating disorders may turn into "how to" sessions [67]. Similarly, destigmatization campaigns emphasizing that mental illness is an illness like any other have been found in some studies to reduce blame for mental illness, but also to increase perceptions that psychiatric illness is marked by dangerousness and unpredictability [95] and possibly increase the desire for social distance from people with mental illnesses [96].

If campus programs are to attract students otherwise unlikely to seek counseling, they clearly must avoid recreating the psychological and cultural barriers that stand in the way of accessing care directly. Talks aimed at international students may, for example, do well to avoid topics with obvious mental health content in favor of programs which focus on pragmatic aspects of acculturation, such as how to approach an advisor, choose a major, compile a resume, and the like. Not only may such talks prove more useful than personal counseling for many international students [97] but they may also serve as an opportunity for these students to get to know counselors in an informal, non-threatening setting, and thereby promote future willingness to contact mental health professionals, if and when they are needed.

Other promising outreach approaches include gate-keeper training, a strategy based on the premise that faculty (especially faculty in writing or small seminar courses), residence hall advisors, coaches, clergy and other members of the campus community who are in almost daily contact with students are best positioned, with proper training and support, to identify students in distress in a timely fashion. Gate-keeper training promotes the notion that the emotional well-being and safety of the campus is a community-wide enterprise. While treatment is the exclusive province of mental health professionals, all members of the wider caring community share a responsibility to recognize the more ostentatious signs of serious psychiatric illness or duress, to know how to approach students in distress, to know where to refer them, and finally, to know whom to consult when students refuse help.

While outreach ordinarily tries to channel students in need of services into the counseling center, a complementary approach places counselors outside the center in settings that lower geographic and psychological barriers to care. For example, stand-alone counseling offices may be situated in residence halls, or in close proximity to academic support services, LBGQT and minority student hubs, career counseling centers and other offices that students do not experience as stigmatizing or intimidating.

Although empirical research is needed to validate their efficacy, residence hall offices may be useful in reaching undergraduates if they remain open well into the evening hours, when students are apt to be in their dorms; adopt a casual look and feel; and operate on a strictly drop-in basis. To the extent that these offices require no prior appointment, or even the resolve and effort required to leave one's dormitory, they harmonize with the affective lability and sense of urgency common in late adolescence [23]. A student despairing alone in her or his dorm room at night might somewhat impulsively walk downstairs to talk with a counselor if one is on-site, but prove less inclined to schedule, much less keep, an appointment a few days hence. Residence hall-based offices may also prove an effective means of reaching out to international students for whom too much loss of face may be involved in visiting a clinic [92] and in reaching under-served minority groups, who may find traditional office arrangements overly formal, reserved, and discordant with their cultural expectations of helping arrangements [44,46].

Partnering with primary care medical services is another clearly logical approach to reaching students who might otherwise not seek help. Somaticization of psychological problems has been found to be common among virtually all ethnic groups in all primary care settings studied [98]. While relatively few patients meet full criteria for somaticization disorder, a great many patients with psychiatric disorders do also have one or more unexplained physical complaints for which they seek medical attention. In addition, somatic symptoms may be used by students, particularly those from Asian backgrounds, as culturally accepted "idioms of distress"; less disposed than students from Western cultures to dichotomize body and mind and naturally reticent about discussing their private lives, these students are inclined to report only somatic complaints in health care settings [99]. However, with sensitive and specific, as opposed to open-ended, questioning truly depressed patients who initially report only physical ailments are likely to endorse depressive symptoms [100]. Thus, at the very least, it makes sense to promote basic proficiency on the part of primary care providers in identifying signs of psychiatric disturbance, and to offer professional development opportunities to nurture their skills in communicating with patients about psychological interventions. Many schools have now also successfully begun to incorporate simple screening instruments, such as the PHQ-9 [85] into their standard medical intake.

Parents and other close family members may be the most over-looked audience for outreach efforts. Like residence hall advisors, faculty and other natural gate-keepers, parents ordinarily have access to substantial information about their college-aged children's mental status but often lack an adequate frame of reference for interpreting the information at their disposal. Materials about common signs of depression and other psychiatric disorders and about on-campus mental health resources may be distributed to parents of incoming students, and counselors may usefully speak to these subjects at Parent

Orientations, Family Days and related events. With proper guidance, parents can be critical allies in connecting students – particularly younger students – with care. It is not uncommon for students who have benefited from psychotherapy and/or psychotropic medications in high school, to discontinue both upon entering college. Anxious to shed what they experience as a debasing need for help and wary of being identified by new peers as "mental patients", they look to college as a fresh start; unfortunately, parents often collude with their childrens' fantasy that the simple act of beginning college will vanquish longstanding psychiatric difficulties, when, in truth, the loss of familial supports and structure together with the psychosocial and academic challenges of transitioning to college are more likely to exacerbate, than relieve, underlying problems. Outreach to parents of incoming students promotes the notion that precisely because college is a fresh opportunity students should do all they can to benefit from this new start, including enlisting supports proactively.

5.10 Concluding Remarks

In this chapter, we have attempted to describe not only a basket of essential services, but also an approach to delivering these services that define college mental health practice, at its best, as a unique subspecialty. Underlying our description of functions as diverse as outreach, arranging access to care, brief psychotherapy, medication management, and referral are the core principles that college mental health practice should be focused, but flexible; active and activating; culturally sensitive; attuned to, and facilitating of, psychosocial development; strategic and efficient in its use of resources; and realistically anchored by the exigencies of campus life. Our approach seeks to emphasize the therapeutic component in all interactions with students. Thus, referral is never regarded as a simple administrative activity, but rather as a clinical process with therapeutic potential, and medication management, even when delivered separately from counseling, is not viewed as just a matter of matching symptoms to drugs, but rather as a potentially evocative, complex emotional experience for students that need be guided by sensitivity to transference and to the psychodynamic meanings of medicine. Perhaps above all else, the approach described here respects the individuality of each student, and while guided by the accumulated wisdom of clinical experience and research, understands each therapeutic encounter as unique and seeks to capitalize on the transformative possibilities intrinsic to therapeutic relationships.

Appendix A: The Relationship Between Predictive Validity and Base Rate

This discussion is based on Domino and Domino [77]; Elwood [86]; and Meehl and Rosen [87].

A test intended to identify a disorder or target behavior can result in one of four outcomes:

- True positive: A person with the target disorder is identified as positive for the disorder

- False positive: A person without the target disorder is identified as positive

- True negative: A person without the disorder is identified as negative

- False negative: A person with the target disorder is identified as negative.

As described in the text, *sensitivity* measures the ratio of true positives to all positives actually in the population (that is, to true positives plus false negatives), while *specificity* measures the ratio of true negatives to all negatives in the population (that is, to true negatives plus false positives).

While the psychometric attributes of an instrument are typically expressed in terms of sensitivity and specificity, what is generally of interest to the clinician is something quite different: Clinicians need to know which people with positive test results are really positive and which with negative results are really negative. The psychometric properties that matter most in clinical practice, then, are *positive predictive value* (the ratio of true positives to all people labeled positive by the instrument – that is, the ratio of true positives to the sum of the true positives plus the false positives) and *negative predictive value* (the ratio of true negatives to all people identified as negative, true and false negatives alike). When the base rate of a disorder in a population is very low, even instruments with outstanding specificity and sensitivity will have very poor positive predictive value; when the base rate increases, negative predictive value declines.

By way of illustration, consider an instrument intended to identify students at risk for suicide attempts that has both a sensitivity and specificity of 0.95 – psychometric properties superior to instruments in widespread use. By self report, 1.2% of college students attempted suicide in a recent 12-month period [3]; applying this statistic to a campus of 10 000 students, let us assume 120 will make an attempt in a particular year, and 9880 will not. Our hypothetical instrument will correctly identify 95% or 114 of the potential attempters, and, given its 0.95 specificity, will also correctly rule out 95% of the non-suicidal students. However, since there are 9880 nonsuicidal students in the population, the 5% that the instrument fails to rule out turns out to be 494 students, creating a situation in which there are many more false positives than true positives: In total the instrument will classify 608 students as suicidal, of whom only 114 or slightly less than 19% are actually so. Thus, our instrument is of very limited value for the purpose of *diagnosis or prediction* since it is wrong more than four times as often as it is correct. However, it can still be quite useful for purposes of *screening*, since, as we have seen, it is able to prune a pool of 10 000 students down to a much more manageable pool of 608 students of interest, while ruling out only six students of concern in the process.

The instrument can, in other words, be used to define a new population in which the base rate of the behavior of interest is higher than in the original population. In our example, a population of 10 000 with a base rate of 1.2% is reduced to a subpopulation of 608 with a base rate of about 19%. Since positive predictive validity rises with increases in base rate, assessing the subpopulation either by clinical interview or with a second, valid instrument will yield much more satisfactory results. For example, a second screening tool with 0.95 sensitivity and 0.95 specificity will identify about 108 of the 114 suicidal students in the new pool, while incorrectly classifying as suicidal 5% or about 25 of the 494 nonsuicidal students. In total, then the second round of screening will identify about 133 students as suicidal, of whom 108, or over 81%, will be classified accurately. This method of *sequential screening* thus increases predictive validity in our example from less than 19% to over 81% – still far from perfect, but much improved!

References

1. Hodges, S. (2001) University counseling centers at the twenty-first century: Looking forward, looking back. *Journal of College Counseling*, **4**, 161–173.
2. International Association of Counseling Services (2005 October 25) Accreditation Standards for University and College Counseling Centers. International Association of Counseling Services. Retrieved February 2, 2009, from: http://www.iacsinc.org.
3. American College Health Association (2009) The American College Health Association-National College Health Assessment Spring 2008 reference group data report (Abridged). *Journal of American College Health*, **57**(5), 477–488.
4. Whitlock, J., Eckenrode, J. and Silverman, D. (2006) Self-injurious behaviors in a college population. *Pediatrics*, **117**, 1939–1948.
5. Rockland-Miller, H. and Eels, G.T. (2006) The implementation of mental health clinical triage systems in university health services. *Journal of College Student Psychotherapy*, **20**(4), 39–51.
6. Rando, R., Barr, V. and Aros, C. (2008) The Association for University and College Counseling Center Directors Annual Survey: Reporting Period: September 1, 2006 through August 31, 2007. Retrieved January 10, 2009 from http://www.aucccd.org/img/pdfs/monograph_2007_public.pdf.
7. Coulter, L., Offutt, C.A. and Mascher, J. (2003) Counseling center management of after-hours crises: Practice and problems. *Journal of College Student Psychotherapy*, **18**(1), 11–34.
8. Schafer, R. (1986) Discussion of transference and countertransference in brief psychotherapy, in *Between Analyst and Patient: New Dimensions in Countertransference and Transference* (ed. H. Meyers), The Analytic Press, Hillsdale, N.J, pp. 149–157.
9. Sullivan, H. (1970) *The Psychiatric Interview*, W. W. Norton and Co., New York, (Originally published 1954).
10. MacKinnon, R., Michels, R. and Buckley, P. (2006) *The Psychiatric Interview in Clinical Practice*, 2nd edn, American Psychiatric Publishing Inc., Arlington, VA.
11. Hansen, N., Lambert, M.J. and Forman, E.M. (2002) The psychotherapy dose-response effect and its implications for treatment delivery services. *Clinical Psychology: Science and Practice*, **9**, 329–343.
12. Gallagher, R. (2008) National Survey of Counseling Center Directors. The International Association of Counseling Centers, Inc. Retrieved January 10, 2009, from http://www.iacsinc.org.
13. Guinee, J. and Ness, M. (2000) Counseling centers of the 1990s: Challenges and changes. *The Counseling Psychologist*, **28**(2), 267–280.
14. Ghetie, D. (2007) The debate over time-limited treatment in college counseling centers. *Journal of College Student Psychotherapy*, **22**(1), 41–61.
15. Brakham, M., Rees, A., Stiles, W. *et al.* (1996) Dose-effect relations in time-limited psychotherapy for depression. *Journal of Consulting and Clinical Psychology*, **64**(5), 927–935.
16. Hilsenroth, M., Ackerman, S.J. and Blagys, M.D. (2001) Evaluating the phase model of change during short-term psychodynamic psychotherapy. *Psychotherapy Research*, **11**(1), 29–47.
17. Kopta, M., Howard, K.I., Lowry, J.L. and Beutler, L.E. (1994) Patterns of symptomatic recovery in psychotherapy. *Journal of Consulting and Clinical Psychology*, **62**(5), 1009–1016.
18. Groves, J. (1996) (ed.) *Essential Papers on Short-Term Dynamic Therapy*, New York University Press, New York.
19. Leichsenring, F. and Rabung, S. (2008) Effectiveness of long-term psychodynamic psychotherapy: A meta-analysis. *Journal of the American Medical Association*, **300**(13), 1551–1565.
20. Shapiro, J.P. (2009) Integrating outcome research and clinical reasoning in psychotherapy planning. *Professional Psychology: Research and Practice*, **40**(1), 46–53.
21. Lambert, M. and Barley, D.E. (2001) Research summary on the therapeutic relationship and psychotherapy outcome. *Psychotherapy: Theory, Research, Practice and Training*, **38**(4), 357–361.

22. Hatchett, G. and Park, H.L. (2003) Comparison of four operational definitions of premature termination. *Psychotherapy: Theory, Research, Practice, Training*, **40**, 226–231.
23. Eichler, R.J. (2006) Developmental considerations, in *College Mental Health Practice* (eds P. Grayson and P.W. Meilman), Routledge, New York, pp. 21–41.
24. Blos, P. (1979) *The Adolescent Passage*, International Universities Press, New York.
25. Erikson, E. (1956) The problem of ego identity. *Journal of the American Psychoanalytic Association*, **4**, 56–121.
26. Erikson, E. (1963) *Childhood and Society*, 2nd edn, WW Norton, New York.
27. Amada, G. (1999) Disqualifying specified students from campus psychological service: Some considerations and guidelines. *Journal of College Student Psychotherapy*, **13**(4), 7–24.
28. Jed Foundation (2008) *Student Mental Health and the Law: A Resource for Institutions of Higher Education*, The Jed Foundation, New York.
29. Miller, W.R. and Rollnick, S. (2002) *Motivational Interviewing: Preparing People for Change*, 2nd edn, Guilford Press, New York.
30. Grayson, P.A. and Cooper, S. (2006) Depression and anxiety, in *College Mental Health Practice* (eds P.A. Grayson and P.W. Meilman), Routledge, New York, pp. 113–134.
31. Schacht, T.E., Binder, J.E. and Strupp, H.H. (1996) The dynamic focus, in *Essential Papers on Short-Term Dynamic Therapy* (ed. J. Groves), New York University Press, New York, pp. 66–96, Originally published 1984.
32. Mann, J. (1996) Time limited psychotherapy, in *Essential Papers on Short-Term Dynamic Therapy* (ed. J. Groves), New York University Press, New York, pp. 66–96, Originally published 1973.
33. Safran, J.D. (2002) Brief relational psychoanalytic treatment. *Psychoanalytic Dialogues*, **12**(2), 171–195.
34. Schafer, R. (1983) *The Analytic Attitude*, Basic Books, New York.
35. Erikson, E.H. (1968) *Identity, Youth and Crisis*. WW Norton, New York.
36. Norcross, J. and Lambert, M. (2006) The therapy relationship, in *Evidence-Based Practices in Mental Health* (eds J.C. Norcross, L.E. Beutler and R.F. Levant), American Psychological Association, Washington, DC, pp. 208–218.
37. Horvath, A. and Symonds, B.D. (1991) Relation between working alliance and outcome in psychotherapy: A meta-analysis. *Journal of Counseling Psychology*, **38**(2), 139–149.
38. Martin, D.J., Garske, J.P. and Davis, M.K. (2000) Relation of the therapeutic alliance with outcome and other variables: A meta-analytic review. *Journal of Consulting and Clinical Psychology*, **68**(3), 438–450.
39. Krupnick, J., Sotsky, S., Elkin, I. *et al.* (1996) The role of the therapeutic alliance in psychotherapy and pharmacotherapy outcome: Findings in the National Institute of Mental Health treatment of depression collaborative research program. *Journal of Consulting and Clinical Psychology*, **64**, 532–539.
40. Horvath, A. and Lubosky, L. (1993) The role of the therapeutic alliance in psychotherapy. *Journal of Consulting and Clinical Psychology*, **61**(4), 561–573.
41. Hilsenroth, M. (2007) A programmatic study of short-term psychodynamic psychotherapy: Asessment, process, outcome, and training. *Psychotherapy Research*, **17**(1), 31–45.
42. Pine, F. (1998) *Diversity and Direction in Psychoanalytic Technique*, Other Press, New York.
43. Coronado, S.F. and Peake, T.H. (1992) Culturally sensible therapy: Sensitive principles. *Journal of College Student Psychotherapy*, **7**(1), 63–72.
44. Sue, D. and Sue, D. (1990) *Counseling the culturally different: Theory & Practice*, 2nd edn, John Wiley & Sons, New York.
45. Cardemil, E. and Battle, C.L. (2003) Guess who's coming to therapy?: Getting comfortable with conversations about race and ethnicity in psychotherapy. *Professional Psychology: Research and Practice*, **34**(3), 278–286.
46. Gloria, A.M. and Rodriguez, E.R. (2000) Counseling Latino university students: Psychosocio-cultural issues for consideration. *Journal of Counseling & Development*, **78**(2), 145–154.

47. Kearney, L.K., Draper, M. and Barón, A. (2005) Counseling utilization by ethnic minority college students. *Cultural Diversity and Ethnic Minority Psychology*, **11**(3), 272–285.

48. Mahler, M., Pine, F. and Bergman, A. (1975) *The Psychological Birth of the Human Infant*, Basic Books, New York.

49. Bernier, A., Larose, S., Boivin, M. and Soucy, N. (2004) Attachment state of mind: Implications for adjustment to college. *Journal of Adolescent Research*, **19**(6), 783–806.

50. Rice, K., FitzGerald, D.P., Whaley, T.J. and Gibbs, C.L. (1995) Cross-sectional and longitudinal examination of attachment, separation-individuation, and college student adjustment. *Journal of Counseling and Development*, **73**, 463–475.

51. Gilbert, S. (1992) Ethical issues in the treatment of severe psychopathology in university and college counseling centers. *Journal of Counseling & Development*, **70**, 695–699.

52. Whitaker, L. and Cooper, S.E. (eds) (2007) *Pharmacological Treatment of College Students with Psychological Problems*, Haworth Press, New York.

53. Gabbard, G. and Kay, J. (2001) The fate of integrated treatment: Whatever happened to the biopsychosocial psychiatrist? *American Journal of Psychiatry*, **158**(12), 1956–1963.

54. Grayson, P., Schwartz, V. and Commerford, M. (1997) Brave new world? Drug therapy and college mental health. *Journal of College Student Psychotherapy*, **11**, 23–32.

55. Kay, J. (2009) Combining psychodynamic psychotherapy with medication, in *Textbook of Psychotherapeutic Treatments* (ed. G.O. Gabbard), American Psychiatric Publishing, Inc., Arlington, Va. doi: 10.1176/appi.books.9781585623648.368017, Downloaded May 15, 2009 from www.psychiatryonline.com.

56. Hollon, S.D. and Fawcett, J. (2007) Combined medication and psychotherapy, in *Treatment of Psychiatric Disorders* (ed. G. Gabbard), American Psychiatric Press Inc., Arlington, pp. 439–448.

57. Schwartz, V. (2006) Medications, in *College Mental Health Practice* (eds P. Grayson and P.W. Meilman), Routledge, New York, pp. 59–78.

58. Schwartz, V. (1994) The panic disorder psychodynamic model. *American Journal of Psychiatry*, **151**, 786.

59. Slaby, A. and Tancredi, L. (2001) Micropharmacology: Treating disturbances of mood, thought and behavior as specific neurotransmitter dysregulation rather than clinical syndromes. *Primary Psychiatry*, **8**(4), 28–33.

60. Winters, K., Stinchfield, R., Henly, G. and Schwartz, R. (1992) Validity of adolescent self report of alcohol and other drug involvement. *International Journal of Addictions*, **25**, 1379–1395.

61. Prince, J. (2006) Pharmacotherapy of ADHD in children and adolescents. *Child and Adolescent Psychiatric Clinics of North America*, **15**(1), 13–50.

62. Schwartz, V. (1988) The somatization of psychiatric disorders. *American Journal of Psychiatry*, **145** (1), 570–571.

63. Singh, S., Crondace, T., Amin, S. *et al.* (2000) Three year outcome of first episode psychoses in an established community psychiatric service. *British Journal of Psychiatry*, **176**, 210–216.

64. Fava, M. (2000) Weight gain and antidepressants. *Journal of Clinical Psychiatry*, **61**(Supplement 11), 37–41.

65. Hirschfeld, M. (1999) Management of sexual side effects of antidepressant therapy. *Journal of Clinical Psychiatry*, (supplement 60), (14), 27–30.

66. Whitaker, L. (2006) Relationships, in *College Mental Health Practice* (eds P. Grayson and P.W. Meilman), Routledge, New York, pp. 95–112.

67. Sheehy, J. and Commerford, M. (2006) Eating disorders, in *College Mental Health Practice* (eds P.A. Grayson and P.W. Meilman), Routledge, New York, pp. 261–280.

68. Golden, B., Corazzini, J. and Grady, P. (1993) Current practices of group therapy at university counseling centers: A national survey. *Professional Psychology: Research and Practice*, **24**(2), 228–230.

69. Yalom, I. and Leszcz, M. (2005) *The Theory and Practice of Group Psychotherapy*, Basic Books, New York.
70. Rutan, J., Stone, W. and Shay, J. (2007) *Psychodynamic Group Psychotherapy*, 4th edn, Guilford, New York.
71. White, J. and Freeman, A. (2000) *Cognitive-Behavioral Group Therapy for Specific Problems and Populations*, American Psychological Association, Washington, DC.
72. Dimeff, L., Linehan, M. and Koerner, K. (2007) *Dialectical Behavior Therapy in Clinical Practice*, Guilford, New York.
73. Richards, P. and Owen, L.A. (1993) A religiously oriented group counseling intervention for self-defeating perfectionism: a pilot study. *Counseling and Values*, **37**(2), 96–105.
74. Kincade, E. and Kalodner, C. (2004) The use of groups in college and university counseling centers, in *Handbook of Group Counseling and Psychotherapy* (eds J. Delucia-Waack and D.C. Gerrity), Sage, Thousand Oaks, California, pp. 366–377.
75. Meyer, G.J., Finn, S.E., Eyde, L.D. *et al.* (2001) Psychological testing and psychological assessment: A review of evidence and issues. *American Psychologist*, **56**(2), 128–165.
76. Clarkin, J., Howieson, D.B. and McClough, J. (2008) The role of psychiatric measures in assessment and treatment, in *The American Psychiatric Publishing Textbook of Psychiatry* (eds R. Hales, S.C. Yudofsky and G.O. Gabbard), American Psychiatric Publishing, Inc., Arlington, Va. doi: 10.1176/appi.books.9781585623402, Retrieved January 22, 2009 from http://www.psychiatryonline.com.
77. Domino, G. and Domino, M. (2006) *Psychological Testing: An Introduction*, Cambridge University Press, New York.
78. Lezak, M.D., Howieson, D.B. and Loring, D.W. (2004) *Neuropsychological Assessment*, 4th edn, Oxford University Press, New York.
79. Walsh, W.B. and Betz, N. (2001) *Tests and Assessment*, Prentice Hall, Upper Saddle River, NJ.
80. Butcher, J.N. and Williams, C.L. (2009) Personality assessment with the MMPI-2: Historical roots, international adaptations, and current challenges. *Applied Psychology: Health and Well-Being*, **1**(1), 105–135.
81. Derogatis, L.R. and Culpepper, W.J. (2004) Screening for psychiatric disorders, in *The Use of Psychological Testing for Treatment Planning and Outcomes Assessment*, vol. **1** (ed. M.E. Maruish), Lawrence Erlbaum Associates, Mahwah, NJ, pp. 65–109.
82. Hamilton, M. (1960) A rating scale for depression. *Journal of Neurology, Neurosurgery, and Psychiatry*, **23**, 56–62.
83. Kroenke, K. and Spitzer, R. (2002) The PHQ-9: A new depression diagnostic and severity measure. *Psychiatric Annals*, **32**(9), 509–516.
84. Saunders, J.B., Aasland, O.G. and Babor, T.F. (1993) Development of the Alcohol Use Disorders Identification Test (AUDIT): WHO collaborative project on early detection of persons with harmful alcohol consumption–II. *Addiction*, **88**, 791–804.
85. Spitzer, R., Kroenke, K. and Williams, J. (2001) The PHQ-9. *Journal of General Internal Medicine*, **16**(9), 606–613.
86. Elwood, R. (1993) Psychological tests and clinical discriminations: Beginning to address the base rate problem. *Clinical Psychology Review*, **13**, 409–419.
87. Meehl, P.E. and Rosen, A. (1955) Antecedent probability and the efficiency of psychometric signs, patterns, or cutting scores. *Psychological Bulletin*, **52**, 194–216.
88. Jacobson, N. and Traux, P. (1991) Clinical significance: A statistical approach to defining meaningful change in psychotherapy research. *Journal of Consulting and Clinical Psychology*, **59**(1), 12–19.
89. Lambert, M. and Hawkins, E.J. (2004) Measuring outcome in professional practice: Considerations in selecting and using brief outcome instruments. *Professional Psychology: Research and Practice*, **35**, 492–499.

90. Maruish, M.E. (ed.) (2004) *The Uses of Psychological Testing for Treatment Planning and Outcomes Assessment*, 3rd edn, vol. **1**, Lawrence Erlbaum Associates, Mahwah, N.J.

91. American Psychiatric Association Practice Guidelines for the Treatment of Psychiatric Disorders: Compendium (2006) Arlington, VA: American Psychiatric Association. Retrieved May 18, 2009 from http://www.psychiatryonline.com.

92. Mori, S. (2000) Mental health concerns of international students. *Journal of Counseling and Development*, **78**, 137–144.

93. Larimer, M.E. and Cronce, J.M. (2002) Identification, prevention and treatment: A review of individual-focused strategies to reduce problematic alcohol consumption by college students. *Journal of Studies on Alcohol*, (supp. no 14), 148–163.

94. Gould, M. and Kramer, R.A. (2001) Youth suicide prevention. *Suicide & Life-Threatening Behavior*, **31**, (supplement), 6–31.

95. Walker, I. and Read, J. (2002) The differential effectiveness of psychosocial and biogenetic causal explanations in reducing negative attitudes toward "mental illness". *Psychiatry: Interpersonal & Biological Processes*, **65**(4), 313–325.

96. Dietrich, S., Matschinger, H. and Angermeyer, M.C. (2006) The relationship between biogenetic causal explanations and social distance toward people with mental disorders: Results from a population survey in Germany. *The International Journal of Social Psychiatry*, **52**(2), 166–174.

97. Nilsson, J., Berkel, L.A., Flores, L.Y. and Lucas, M.S. (2004) Utilization rate and presenting concerns of international students at a University counseling center: Implications for outreach programming. *Journal of College Student Psychotherapy*, **19**(2), 49–59.

98. Kirmayer, L. and Young, A. (1998) Culture and somatization: Clinical, epidemiological, and ethnographic perspectives. *Psychosomatic Medicine*, **60**, 420–430.

99. Lin, K. and Cheung, F. (1999) Mental health issues for Asian Americans. *Psychiatric Services*, **50**(6), 774–782.

100. Parker, G., Gladstone, G. and Chee, K.T. (2001) Depression in the planet's largest ethnic group: The Chinese. *American Journal of Psychiatry*, **158**(6), 857–864.

101. Gyorky, Z.K., Royalty, G.M. and Johnson, D.H. (1994) Time-limited therapy in university counseling centers: do time-limited and time-unlimited centers differ? *Professional Psychology Research and Practice*, **25**(1), 50–54.

102. Brown, J., Fischo, M. and Hanna, G. (1993) Nelson–Denny Reading Test, Form H. Chicago, IL: Riverside Publishing Co; [76–79].

103. National Center on Addiction and Substance Abuse at Columbia University, 2007, www.casacolumbia.org/absolutenm/articlefiles/380-Wasting%20the%20Best%20and%20the%20Brightest.pdf.

6 The Counseling Center Team

Paul Grayson

Counseling and Psychological Services, Marymount Manhattan College, New York, NY, USA

6.1 Introduction

When I directed a large counseling center, during my "state of the union" address at our annual retreat I liked to compare the staff to an all-star team. Allowing for a bit of hyperbole on these morale-boosting occasions, the baseball metaphor seemed apt, since all the staff members were fine clinicians, and in complementary ways. We had the equivalent of infielders and outfielders and pitchers and catchers, every one of them quite good. During my remarks I also played up the staff's teamwork and positive attitude, values I wanted to reinforce. With several dozen clinicians in all, from varied professional disciplines and diverse backgrounds and working at separate campus locations, teamwork and positive attitude were by no means a given. That by and large the staff maintained its camaraderie and spirits in spite of the differences and the work pressures was, I felt, something to celebrate. We were more than capable clinicians. We were a team.

This chapter is about the constituent parts of the counseling center staff and the fine art of putting them all together and achieving staff harmony. I begin by looking one by one at the various units – director, therapists, prescribers, and the rest – sketching out their duties, roles, pressures and points of view. Mid-sized and especially large-sized centers, as we shall see, are rather complex enterprises. The second section considers the precariousness of morale and cohesiveness, the challenge of keeping all these units motivated and smoothly working together. The final section cautiously ventures some responses. You cannot expect every staff member to be contented all the time. Directors certainly are not. Experience teaches, however, that certain practices by directors can contribute to staff morale and a culture of teamwork.

6.2 The Team

6.2.1 Director

The director's duties depend on the size of the service. At one-person counseling centers the director necessarily functions primarily as a therapist, somehow squeezing in between patients everything else that needs doing: record keeping, reports, outreach, meetings, supervising a trainee, perhaps a receptionist shift or two. At two- and three-person centers other therapists share the clinical workload, but still the director's time is largely devoted to

Mental Health Care in the College Community   Edited by Jerald Kay and Victor Schwartz
© 2010 John Wiley & Sons, Ltd.

seeing patients. When we get to mid-sized and large centers (the largest boast 30 or more clinicians), the director's management and administrative responsibilities grow, which is to say the director spends more time directing. Still, almost all directors continue seeing patients, partly out of inclination and partly from necessity, since it is a rare center that does not need all hands on deck to meet the relentless demand for appointments. And so while at small institutions (under 2500 students) directors report seeing an average of 17.7 patients per week, directors at large institutions (over 15 000 students) see a not inconsiderable average of 7.8 patients per week [1].

The number of patients does not fully tell the tale, however. A director's case load is less likely to consist of garden-variety cases than of high-stakes evaluations following a suicide threat or psychiatric hospitalization, recommendations for medical leave of absence, or difficult referrals from within the counseling center or the campus community. Further, directors' clinical hours are not in lieu of administrative tasks – they are in addition to them. As a student health center director explained at a conference, speaking as much for counseling directors as for his own position, 70% of his time was spent seeing patients – and 70% was spent on administration [2]. The life of a college counseling director consists of arriving early at the office, staying late, taking work home, and checking e-mail on weekends and holidays.

As for what precisely directors do when not seeing patients, when they are "directing", the list is long. A respected accrediting organization specifies, among other duties, recruiting and evaluating staff members, preparing and administering budgets, writing reports, monitoring the quality of services, and overseeing the crisis management system and outreach program [3]. Other tasks we might add are attending to computers and the electronic health record, student insurance policy issues, community treatment and hospitalization options, training program concerns, and such Solomonic decisions as to which staff member merits the one available windowed office. Directors are tethered to their phones and e-mail accounts, continually consulting with staff members, student affairs administrators, faculty, housing personnel, parents, outside providers and hospitals. Most directors lead committees and directly supervise staff and/or trainees. Some teach and conduct research; and all attend meetings. Regarding the last activity, I remember very many years ago, before becoming a director, thinking it would be stimulating to attend more meetings. Be careful what you wish for. After becoming a director, many were the times I surreptitiously checked my watch during my second or third consecutive meeting wondering when I could get back to the office to catch up on work.

What most distinguishes directors from everyone else on staff can be summed up in two words: ultimate responsibility. It is the director's job to view the counseling center holistically, to plan and set goals and ensure the center runs well and fulfills its mission, and it is the director's job to assess campus mental health needs and respond to student affairs vice presidents and the like. The director is the one who is in charge. By contrast, staff therapists, no matter how loyal, team-oriented, and supportive of the center's mission, look through a narrower lens. Their natural focus is on the welfare of their own patients, not the overall clinic or campus. A key challenge for the director, therefore, is to persuade staff therapists to widen their attention beyond individual and group treatment and think in terms of community mental health.

To cite a common example, directors squirm when the demand for appointments swells and a waiting list builds up, since some students may grow discouraged and give up on treatment, acute cases won't be assessed in time (although prompt intake arrangements such as a phone triage system help address this concern [4]), and, to be honest, it just looks bad. No director wants to preside over a center with a reputation for putting off students. In reaction, directors naturally push for measures to free up slots for new cases: strict session limits, referrals of current cases into the community, mandated spacing out of sessions, suspension of staff therapists' administrative hours, assignment of cases even when staff members have no openings. Now how do staff therapists feel about all this? They are immersed in the concrete reality of current patients, not the abstraction of potential future patients. Hearing their patients' stories and struggles, they understandably balk at measures that threaten to water down treatment – or pile on still more work. As a therapist as well as a director, I personally was on both sides of this struggle. Wearing my leadership hat, I took steps and made appeals to ward off a wait list. But with my own patients I strained to play by the rules. Even during the busiest times I held onto a few cases longer than strictly necessary, because from a therapist's perspective there are always valid reasons why a given student needs extra clinical attention.

Let us now take a snapshot of directors. According to two surveys of counseling center directors [1,5], female directors outnumber males, a reversal from 1994 [6], the first year this question was asked (Table 6.1). The rise in female directors is unsurprising, since women are ascendant throughout the mental health field: female psychologists, once a small minority, now receive more than 70% of new doctorates [7]; female psychiatric residents, a novelty in the past, caught up to men in 2000 [8]; and social work is, and always has been, a predominately female profession. Despite the increase in female directors, however, we should not assume college mental health has torn down the glass ceiling, since anywhere from 65% [5] to a huge 75% [1] of *staff* members are female. Female directors may be in the majority, but male therapists are still proportionately likelier than their female colleagues to be promoted to director.

It's tempting to speculate on the implications of the increase in female directors. Have there been subtle changes in directors' leadership style or priorities, or in the position's prestige or financial compensation? The only evidence on these matters I am aware of is the disquieting finding that new male directors report earning more money on average than new female directors [1,5]. Again, women may predominate among directors, but that does not prove equal treatment.

Racial minority directors make up about 9% of the total on one directors' survey [1] and 15% on the other [5], compared to 11.5% in 1994 [6] (see Table 6.1). For a field that prides

Table 6.1	Directors' self-reported gender, racial identity and sexual orientation [1,5,6]		
Year (and survey)	**[1]**	**[5]**	**[6]**
Males	45%	46%	57%
Females	55%	54%	43%
Black/African American	3.9%	7.2%	6.8%
American Indian/Native American	0.0%	0.3%	0.3%
Latino/Hispanic	2.5%	2.0%	1.0%
White/Caucasian	90.8%	85.2%	88.4%
Multiracial	—	1.0%	—
Other	2.1%	1.8%	1.0%
Gay man	—	4%	—
Lesbian	—	5%	—
Bisexual	—	2%	—
Heterosexual	—	88%	—

Table 6.2	Directors' professional identity	
Survey	Gallagher and Taylor [1]	Rando and Barr [5]
Clinical psychologist	23%	27%
Counseling psychologist	42%	44%
Psychiatrist	0.7%	0.5%
Mental health professional	6%	5%
Professional counselor	15%	13%
Social worker	7%	7%
Student personnel administrator	1.1%	0.5%
Other	5%	2%

itself on cultural sensitivity and respect for diversity, and where 34% of professional staff positions self-identify as from a minority group [5], this is not heartening news. Perhaps more encouraging is the total of 11% who identify as being gay, lesbian, or bisexual [5]. Lesbian/gay/bisexual/transgender (LGBT) directors certainly seem to be more open today than in the past, as witness the LGBT luncheon held at the annual conference of the Association for University and Counseling Center Directors (AUCCCD) and the very fact that sexual identity is now included as a question on the director's survey.

According to both directors' surveys (Table 6.2), most directors identify themselves as doctoral level psychologists, and most of these psychologists identify as counseling psychologists. The figures in Table 6.2 under-represent both psychiatrists, who rarely join AUCCCD and so do not fill out the organization's survey, and non-doctoral directors, who often work at the smallest, limited-budget centers and so are also less likely to join the directors' association and fill out the survey. Still, we are on safe footing concluding that most directors are psychologists. Not coincidentally, many counseling centers were originally sponsored by counseling psychology departments, and to this day many have affiliations with departments of counseling or clinical psychology.

Directors' professional background matters, but less than one might think. Yes, there are significant differences in salary. Psychiatrists on average make considerably more money than psychologists, and psychologists on average make more than social workers and especially masters level counselors. When colleges decide which profession to pursue for counseling center director, the budget is a consideration. Differences also exist in training programs' admissions standards, years of training, courses and training experiences; psychiatrists, of course, specialize in prescribing medications, psychologists in psychological testing, and social workers in concrete services. There are also differences in core philosophy. To grossly simplify, psychiatrists espouse the medical model, believing in applying the right specific treatments for diagnosed psychiatric illnesses. Counseling psychologists concentrate on facilitating "normal and optimal development" and are attuned to the relevance of cultural factors [9]. Clinical psychologists fall somewhere in the middle, focused more on psychopathology than counseling psychologists but less wedded to the disease model than psychiatrists. Social work teaches clinical skills in the context of a social welfare philosophy, explicitly emphasizing caring and empathy [10].

But again, these capsule descriptions are overgeneralizations, and fail to reflect the diversity of training programs within each profession or the unique experiences and outlook of each individual undergoing the training. What is more, differences in professional background come to count less over time as directors encounter the distinctive features of college mental health. Thus all directors learn about college students as patients, whose distress reflects a combination of acute college stressors, the growing pains of late adolescence and early adulthood, familial and societal pressures, and emerging or pre-existing psychopathology. All directors learn how the academic calendar frames the course of treatment and students' rapidly changing lives thwart tidy treatment plans. All directors learn about the influence of the college setting, which requires balancing the rights of students against the rights of the community; the need for confidentiality and patient privacy against the need to protect patients' safety; and again the need for confidentiality against the right to information claimed by parents, vice presidents and deans, housing personnel and faculty.

In short, college counseling is a specialty, and the director's job is a specialty within a specialty. All directors, regardless of professional background and identity, undergo a common experience, postgraduate training in being a director; they come to think of themselves first and foremost as counseling center directors, and secondarily as psychologists or psychiatrists or social workers. A clinical psychologist myself, I feel more in my element at a multidisciplinary directors' gathering than at 95% of the programs at the American Psychological Association conference.

6.2.2 Other Administrators

Larger counseling centers generally have an intermediate layer of administrators between director and therapists. Associate, assistant and training directors are the most common titles, sometimes unmodified and sometimes tied to an area of responsibility, such as "associate director of clinical services" or "assistant director, outreach and consultation". Centers also may use coordinator titles to acknowledge particular duties: peer education program coordinator, intern program coordinator, coordinator of student development, coordinator of group programs.

With so many ways of slicing the administrative pie, no consensus exists about the ideal structure, but clearly it makes sense to carve out special areas of responsibility. Directors at large centers cannot possibly run every program, nor are they most qualified to do so. Staff members who take over special programs – groups, training, eating disorders, liaison to a school or organization – have the satisfaction of running their own show, developing skills, and concentrating on an area of interest.

The perspective of associate and assistant directors falls somewhere between that of directors and staff therapists. The wider their scope of responsibility, the closer these administrators come to the director's holistic, community-minded point of view.

6.2.3 Therapists

Therapists' job is to provide individual and group counseling, manage crises, do outreach, consult, train and supervise, and perform "other assigned functions that contribute to the service offerings of the center and the academic mission of the institution" [3]. It helps too if each therapist can be a specialist, making special clinical contributions and contributing to a well-rounded team. Top priorities for specialization are substance abuse, eating disorders, sexual assault and trauma, and the concerns of racial minorities and LGBT students. Also of value are the ability to speak Spanish and other languages of international and immigrant students, and expertise in group treatment, cognitive behavioral therapy (CBT), mindfulness and relaxation techniques, attention and learning difficulties, and dialectical behavior therapy (DBT). But there are limits to the expertise even large, resource-rich centers can provide. A student who insists on a specialist in trichotillomania or an Italian speaking therapist probably must accept a referral in the community, if such a person exists.

Filling special needs is a challenge, particularly for smaller centers. One solution is to select therapists who meet several needs at once. The joke at our office was we would hire a disabled, Korean-speaking, African-American, lesbian EMDR specialist. While we never pulled off that five-in-one coup, it is not unusual for staff members to do double or triple duty, like one social worker who speaks Spanish and is trained in group treatment and DBT. To optimize therapists' clinical reach, new hires can be asked to specialize in an area. You cannot train to be gay or African-American or a native Japanese speaker, but any enterprising therapist can develop expertise in eating disorders, substance abuse, or CBT.

Trying to fill the gaps in clinical offerings can create hiring dilemmas. What do you do if the strongest candidates in a search do not fulfill the need in question? Should you compromise on overall counseling quality for the sake of putting together a well-rounded staff? There are arguments to be made on both sides. In favor of prioritizing special expertise, some counseling center patients clearly benefit from seeing a specialist and may refuse treatment without one. Staff members benefit too from the opportunity to consult with a specialist. A diverse counseling staff sends the inclusive message that all students on campus, regardless of race or sexual orientation or presenting problem, are welcome. For all these reasons, a center making hiring decisions has no choice but to give precedence to missing ingredients. Not to put too fine a point on it, it is not appropriate for a larger center to assemble a therapy staff of exclusively Caucasian, heterosexual, psychodynamically oriented females.

And yet, all college therapists end up as generalists anyway, working with the full range of problem areas. Partly this is due to scheduling factors, since logistically it is impossible to match every student who has Problem A with a therapist who specializes in Problem A. But the main reason is that students' problems are too complex and tangled to be neatly slotted into discrete categories. Students who have eating disorders often abuse substances, and vice versa, and on top of that may simultaneously present with suicidal ideas and self-mutilation, sexual or ethnic identity concerns, academic paralysis, clinical depression and an anxiety disorder. Understanding such cases as a whole and helping them get untracked in all domains of their lives calls for the perspective and skills of a generalist. Further, on issues of race, ethnicity and sexual orientation, some students prefer *not* to work with a therapist like themselves, fearing this person would have preconceived notions and stunt their self-expression.

So to return to our dilemma, sometimes the fates are kind and there's an applicant who shines as both a generalist and a specialist, but not infrequently the center has to settle for less-than-ideal on one dimension or the other, either a relatively inexperienced therapist who brings special skills, or an experienced and talented generalist who doesn't fulfill a particular need. Complicating matters further, centers also need to make subtle judgments about how newcomers will fit in with the team. Whether someone is male or female, older or younger, introverted or sociable, liberal or conservative, psychoanalytically or behaviorally minded has an unpredictable effect on team dynamics. Every addition to staff shakes up the status quo and represents a gamble in terms of morale and cohesiveness.

As stated earlier in connection with directors, differences among psychologists and social workers and professional counselors tend to blur over time as new staff therapists get a taste of working with college students. Some centers are made up entirely or almost entirely of therapists from a single professional background, for reasons having to do with the payroll, the center's history or current departmental affiliations, or the director's preference. Other centers are truly multidisciplinary, the various therapy disciplines working side by side and essentially performing the same duties. Counseling centers tend to be less professionally hierarchical than hospital settings. When rifts appear among staff members, generally the reason has nothing to do with professional training background.

6.2.4 Psychiatrists

In the past, staff psychiatrists at certain centers did psychotherapy, and in some centers were the main psychotherapists [11]. Not so today. College psychiatrists these days may conduct medical leave or safety evaluations, facilitate hospitalizations, and consult with counseling staff, but most of their time is spent churning out medication consultations for the ever growing number of students who already take psychiatric medications or are referred by college therapists for psychiatric evaluations. It doesn't help that there aren't enough psychiatrists. According to counseling directors, psychiatric services are "woefully inadequate or nonexistent" on 32% of college campuses and insufficient on an additional 41% of campuses [1].

To meet the insatiable demand for medication consults, centers have had to scramble. Psychiatrists may see two, three or more students in an hour – no mean feat given the instability of many cases. Many centers economize by hiring comparatively inexpensive nurse practitioners in addition or instead of psychiatrists, or by having counseling center psychiatrists evaluate and start students on medication and then referring straightforward, stable cases to primary care physicians and nurse practitioners at the health center. While using nurse practitioners and primary care health professionals makes for more medication hours, these practices place an extra burden on staff psychiatrists, who must be available to consult with the non-psychiatrist prescribers and if necessary personally conduct further evaluations.

The coexistence of psychiatrists and therapists within the counseling center has the obvious advantage of making possible both medication treatment and psychotherapy, but the benefits go further. Two heads are better than one in assessing confusing cases (often students reveal problems or aspects of themselves to one provider they withhold from the other), and two are a comfort in sharing difficult cases. Even if both therapist and psychiatrist are stumped by a case, as happens, it's reassuring to know another clinician is equally perplexed. A therapist and psychiatrist can be an effective tag team convincing reluctant students to take an off-campus referral, go on medical leave, or go to the hospital. Therapists and psychiatrists can support one another's treatment, the therapist by referring students for psychiatric evaluations, encouraging medication compliance and hearing students' concerns about taking pills, and the psychiatrist by advocating psychotherapy and reinforcing therapeutic goals. It helps both treatments when each clinician monitors worrisome symptoms and endorses the same coping methods.

For certain troubled students who seem to need more than a single clinician can give, the psychiatrist-therapist partnership is truly a godsend, like two parents taking turns managing a demanding child. Sometimes even two clinicians can't contain a student, and a center finds itself, not necessarily by design, conducting a collective, it-takes-a-village treatment. One episodically suicidal, perennially miserable senior accrued an *ad hoc* team of individual therapist, psychiatrist, group therapist, walk-in counselors and on-call counselors, each one feeling somewhat ineffectual but as a team somehow keeping her going. When at last the day arrived for her to march with her graduating class, half a dozen clinicians exhaled in relief.

The psychiatrist–therapist collaboration does pose challenges, however, notably the risk of miscommunications and unrelated, potentially contradictory treatments. Years ago at our center a part-time psychiatry resident tried to refer a student she was medicating to her hospital's mental hygiene clinic, unaware that the student's psychotherapist, a psychology trainee, had embarked on a course of on-campus counseling. This unwitting tug of war lasted for several weeks, greatly confusing the student [12]. Such uncoordinated treatments are now less likely with the advent of an electronic health record, but an electronic health record only works if clinicians use it properly. The onus is on therapists and psychiatrists to take precious moments to read each others' chart notes and then communicate when questions arise about diagnosis and assessment, treatment goals and methods, and referral plans.

Combined treatments have implications for all three participants. Yes, some students thrive on attention from both therapist and psychiatrist, but others favor one clinician over the other. The psychodynamically resonant therapy triad, like the Oedipal triangle, causes some patients to choose sides and split treatment into good and bad treaters. As for the providers, hints of professional and personal rivalry and insecurity may seep in, therapists secretly feeling skeptical of drug treatment or conversely in awe of the psychiatrist's prescribing power, and psychiatrists secretly feeling dismissive of talk therapy or envious that they can't do psychotherapy themselves. A therapist may fear the psychiatrist will encroach on psychotherapeutic material. A psychiatrist may question the direction the therapist is taking.

We must not exaggerate. For the majority of patients, accustomed to guidance from many sources – parents, teachers, coaches, resident assistants, advisors, and physicians, having two more helpers, a therapist and psychiatrist, is no big deal. And for therapists and psychiatrists the collaboration almost always does go well, with at most occasional small doubts creeping in, as happens in any human relationship. Again, one of the hallmarks of college counseling centers is their non-hierarchical atmosphere and the mutual respect that obtains across disciplines.

6.2.5 Trainees

Seventy percent of centers report having some form of training program [5]. The advantages are clear. Trainees increase the supply of counseling hours at little or no cost, and, if my own center's surveys are any guide, with no drop-off in student satisfaction (a humbling finding for those of us who cherish the belief that clinical experience matters). Trainees can enhance a center's ethnic, linguistic and sexual diversity. With their youth, enthusiasm and willingness to work evenings and weekends, trainees are ideal choices to give workshops and be liaisons to student groups. Trainees give staff members a break from the clinical grind. After a run of depressed and anxious and demanding cases, it's a treat to shift gears and spend an hour doing supervision.

But running a trainee program is not without drawbacks. By the time you subtract the hours spent communicating with training programs, reviewing trainee applications, interviewing candidates, conducting trainee orientations, providing supervision, planning

and conducting didactic programs, and filling out evaluations and writing recommendations, the net gain in therapy appointments is modest. There's also the risk that
trainees will be assigned cases they are not prepared for. Intake procedures such as a phone
triage system or in-person interviews are supposed to match trainees with relatively
straightforward cases, but risky students often underreport pathology during intakes.
Sooner or later, every trainee, heart pounding, sits across from a suicidal, substance
abusing or borderline patient. Centers prepare for these mismatches – a supervisor may
be called in during the session; the patient may be transferred to a senior therapist – but
better if the riskiest cases saw seasoned professionals from the beginning. The other
considerable drawback is trainees' brief tenure at the center. Just when trainees have
mastered the center's procedures and developed a feel for college counseling, their placement
finishes.

Trainee is a broad category, of course. While psychology practicum students are most
common [5], you can find trainees from doctoral psychology, masters counseling, social
work, nursing, and psychiatry residency programs, ranging in experience from raw first-year
graduate students to advanced postdoctoral psychology fellows. The trainees a center
chooses to recruit partly depend on availability – which programs exist within the university
or surrounding community. Another consideration is the center's mission, its emphasis on
training for its own sake. Within the field of psychology, pre-doctoral internship programs
make a splendid *training* contribution, providing interns a rich mixture of individual and
group counseling, outreach, intensive supervision, and in-service seminars – an excellent
preparation for a college counseling career. But predoctoral internships are rather high
maintenance; getting and maintaining accreditation from the American Psychological
Association, however valuable an endeavor in itself, steals time from clinical services.
Strictly from the standpoint of *service*, postdoctoral psychology fellowship programs, which
generally bypass the accreditation process, are the better investment. Though postdocs earn a
higher stipend than predocs, their pay is a bargain compared to regular staff members, and
they see far more patients and are more advanced than predocs, who in turn are more
advanced than practicum students.

6.2.6 Others

This grab-bag category is for professionals whose duties fall outside our usual understanding of psychotherapist or counselor. Examples are staff members who do disabilities
accommodations, evaluations for attention deficit disorder and learning disabilities,
health education and promotion, and career counseling and vocational assessment
inventories. A recent trend is care or case manager positions, responsible for ensuring
students' compliance with treatment recommendations, making referrals, and providing
concrete services. At least one student health center has formed an in-house mobile crisis
team of clinical social workers, who are available around the clock to evaluate students in
distress, arrange hospitalizations, and follow up afterward with students, their roommates
and friends.

These quasi-counseling roles enrich a center's menu of services, and, in the case of
care managers and the mobile crisis team, free therapists to concentrate on doing therapy.
But they also add layers of complexity to what are already complex units. The challenge
of pulling everyone together and ensuring morale across all units becomes that much
greater.

6.2.7 Support Staff

I come last to the support staff or clinical aides, and last is surely how they see themselves, and are seen, within the system. Clinical aides rank lowest in salary, grade level, status, and educational attainment, and they are, in a sense, outsiders, the only center staff members with no official role in treating students. Because it is their thankless task to make appointments when available hours are running out and when therapists are feeling stretched, they are subject to poor treatment. I have overheard students scolding an aide because they could not get specific appointment times or their appointment was canceled due to the therapist's illness, and I have learned of therapists grilling an aide because an appointment was scheduled during a formerly free hour. Never once did I hear of a clinical aide lashing out in response, sadly as if putting up with rudeness were part of the job description.

Mistreatment aside, the job is stressful. Clinical aides can be suddenly confronted with several phone lines lit up at once, a line of students waiting to check in or reschedule appointments, and a hovering trainee or staff member expecting immediate assistance. Aides are responsible for receptionist duties, scheduling, ordering supplies, miscellaneous counselor requests and questions, and the dozens of small glitches (copy machines, computers, dead light bulbs) that bedevil any office. At my center, whenever a good-hearted counselor helps out at the front desk, the unfailing comment afterward is, "I'm glad I don't do *that* all day long".

While aides do not do therapy, students associate them with the experience. Theirs is the voice when students call for an appointment and the first face seen when students arrive for the visit. Whether they seem friendly or cold, discreet or careless about privacy, leaves a strong impression. Without clinical training, aides are also a *de facto* part of the assessment team, picking up from a student's distress on the phone the need for an immediate assessment. Because of their critical role in supporting treatment, the front-line staff needs careful training on communication skills, professionalism, confidentiality and the signs of urgent situations.

6.3 Challenges to Morale and Teamwork

It would be nice to think mental health professionals were above feeling resentment, envy, and the other seven deadly sins of poor office morale, but it wouldn't, of course, be realistic. Counseling center employees are generally good people – there is a reason they chose a helping profession – but they are, none the less, people. When they have morale problems, partly it is because of work conditions, above all the toll of dealing with distraught 19-year-olds for a living. But fissures and discontent are also the expectable byproducts of individual dispositions and interpersonal dynamics, of the predictable ways human beings react in groups and with authority figures.

First a word about the work conditions. College students' problems are more severe these days than in the past, at least in the near-unanimous opinion of counseling center directors [1]. Treating even one suicidal or substance abusing or near-psychotic student can be nerve-racking and sleep-depriving, causing therapists to anxiously replay their actions: "Should I have let that student leave my office?" Then there's the pressure of doing therapy all day long, with hardly a break. Staff members who must give away administrative and lunch hours to squeeze patients in and then stay late catching up on notes can be forgiven if they do not leave the office with a smile.

Counseling center salaries range, as far as I can tell, from reasonable to risible. Those who cannot make ends meet must see private patients in their non-center hours, and enjoy little down time. Centers offer limited possibilities for job advancement. Depending on the structure you can aspire to be the director or an assistant or associate director, but there are only so many administrative plums to go around; many staff members work in the same position – some contentedly, it must be said – for as long as they are on the staff.

Mind you, counseling center positions can't really be so dreadful, or else how do you explain the dozens of applications whenever one becomes available, or the fact that staff members, once hired, tend to stay on? Balancing out the negatives are ample rewards – interesting patients, interesting colleagues, the academic atmosphere, a steady if unspectacular paycheck, good vacation benefits, work lulls during the summer and winter intersession. But acknowledging these benefits requires perspective, and college therapists are not immune from the perverse human tendency to treat the good as a right and the bad as an injustice. When something rankles, it is easy to lose sight of all that's going well.

Staff morale particularly takes a beating when some employees seemingly have it better than others. I recall a number of conversations through the years with unhappy staff members who compared their salaries to others they assumed made more money, or their schedules to others they felt worked less hard. Not once did someone call attention to others who perhaps earned less or worked harder. A sense of unfairness, for those so inclined, is selective about the evidence.

Another drain on morale is certain leadership styles. Directors and administrators perceived as uncommunicative or autocratic spur resentment; two of the commonest staff complaints are "we weren't told" and "we weren't consulted". Rigidity and inflexibility, a refusal to bend the rules when circumstances dictate, are likewise turn-offs. While these sound like easy failings to avoid – what director *wants* to be viewed as secretive, dictatorial or rigid? There is danger in going too far in the opposite direction. A director who tells staff members about every administrative detail, or worse, wants approval for every decision, will not come across as – or be – an effective leader. The same applies to a director who in the name of flexibility hastily suspends or inconsistently applies policies. The analogy with parenting is clear. Directors and administrators must strive for the right balance between communicativeness, collaboration and flexibility on the one hand and circumspection, decisiveness and consistency on the other, and then prepare for grumbling wherever the line is struck.

On the topic of parenting, you need not be a card-carrying Freudian to see that directors, as authority figures, are the object of parental transference reactions, whatever their personality style. This lesson was brought home for me many years ago by the skewed reactions of a septuagenarian staff therapist when I took over as director. Though I was 20 years his junior and tried to put him at ease, he was fearful and ingratiating in my presence, so uncomfortable he could not wait to walk away from me, not at all like his puckish, playful manner with everyone else. I can only imagine what childhood humiliations my directorial presence evoked. Meanwhile, directors have their own internal responses, some merited and some prewired, to staff members. I recall years ago a quite competent psychologist whose slowness at times to get a point would get under my skin, much as I tried to hide it, and who, yes, in this way reminded me of a central figure from my past. The interactions between director and staff members always contain private meanings for each.

On the level of group dynamics, we know that employees in any office gossip about their jobs and the boss. If you're a director and you think the staff talks about you, you are not being paranoid. Criticizing the boss actually can be a healthy release and a constructive bonding experience; in my first counseling center job, comparing notes about our larger-than-life director brought me closer to a colleague. Past a certain point, however, complaining about work or the director becomes destructive; there is socially lubricating gossip, and there is corrosive gossip.

Staff employees also may resent or come into conflict with one another. In my experience, divisions among the counseling staff are rarely provoked by the usual suspects of race, ethnicity, age, gender, and sexual orientation, or by professional discipline or theoretical orientation. More often it is a question of one group or individual feeling mistreated or looked down upon by others, as mentioned above in connection with clinical aides, or of certain personalities just not hitting it off. Another source is simply who works where and when. Generally, people get closest to their neighbors. At my center, a minority of therapists are based in satellite offices within academic schools, and it is they who historically have been likeliest to feel apart from the rest of the staff and, not coincidentally, to have lower morale. The same applies to part-time work schedules. As a rule, part-timers conscientiously do their shifts but are less likely than full-time therapists to identify with their counseling center jobs and bond with their colleagues.

6.4 The Director's Responses

When it comes to assessing morale and cohesiveness, the director isn't always in the best position to judge. Unhappy staff members may brood in private or gripe to one another without saying a word to the boss. There is also only so much directors can do about staff members' feelings, since work conditions are largely–and human nature entirely – beyond a manager's control. Still, certain practices are conducive to morale and cohesiveness, and others likely make matters worse. The following suggestions do not articulate lofty principles or draw on empirically based studies, but, rather, express opinions derived from close to 25 years in the director's hot seat.

6.4.1 Hiring

The first rule with morale and togetherness is to hire candidates with the right attitude. Positive people tend to stay that way, whereas those predisposed to be unhappy always find their justification. Assessing attitude is tricky, however, since all savvy candidates smile and tout themselves as team players. In the romantic arena people spend years checking out potential spouses and still make the wrong call half the time. What then can we hope to learn about a job applicant from an hour's interview?

Fortunately, there are ways to tease out attitude. The first is to be alert to and respect first impressions, because even in a single interview candidates do send out telltale signs. Take seriously a hint of prickliness or rigidity or entitlement or inauthenticity or ambivalence about the job, even if you can't put your finger on what's troubling. Experience teaches that discounting initial misgivings because the candidate looks good on paper can lead to headaches later. Second, ask how the candidate handled prior problems in three specific areas: (1) treating students, (2) working with colleagues and supervisors, and (3) dealing with stress. Candidates are unlikely to have prepared canned answers to these questions, and their responses may reveal their tendencies in morale-testing situations. Third, be candid about job features and drawbacks – stress, student pathology, salaries, limited prospects for advancement – to weed out those with rosy notions about college mental health. Last, ask for candid feedback from people who've worked with this person before – and listen closely for faint praise and veiled reservations.

One way to cut down on guesswork is to fill staff positions with ex-trainees. Former trainees know what they are signing up for when they're hired, and you have a good idea who you are getting.

6.4.2 Communications

An inescapable complaint in any organization is lack of communication and transparency, the perception that leadership keeps the staff in the dark about decisions and developments and doesn't value their opinions. The truth is, counseling center leaders *should not* discuss every matter with staff – it would not be practical (there is no time), appropriate, or even of interest. That said, morale does benefit when the staff trusts leaders to disclose necessary information, report truthfully, and be open to staff input. A good rule of thumb is: Tell staff what you'd want to know if you were in their position.

Equally important is a reciprocal rule: Tell staff what you *want* them to know. Staff members can't be expected to sympathize with, let alone share, the director's community perspective if kept uninformed about clinic-wide and campus issues. Returning to the wait list example, therapists are likelier to go along with unpalatable measures to reduce the wait list if they learn the student newspaper has written a critical editorial about students kept waiting for counseling. Also key is clarifying job expectations. Unless the director spells out elements of good performance, staff members cannot be expected to fulfill them.

As for the nuts and bolts of communication, a combination of formal and informal channels works best: staff meetings, committees, reports, retreats, e-mail updates, and simply keeping one's door open to answer questions and hear concerns. It helps too to divide larger staffs into subunits, so each employee has a voice in small group discussions.

6.4.3 Decision Making

Counseling centers cannot run as a democracy, with every decision and policy subjected to a majority vote. But employees do enjoy work more when they have a say in decision making and feel a sense of autonomy [13]. One way to accomplish this goal is to appoint representatives to weigh in on job searches and other major decisions. Another strategy is to encourage everyone to take charge of an area, to become the coordinator – the chief decision maker – in one or more aspects of the center's functioning.

6.4.4 Supportive Meetings

Staff meetings are ostensibly about exchanging information, clarifying policies and the like, but they're also, no less crucially, social and team-building occasions. Large, far-flung staffs in particular need the experience of sitting side-by-side in one room, everyone literally coming together, to gel as a staff.

Meetings are a must during crises. After the World Trade Center attacks in New York in 2001, just a mile from my university's campus and mere blocks from two residence halls, the counseling staff was pushed to the limit tending to devastated students while trying to keep a lid on their own anxieties. Though time was very scarce, we set aside a half hour each morning to check in, let our hair down, and exchange support.

6.4.5 Supervision and "Schmoozing"

Formal arrangements like supervisory relationships, mentorships and peer supervisory meetings can create bonds among staff members. Even an initial supervisory period for a month or two helps welcome newcomers into the fold.

But formal mechanisms or no, staff members naturally seek out their fellows. Signs of a healthy center atmosphere are informal case consultations in offices, laughter in the staff lounge and groups stepping out for lunch or coffee. At my center, one counselor plans farewells for departing staff members and showers for expecting parents, another celebrates birthdays with cookies, and a third runs a pool during the college basketball championships. A giggly contingent (one of the ringleaders being a senior psychiatrist) used to take turns playing practical jokes and then turning to me, their foil, in feigned protests against the others.

And what is the director's role in all of this? In my view it is mostly benign non-intervention – refraining from pouring cold water on lightheartedness. You may not join every outing or be in on every prank – better with some pranks if you are not – but the staff should not tense up and feign seriousness when they see you coming.

6.4.6 Relationships with Staff Members

It can be lonely at the top. A director can crack jokes at meetings and loosen up at staff parties, but socializing outside of work, to say nothing of sexual encounters, smacks of favoritism and is playing with fire. A director may be tempted to complain to a trusted staff member about job dissatisfaction or about other staff members, but should not. For the sake of morale, the director must come across as even-handed, looking out for everyone's best interests, and as reasonably confident and stable, up to the challenge of leading the center.

At times, an impartial, on-top-of-it-all stance can feel like a performance. But performances matter. Managing self-presentation, as Goffman [14] explained in detail, is a critical component of work success. A director's ability to more or less stay in role steadies and reassures a staff.

6.4.7 Feedback

At one time I reported to a vice president who had a genius for appreciation. Her gift was to make everyone reporting to her feel special, which of course inspired everyone to work hard and continue earning her favor. Her praise never felt like a technique or handling or flattery, but instead came across as genuine delight in noticing and acknowledging good performance. She closely listened to subordinates' opinions and took the trouble to read their reports – not, I have observed, universal practices. She spoke too not like someone who mistook her place on the organizational ladder for superiority, but as one professional to another, with the implication that "I'm not the expert in this area – you are". Such accurate, sincere, respectful praise is of course something counseling directors should strive for to motivate the staff. People work best when their efforts are appreciated.

Positive feedback can be given generously, but negative feedback should be dispensed with caution. Sometimes there is no alternative. A pattern of lateness, failure to write clinical notes, non-compliance with center policies – problems like these must be addressed, and promptly. An individual meeting should be set up with the staff member. (I have queasily witnessed several inquisitions where a group of senior university administrators ganged up on an out-of-favor employee.) The tenor of the meeting should be problem solving, neither blaming or threatening the employee nor making excuses for the person or getting bogged down in his or her personal problems. The goal is to be direct and honest, spelling out concrete examples of unsatisfactory performance and clear expectations for future performance. If the problem has come up before, the director should document the meeting and consult with the human resources department about proper procedure.

With minor transgressions or with ingrained personality traits, though, it's often better to say nothing, lest the director appear to be fault-finding and staff members fearfully look over their shoulder. The better part of leadership is sometimes to bite one's tongue and let a small matter pass. One therapist's edgy style periodically rubbed other staff members the wrong way. When I raised this issue with him a couple of times, he responded, predictably, with edginess, but vowed to change and in fact appeared to make the effort. But resolving the problem would have required a personality makeover. From that point on, I decided barring serious disruptions to leave him in peace; he was already mistrustful of me, and no further words on my part would sandpaper his rough edges. In the same vein, I learned to slow down upon hearing breathless reports from one employee about supposed misbehavior by another. While informants need to know their reports are taken seriously, it is a mistake to rashly confront the other employee until the facts are in and you have thought through what, if anything, needs saying.

6.4.8 Forbearance

The last point, about avoiding overreaction, deserves elaboration. Even in healthy offices, staff members sometimes feel disgruntled about their jobs, irritated with a colleague, and less than enthralled with the director. Nobody is pleased all the time. A wise director therefore assumes the existence of subterranean grumbling and doesn't overreact when it comes to the surface. I never exactly took delight in hearing staff complain at a meeting, but I consoled myself that it was good to know what bothered people, and a positive sign that they felt safe to speak up. The director's task when staff members vent is not unlike sitting with an angry patient. You want to validate what is being said, react non-defensively, and strive to give an objective, empathic response. And, oh yes, it helps to remember that staff complaints may be well-founded and, if it is in your power to correct the problem, to do so.

6.4.9 Rewards and Incentives

Salaries carry meaning beyond ability to pay the bills. Paychecks can be a measure of self-worth and perceived value to the institution, an index of one's status in comparison to other staff members. For symbolic as much as practical reasons, therefore, monetary rewards – generous starting salaries, raises, annual merit increases, bonuses – are a morale-booster for those who get them, and a downer for those who feel left out.

One of my more delicate directorial tasks was allotting merit salary increases for the upcoming year – deciding if employee X should get a 2.5%, 3.0% or 3.5% raise. The actual dollars in question were dwarfed by the emotional significance of getting more or less than the baseline increase. My difficulty was that some staff members perhaps stood out as especially deserving, but no one was undeserving. If I followed the directive to penalize some employees with minimal increases in order to free up extra funds for the worthiest, I risked alienating and demoralizing people who had done good work. The alternative, and my preference, was to give a reasonable amount to everyone – we were an all-star team, weren't we? – with perhaps a token additional compensation for a few. Across-the-board increases minimize hurt and envy and reinforce a "we are-all-in-this-together" mindset. By the same reasoning, whenever a pot of extra money became available, I campaigned to reward everyone, for example in the form of a center party or retreat, rather than singling out a few individuals.

Non-monetary rewards for good performance include approving flexitime requests and granting time for research, conferences, taking or teaching a class. Here the challenge is to be flexible and reward good performance without playing favorites. Once one employee is allowed to change his or her schedule, others will feel entitled to the same privilege and feel resentful if it is denied.

6.4.10 Evaluation

In recent years, my center adopted a numerical staff evaluation form that asked supervisors to assign rankings of "unsatisfactory", "needs improvement", "meets expectations" or "exceeds expectations" on a series of performance criteria. These forms had the advantages of specifying strengths and weaknesses and providing a paper trail for employees' personal files, which pleased the Human Resources department, but just like the merit increase exercise they stirred up bad feelings. Too often conscientious staff members tallied their "exceeds expectations" and wondered why they did not get a higher score. Such employee report cards, I suspect, cause more harm than good. In their stead, I favor a candid face-to-face evaluative discussion or, if the director must put something in writing, a qualitative written evaluation describing the employee's strengths, good performance, and realistic areas for growth and improvement, which gets the necessary points across without the bruised feelings. A related idea is to ask employees to submit their own written evaluations, listing, for example, notable accomplishments and goals for the upcoming year (J. Kay, personal communication, May 7, 2009).

An evaluation process ideally should be a two-way communication. Staff members should be encouraged to give the director feedback about job satisfaction and suggestions for improving the center. Many will hesitate to speak openly – it takes courage to speak truth to power – but merely to invite feedback sends staff members an empowering message.

6.4.11 Professional Development

Stagnation deadens morale. Therapists who feel at a professional standstill lose passion for their work and start going through the motions. A clinic-wide answer is to use staff meetings to bring in speakers or exchange ideas about cases. For individual clinicians, the remedy is to tackle something fresh – taking courses, attending conferences, conducting research, writing papers, teaching a course, achieving licensure, adding credentials, or earning a more advanced degree. Directors can support these efforts through enthusiasm and interest, and, when appropriate and feasible, approving time away from the office and supplying funding.

Ideally, professional development coincides with clinic needs. That is why my center invites all therapists to delve into and take ownership of a clinical or administrative area; they then feel engaged and empowered and the center gains expertise. One psychologist, hired to head the eating disorders program, later trained in and co-led a new program in DBT for borderline patients. Another coordinated the group and workshop program for several years, then took on a new challenge as coordinator of the psychology externship program. An interdisciplinary team – a psychiatrist, psychologist and social worker – intensively trained over the summer in mindfulness techniques and then inaugurated a program of workshops, on-line offerings and staff stress relief hours.

6.4.12 Major Problems

In a quarter century as director I faced a handful of unsolvable staff problems. A clinician with declining health stopped making the effort to listen to patients. Another who showed unmistakable signs of substance abuse persistently denied anything was wrong. A third repeatedly and blatantly was rude to colleagues, including myself. In these instances, efforts to work things out failed, until eventually the employee left voluntarily or, in accordance with Human Resources guidelines, was let go. Sometimes staff members must leave the team, if for no other reason than so the rest can concentrate on their jobs without distractions.

Major problems do not have to end in separation. I have also seen profoundly impaired therapists, far too distraught to perform at work, take a leave of absence, undergo treatment and make a successful return. These rewarding outcomes hinged on their admitting to a problem and seeking professional help. As with therapy cases, impaired employees must be motivated to change. But just as importantly, the staff was taking their side. Though they had taxed colleagues' patience by demanding support and not pulling their weight at work, they had not alienated themselves. They were like troubled family members – troubled, but still family. And this leads to my final observation about morale. When an impaired staff member is still viewed as part of the team, the rest closely watch what happens. A humane and patient response to the wounded individual is a reassurance to everyone – "this is how I would be treated if I were in trouble" – and a morale-boosting affirmation of team togetherness.

References

1. Gallagher, R.P. and Taylor, R. (2008) *National Survey of Counseling Center Directors*, International Association of Counseling Services, Alexandria, VA.
2. Lawrence, L. (2008) Self-management team presentations, New York: National College Depression Partnership, Learning Session, 2.
3. International Association of Counseling Services (2000) Accreditation Standards for University and College Counseling Centers. Retrieved February 15, 2009 from http://www.iacsinc.org/IACS%20STANDARDS.pdf.
4. Rockland-Miller, H.S. and Eells, G.T. (2006) The implementation of mental health clinical triage systems in university health services. *Journal of College Student Psychotherapy*, **20**(4), 39–52.
5. Rando, R.R. and Barr, V. (2008) The Association for University and College Counseling Center Directors Annual Survey. Association for University and College Counseling Center Directors.

Retrieved May 7, 2009 from: http://www.aucccd.org/img/pdfs/aucccd_monograph_public_2008.pdf.

6. Gallagher, R.P. (1994) *National Survey of Counseling Center Directors*, International Association of Counseling Services, Alexandria, VA.

7. Cynkar, A. (2007) The changing gender composition of psychology. *Monitor on Psychology*, **38** (6), 46.

8. Bogan, A.M. and Safer, D.L. (2004) Woman in psychiatric training. *Academic Psychiatry*, **28**, 305–309.

9. Teachers College, Columbia University (2008) Counseling psychology, PhD. Program Description. Retrieved February 2, 2009 from http://www.tc.columbia.edu/CCP/CounPsych/.

10. NYU Silver School of Social Work (2008) Innovation and education in the spirit of Service. Retrieved September 10, 2009 from http://www.nyu.edu/socialwork/.

11. Blaine, G.B. Jr and McArthur, C.C. (1971) *Emotional Problems of the Student*, Appleton-Century-Crofts, New York.

12. Grayson, P.A., Schwartz, V., and Commerford, M. (1997) Brave new world? Drug therapy and college mental health. *Journal of College Student Psychotherapy*, **11**, 23–32.

13. Eells, G.T., Seals, T., Rockett, J. and Hayes, D. (2005) Enjoying the roller coaster ride: Directors' perspectives on fostering staff morale in university counseling centers. *Journal of College Student Psychotherapy*, **20**(2), 17–28.

14. Goffman, E. (1959) *Presentation of Self in Everyday Life*, Doubleday, New York.

7 Legal and Ethical Issues in College Mental Health

Karen Bower[1] and Victor Schwartz[2]

[1]Judge David L. Bazelon Center for Mental Health Law, Washington, DC, USA

[2]Yeshiva University, Albert Einstein College of Medicine, New York, NY, USA

7.1 Introduction

The legal and ethical principles that frame the management of mental health services on university campuses present campus clinicians and administrators with multiple challenges. In the following discussion we will present a theoretical framework that explicates the sources of these challenges and seeming conflicts. We will then analyze the statutory and case law around these issues. And finally, we will make some general recommendations to those managing these challenging issues.

7.2 Conceptual Framework

The statutory, case law and ethical principles relevant to university mental health can be generally grouped into two overarching categories. On the one hand, there is strong support for the privacy and autonomy of the individual student. In line with this is the idea (supported by legislation such as the Americans with Disabilities Act (ADA)) that universities should make every effort to support the ability and right of a student with disabilities, including mental illness, to attend and succeed in college. On the other hand, there has been an increase in attention to community safety and an increased sensitivity to parental expectations of involvement with their children. Administrators and clinicians have felt increasing pressure to anticipate and prevent tragic outcomes, even when this might mean taking steps that might limit student autonomy and privacy.

7.2.1 Privacy/Autonomy

An expectation of privacy is a fundamental ethical standard in a free society [1]. Beyond this, the concept of *confidentiality* in the mental health setting is absolute bedrock upon which the therapeutic relationship must rest [2]. Creating an environment where students feel that it is safe to seek help is essential. The practice of psychotherapy is founded on the notion that people will feel safe in sharing personal and at times embarrassing information.

Mental Health Care in the College Community   Edited by Jerald Kay and Victor Schwartz
© 2010 John Wiley & Sons, Ltd.

This can only occur when the student has confidence that being in mental health treatment and what transpires in therapy will not be shared with others. This expectation and the fear of its breach are immediate and intense in small and self-contained communities such as universities where many members have personal interconnections.

It would not be surprising that many students coming to college mental health services (CMHSs) for help might worry about whether clinicians are sharing information with college personnel outside of the service and wonder under what conditions their parents might be contacted by the service or the university. If the CMHS has not succeeded in establishing a fundamental relationship of *trust* with the student body, its effectiveness in engaging students in need of help and in achieving good clinical outcomes will be severely undermined [3]. It is also important to note that students come to university to promote their future success. So it is not a simple matter to confide in the people on whom one's future may rest that one is having a serious problem. Again, the establishment of trust is a crucial and at the same time fragile matter.

7.2.2 Campus Safety/Parental Involvement

Although college students are young adults and in almost all cases are also legally adults, parents typically remain highly involved in their lives and university careers. (The reasons for this are complex and will be taken up in greater detail in Chapter 10). Accordingly, there may be an expectation by parents that information about their college-attending child ought to be available to them, particularly in circumstances where a student is struggling with academic, personal or emotional problems. Many parents assume that they should be part of whatever discussion or plan may ensue in the course of addressing this concern. While there are many situations where parents can be involved in these discussions, there are also legal and ethical constraints that need to be weighed. These will be addressed in detail later in the chapter.

Paralleling parents' concerns about their children's lives while in college, there has developed a sense among university administrators that students are in regular and consistent need of supervision and oversight. This trend has been heightened dramatically subsequent to recent campus tragedies and several well publicized lawsuits involving universities [4]. University administrators have felt growing pressure to safeguard their campuses from tragedies, mishaps, and resultant lawsuits.

Certainly, universities can be expected to take sensible (and often legally mandated) steps to protect their campus communities. Fire and building safety codes and conformity with basic law enforcement and security practices must be in place and, should untoward events occur, universities should strive to reduce the likelihood of reoccurrence. Nevertheless, there is a sentiment among parents and university personnel that universities ought to do more to safeguard their communities. Moreover, as discussed later in the chapter, certain elements of law (i.e. Virginia law re: parental notification, [5]) highlight affirmative steps colleges should take to safeguard their students and communities.

7.2.3 Conflicting Incentives and Players

These conflicting trends are not surprising. Every society or community must consider how it balances the sometimes conflicting values of individual rights (including the right to be different, strange or troubling to others) against the need for order, structure and even some degree of conformity, so that the community can function effectively and people are able to live with each other in safety and comfort. Colleges are special communities in two important ways. First, many of the members of these communities are young people who have never before lived independently and continue to have close, quasi-dependent ties to parents. College may be their first major experience at trying their adult wings and parent–child roles may be in a period of redefinition. Second, as noted above, students are living in these communities because they are pursuing a specific series of goals: to become educated and acquire tools for ongoing success in life.

On the one hand, students want to maintain the greatest latitude of freedom, privacy and independence for their participation in university life. Their families want university faculty and administrators to maintain communities that are most conducive to free, interesting and exploratory discourse and thought. Parents want their children to succeed, and often want to participate in their children's educational life and experience. University therapists and students want to create systems that allow them the greatest sense of privacy so that therapeutic work can be done. Clinicians don't want policies that erode privacy and discourage students from seeking or receiving treatment. Everyone wants our university communities to be safe.

Statutory and case law may be seen as a broad attempt to find balance among these varied considerations and principles. The law here is best viewed as a dynamic system that is working to set and maintain this balance. Yet, while the law may provide outer boundaries beyond which actions would be unlawful or unethical, it often does not provide clear answers for the resolution of mental health crises on college campuses.

In the following discussion of the specifics of statutory and case law it would be helpful to keep this framework in mind. In reading this chapter, it may be useful to consider the ethical principle or problem the law or case is addressing and how the various concerns find balance within the system as a whole. We will first lay out the details of the laws and conclude with recommendations and suggestions for practice.

7.3 Legal Framework

7.3.1 Confidentiality

In colleges and universities, the circumstances under which mental health information and records can be disclosed are governed by professional licensing standards and ethics, state law, and federal law. More than one law can apply to any given situation, so individuals in possession of confidential information are obliged to comply with the most restrictive among these requirements. Generally speaking, state laws afford the greatest protection and therefore, will be broadly applicable. Both state and federal laws allow disclosure of mental health information when there is a specific danger to self or others.

It is important to remember that in the education context, privacy is critical. In this regard, the education context is no different than any other setting involving mental health treatment. Students are often fearful that they will be denied jobs, housing or educational or social opportunities if they disclose their mental illness. To encourage students to seek treatment, schools must ensure confidentiality. Failure to adequately protect mental health information can result in negative consequences for students, can erode confidence in university health care clinics and counseling centers, and may discourage students from using available services and getting needed treatment.

Limitations on confidentiality, for example regarding danger, duty to warn, and so on, are not unique to the campus mental health setting and are negotiated daily within all mental health service contexts. These limitations may be a disincentive to seeking treatment. Schools have recognized that:

> [i]f students believe that college staff may notify their parents or seek to hospitalize them if they disclose their mental problems or suicidal thoughts, they may decline to provide important information about their mental health history, they may entirely avoid seeking help for their problems, or, if they do make an effort to get help, they may not be fully honest.

Amici Curie American Council on Education, American Association of Collegiate registrars and Admissions Officers, American Association of Community Colleges, American Association of State Colleges and Universities, Association of American Universities, National Association of Independent Colleges and Universities, National Association of State Universities and Land-Grant Colleges, and National Association of Student Personnel Administrators in support of Petition for Relief Under G.L.C. 231, § 118 (First Paragraph) by MIT Administrators Arnold Henderson and Nina Davis-Millis.

Key to developing a successful therapeutic relationship is an understanding by any consumer of the scope and limitations of the privacy considerations guiding the therapeutic interaction.

When disclosure is necessary, it is always preferable to obtain consent to a voluntary disclosure of confidential information. Schools can ask students upon matriculation and upon becoming a client of the counseling center to voluntarily identify individuals whom the school can contact in case of an emergency. Colorado wrote this option into law, as a pilot program allowing schools to offer students the opportunity to complete a consent form designating a contact person who the school can contact if the school believes the student is considering suicide or may be a danger to him or herself [6]. The University of North Carolina at Chapel Hill is researching use of psychiatric advance directives in the college setting to address this and similar matters (see http://www.miwatch.org/2008/09/helping_college_students_pads.html).

State law

Since state confidentiality laws address the treatment of mental health information and records wherever they are maintained, they are applicable to both clinicians and school personnel generally. State laws governing health records provide for confidentiality but vary from state to state in their terms, scope, requirements, and application. The following discussion therefore addresses state law confidentiality principles generally. Schools should seek legal counsel for state specific information.

Most state statutes broadly define protected mental health information to encompass identifying information about clients, oral communications made to therapists or others, and written records. Depending on the jurisdiction, confidential information shared with a mental health treatment provider may be disclosed without the patient's consent only in very limited situations. The legal precedent for a mental health professional's disclosure of confidential information lies in the duty to protect or warn which was established by the California Supreme Court's decision in *Tarasoff v. Regents of the University of*

California [7]. In *Tarasoff*, a University of California student told his psychologist that he intended to kill an unnamed but readily identifiable woman. The psychologist believed the patient met the commitment standard and informed police, who detained him briefly, but did not inform the intended victim. The patient subsequently killed the woman. Her parents sued the psychologist for failing to warn them or their daughter about the impending danger. The California Supreme Court rejected the psychologist's claim that he owed no duty to the woman because she was not his patient, holding that:

> when a therapist determines, or pursuant to the standards of his profession should determine, that his patient presents a serious danger of violence to another, he incurs an obligation to use reasonable care to protect the intended victim against such danger. The discharge of this duty may require the therapist to take one or more of various steps, depending upon the nature of the case. Thus it may call for him to warn the intended victim or others likely to apprise the victim of the danger, to notify police, or to take whatever other steps are reasonably necessary under the circumstances.

Since the *Tarasoff* ruling, most states have created, through case law or statute, a duty of mental health professionals to protect or warn third parties of a serious risk of injury [8]. Generally speaking, privacy may be breached and confidential information shared without consent when the treatment professional believes there is a substantial and imminent risk that his or her failure to disclose information will result in serious physical harm to others. In those circumstances, a mental health professional may disclose confidential information as part of a duty to protect or warn the intended victim of harm [8]. However, this exception to confidentiality is very limited and narrowly proscribes the individuals with whom confidential information may be shared.

Most state statutes provide for disclosure of confidential information without consent on an emergency basis to law enforcement officers and emergency medical personnel when the patient presents a serious risk of violence to self or others. These statutes often do not allow disclosure to a parent or other relative or to individuals such as a school dean or administrator unless they are individuals who can prevent a specific threat of violence. For example, the California Confidentiality of Medical Information Act includes a list of parties to whom information may be disclosed for safety reasons [9]. There are protections and limitations for disclosure even when authorized by law [9].

New York's Mental Hygiene Law allows non-consensual disclosure of mental health information to an endangered individual and a law enforcement agency when a treating psychiatrist or psychologist has determined that a patient or client presents a serious and imminent danger to that individual [10]. Texas limits disclosure of confidential information to judicial or administrative proceedings and without consent to, among others, medical or law enforcement personnel if the professional determines that there is a probability of imminent physical injury by the patient to the patient or others [11]. Virginia recently passed a law requiring state colleges to notify a parent of a dependent student who receives mental health treatment at the school's counseling center when there exists a substantial likelihood that the student will cause serious physical harm to himself or others, unless the student's treatment provider, in the exercise of professional judgment, indicates that notification would be reasonably likely to cause substantial harm to the student or another person [12].

Confidential information that has been disclosed by mental health treatment providers in a health and safety emergency retains its protection as a mental health record. State laws prohibit re-disclosure of confidential information except to the extent that re-disclosure is consistent with the initial purpose for which disclosure was authorized. Therefore, school personnel who receive confidential mental health information in an emergency situation must take precautions to safeguard privacy of the information except as necessary to respond to the emergency. State laws generally require a treatment provider to record non-consensual disclosures. Most state statutes provide for damages, fines or imprisonment for privacy violations.

Given the differences among state statutes, it is important to consult with counsel for state specific information.

Federal law

In addition to the state law protections afforded to mental health information, the sharing of student information is also governed by federal law – primarily the Family Education Rights and Privacy Act (FERPA) [13]. The Department of Education has issued implementing regulations, which can be found in the United States Code of Federal Regulations (CFR) at 34 CFR Part 99 [14]. FERPA applies to colleges and universities that receive federal funds under any program administered by the Secretary of Education [14]. "Receipt of federal funds" is broadly interpreted, and includes receipt of grants, or contracts and the enrollment of students who receive federal financial aid, Pell grants, or guaranteed student loans [14,15]. Some schools, including those that do not receive any federal funds, or that have university hospitals, may also be governed by the Health Insurance Portability and Accountability Act (HIPAA). Each of these laws is addressed below.

1. Family Education Rights and Privacy Act (FERPA). FERPA governs disclosure of student educational records and information contained in those records, and establishes when such records and information may be disclosed. FERPA has limited applicability to clinical personnel since, as discussed below, they are subject to strict standards under licensing and ethical codes and state law. Its protections primarily apply to non-clinical personnel. FERPA prohibits disclosure of educational records and information contained in those records without consent. FERPA has several enumerated exceptions which allow – but do not require – disclosure of student information without consent to specific categories of individuals.

Education records protected by FERPA are broadly defined as: records, files, documents, and other materials that: (a) contain information directly related to a student; and (b) are maintained by an educational agency or institution [15]. A record is "directly related" to a student if it identifies the student on its face, or if the student's identity can be deduced from the demographic, descriptive or other information, either alone or in combination with other publicly available information. This definition is broad enough to encompass virtually all records maintained by a college or university, including transcripts, academic records, exams, financial aid records, disciplinary records, housing contracts, disability services records, e-mail messages and handwritten notes.

FERPA allows students to inspect and review their education records for accuracy, provides a procedure for challenging the accuracy of education records, and prevents personally identifiable information from being disclosed to third parties without consent. If a student requests his or her educational record, it must be provided within 45 days [16].

The definition of education records specifically excludes personal notes created solely for an individual's personal use that are not accessible or shared with others, law enforcement records for a law enforcement purpose, certain employment records, and treatment records [17]. "Treatment records" are defined as "records that are (a) made or maintained by a physician, psychiatrist, psychologist or other recognized professional or paraprofessional acting in his or her professional capacity or assisting in a paraprofessional capacity, (b) made, maintained or used only in connection with treatment, and (c) disclosed only to individuals providing treatment" [18]. Progress notes by a physician, social worker, psychiatrist or psychologist are treatment records. Records detailing a student's health, "including mental illness or disability," that are created or maintained by school officials who are not treatment providers (including teachers, deans, administrators, and resident advisors), or are used for purposes other than treatment, are education records and thus are governed by FERPA [19]. Note that since these records contain information about a student's mental health, they may also be governed by state mental health law and, in limited circumstances, by the Health Insurance Portability and Accountability Act of 1996 (HIPAA). A school must comply with the state or federal law with the strictest requirements.

It is important to note that FERPA's protections apply to oral and written disclosure of information contained in education records. Observations by school personnel other than mental health personnel (faculty, student affairs directors, deans, resident advisors) are not educational records, and are not governed by FERPA. University administrators can disclose their observations to others without consent [20]. However, any *written* notes that contain personal observations are education records protected by FERPA and can only be disclosed by consent or pursuant to one of the FERPA exceptions.

The FERPA exceptions that allow disclosure without consent include:

- **Directory information**: Directory information includes information contained in an education record of a student that would not generally be considered harmful or an invasion of privacy if disclosed [22]. Examples of directory information include the student's name, address, phone number, e-mail address, photograph, date of birth, field of study, sports participation, awards received, and other schools attended, among other examples [23]. If a college or university wishes to designate certain classes of information as "directory information" that will be released without the student's consent, it must first afford the student an opportunity to opt out and prevent the release of directory information [25].

- **Legitimate educational interest**: Under this exception to consent, a school official may release non-directory information and education records to another school official within the same educational institution who has a "legitimate educational interest" in the material [26]. If a school does disclose records under this exception, it must define and give notice to its students of who qualifies as a "school official" and what constitutes a "legitimate educational interest" [26]. However, since FERPA does not require a postsecondary school to make education records available to anyone other than an eligible student, a school can determine that certain records cannot be shared without consent even when a legitimate educational purpose exists [27].

- **Health or safety emergency**: FERPA permits disclosure without consent to appropriate persons in connection with an emergency when information is necessary to protect the health or safety of the student or other persons [28]. Appropriate persons typically include law enforcement officials, public health officials, trained medical personnel and a student's parents [29]. Schools may disclose information to such third parties if there is an articulable and significant threat to the health or safety of the student or others [30]. The US Department of Education has interpreted the health and safety emergency exception to allow disclosure only if the school has determined, in a specific case, that there is immediate need to disclose information in order to avert or diffuse a serious threat to the safety or health of the student or other individuals [31]. Further, any release must be narrowly tailored, and be made only to parties who can address the specific emergency in question [32]. "The Department [of Education] will not substitute its judgment for that of the agency or institution if, based on the information available at the time of the determination there is a rational basis for the agency's or institution's determination that a health or safety emergency exists and that the disclosure was made to appropriate parties." US Department of Education Final FERPA, Federal Register, vol. 73, No. 237, at 74837, December 9, 2008 (available at: http://www.ed.gov/policy/gen/guid/fpco/ hottopics/ht12-17-08.html), see [33] for more information. The health and safety exception is "limited to the period of the emergency and generally will not allow for a blanket release of personally identifiable information from a student's education records" [32].

- **Parents of dependents**: Disclosure of education records to parents of students who have been declared dependant for federal tax purposes is permitted without consent [34]. Schools can determine if a student is a dependant by asking students to submit redacted copies of their parents' tax returns, or one of the model forms created by the Department of Education. http://www.ed.gov/policy/gen/guid/fpco/ferpa/safeschools/modelform.html or http://www.ed.gov/policy/gen/guid/fpco/ferpa/safeschools/modelform2.html (including a consent section for students who are not dependent).

- **Judicial order or subpoena**: Release of records without consent is allowed in order to comply with a judicial order or lawfully issued subpoena [35].

- **Other exceptions**: school officials are permitted to share education records in certain circumstances with: officials of another school for purposes related to enrollment or transfer; authorized representatives of the Comptroller General of the United States, the Attorney General of the United States, the United States Secretary of Education, or state and local educational authorities; in connection with the student's financial aid; organizations conducting certain studies for the educational institution; accrediting organizations to carry out their accrediting functions; or the student him or herself [36]. Further, FERPA allows disclosing information to parents without a student's consent if the student has violated any Federal, State or local law, or any school rule or policy governing the possession or use of alcohol or a controlled substance, if the student is under age 21 and the use or possession constitutes a disciplinary violation [37]. It also allows a school to disclose results of disciplinary proceedings for crimes of violence or non-forcible sex offenses to a victims or others if the crime violated schools rules or policies [38].

A school that discloses information pursuant to one of the enumerated exceptions must inform the recipient that the information may not be re-disclosed unless the recipient obtains consent or the subsequent disclosure falls within one of the FERPA exceptions [39]. Before a FERPA disclosure is made, state mental health privacy law protections must be considered. A school should comply with the state or federal law with the strictest requirements.

Schools must record all requests for access and all disclosures and re-disclosures of personally identifiable information, and the basis for the release (i.e. the recipient's legitimate educational interest) [40]. Schools must also, upon request, provide a copy of the released records to the student and an opportunity to challenge the content [41]. Similarly, if a school discloses information under the health or safety emergency exception, schools must record the articulable and significant threat to health or safety that formed the basis for disclosure and the parties to whom information was disclosed [42].

While there is no cause of action against school personnel for violation of FERPA (i.e. individual clinicians or administrators cannot be sued for FERPA violations), students may file a complaint with the Department of Education Office of Family Policy Compliance against a school that violates the FERPA requirements. Sanctions may include loss of federal financial assistance. Students may also file complaints with the state Department of Higher Education. Even though a disclosure may be permissible under FERPA, it may violate a state re-disclosure law or other privacy law. While it may be time consuming to obtain consent, when mental health information is at issue it is always preferable to obtain consent to a disclosure of confidential information, and as discussed above, it is potentially legally risky not to do so.

2. Health Insurance Portability and Accountability Act (HIPAA). In the majority of cases, the Health Insurance Portability and Accountability Act (HIPAA), Pub. L. No. 104–191, 110 Stat. 1936 (codified as amended at 45 CFR. §§ 160, 164 (1996)), will not apply to the records maintained at postsecondary institutions. HIPAA was enacted to provide national standards for privacy and access to identifiable health information, and to standardize the communication of electronic health information between health insurers and health care providers such as: hospitals, health care clinics, physicians' offices, pharmacies, clinical social workers, psychologists, nurses, and any person or organization that furnishes bills, or is paid for health care in the normal course of business. As such, most communication in campus settings is outside the domain of HIPAA [43].

HIPAA applies only to "covered entities"-health plans, health care clearinghouses, and health care providers that transmit health information in electronic form in connection with certain "covered transactions". A HIPAA covered transaction is "the transmission of information … to carry out financial or administrative activities related to health care". HIPAA specifically enumerates 11 HIPAA transactions such as processing health claims, billing third-party payers, transmitting encounter information, payment and remittance advice, health plan eligibility, and premium payments [44].

Schools may be "covered entities" under HIPAA if they have a health program or clinic and staff that transmit health information in electronic form in connection with health care billing, payment and remittance advice, claims or encounter information. While many schools do provide health care services, if they do not engage in the enumerated transactions in electronic form, they are not covered entities.

However, even if a school that receives federal funds is a covered entity, education records and medical and mental health records are *specifically exempted* from the definition of protected health information in the HIPAA privacy rule [45]. However, since the reasoning for exclusion of treatment records from HIPAA protections in the postsecondary school context is questionable, the regulations are legally vulnerable (see HIPAA Privacy Rule preamble [46]).

Note, however, that treatment records of hospitals affiliated with universities are not FERPA education records (directly related to a student and maintained by an educational institution or party acting for the institution) and are therefore governed by the HIPAA Privacy rule.

Like FERPA, HIPAA has exceptions to comply with law enforcement and to uphold other laws, such as those addressing public health, child abuse or neglect, domestic violence, criminal investigations, and judicial or administrative proceedings [47]. The HIPAA privacy rule has an emergency exception, which allows disclosure of protected health information without consent to prevent or lessen a serious and imminent threat to the health or safety of a person or the public, and disclosure is to a person reasonably able to prevent or lessen the threat, such as the target of the threat [48]. Such disclosure must be consistent with applicable state law, as discussed above. A school must comply with the state or federal law with the strictest requirements.

HIPAA does not give people the right to sue. Instead, someone aggrieved by violation of HIPAA may file a written complaint with the Department of Health and Human Services Office for Civil Rights, which has the authority to impose civil and criminal penalties if they find a violation of the law.

Other laws also apply to certain student health records, such as substance abuse records. Section 543 of the Public Health Service Act, 42 USC. 290dd-2, and its implementing regulation, 42 CFR Part 2, establish confidentiality requirements for patient records that are maintained in connection with the performance of any federally-assisted specialized alcohol or drug abuse program. Publically operated schools are also subject to any protections for privacy that may exist in state constitutions.

As described above, in most cases the mental health treatment records of a university counseling center will be exempt from federal law (i.e. they are excluded from the definition of education records under FERPA and the definition of protected health information under HIPAA). Instead, a counseling center's mental health treatment records are primarily governed by state law, and professional licensing requirements, and codes of ethics.

Licensing and professional ethics

In addition to legal duties to protect confidentiality, treatment providers have an ethical obligation not to disclose confidential information. The American Psychiatric Association, American Psychological Association, National Association of Social Workers, American Counseling Association, American School Counselor Association, and American Medical Association, among others, all have codes of ethics that prohibit disclosure of confidential information except in limited circumstances.

For example, the American Medical Association's code of ethics holds as a central tenet that a physician shall safeguard patient confidences and privacy within the constraints of the law [49]. It also provides that:

> [w]hen a patient threatens to inflict serious physical harm to another person or to him or herself and there is a reasonable probability that the patient may carry out the threat, the physician should take reasonable precautions for the protection of the intended victim, which may include notification of law enforcement authorities [50].

However, the Code stresses that when disclosure is necessary, only the minimal amount of information required by law should be divulged [50–53]. Family members may be appropriate individuals to whom confidential information can be released in an emergency situation, however, treatment providers must exercise professional judgment and consider whether disclosure to family members will exacerbate the problem or damage the therapeutic relationship.

Several Codes also include an ethical obligation for mental health treatment providers to inform their clients of the nature and limits of confidentiality, and the circumstances in which confidentiality will be breached. See for example [53].

It is appropriate for counselors to assist a student in seeking a leave or accommodations, at the student's request. But, it is a breach of professional ethics for a therapist to have a "dual relationship" with a client, simultaneously acting as a treatment provider to a student and a decision-maker for the university. A counselor cannot provide treatment services to the student and simultaneously use information gathered in treating the student to make an administrative determination on behalf of the university. When a counselor is in a treatment relationship with a student, participating as a decision-maker on behalf of the university to determine, for example, whether the student should be placed on an involuntary leave of absence presents a conflict of interest and is unethical. Of course, in a situation in which the student may present significant danger to self or others, the therapist is obligated to take necessary steps to protect the student and the community (more on this later).

Recommendations

- Policies should be developed so as not to discourage students from seeking treatment, for example forcing students to take a medical leave solely on the basis of seeking treatment for suicidal thoughts or attempts.

- Confidentiality is critical. Efforts to relax confidentiality and mandate parental notification are likely to have an unintended deleterious impact on the care of college students.

- A school should comply with the state or federal law with the strictest requirements.

- State and federal law and codes of ethics allow disclosure to appropriate persons in connection with an emergency. Perceived impediments to information – sharing seem to be the result of limited or mis-understanding of FERPA and other relevant laws and regulations. The applicable laws actually provide an adequate framework for thoughtful clinical decision-making.

- As described above, schools should ask students to identify individuals whom they wish to be contacted in case of a medical or psychiatric emergency.

- Student mental health services need to be clear with students and families when they are not in a treatment relationship but are acting as an agent of the university, for example when doing assessments about whether a student may re-enter the university after a medical leave.

7.3.2 Liability for Suicide

As noted earlier, in recent years, schools have felt growing pressure to disclose student information to family members or others. Such pressure has been fueled in part by exaggerated fears of potential liability for failure to prevent suicide [4].

Although there is fear of liability for failure to prevent suicide on college campuses, to date, no court has found a school liable for failure to prevent suicide. Cases involving failure to prevent suicide are governed by state tort law. In order to have liability for the negligent failure to protect, there must be a duty, a breach of that duty which results in a foreseeable harm, and causation. Historically, suicide was seen as an intentional intervening act, which broke the chain of causation and prevented liability (see discussion in [54]). Further, the general rule is that there is no duty to prevent harm to third parties, except where there is a special relationship between the parties and the harm is reasonably foreseeable [55]. Such a special relationship giving rise to a duty to protect is usually found in custodial settings such as a jails or psychiatric hospitals [55].

For years, the leading case involving failure to prevent suicide in an educational setting was *Jain v. State* [54]. In that case, student Sanjay Jain admitted to the resident assistant (RA) that he was planning to kill himself by inhaling exhaust fumes from his moped. After speaking with the RA, he agreed to remove his moped from his room and assured the RA that he would seek counseling. Jain refused the RA's request to speak with his family. Several weeks later, Jain killed himself in the manner he had previously described. Jain's father brought suit against the University of Iowa, claiming that the University's knowledge of Jain's mental condition created a special relationship and the university failed to exercise reasonable care in exercising its duty to protect his son by informing his parents of his suicide attempt.

The Iowa Supreme Court disagreed, finding that:

> it is undisputed that the RA appropriately intervened in an emotionally-charged situation, offered Jain support and encouragement, and referred him to counseling. [The RA] likewise counseled Jain to talk things over with his parents, seek professional help, and call her [the RA] anytime, even when she was not at work. She sought Jain's permission to contact his parents but he refused. In short, no action by university personnel prevented Jain from taking advantage of the help and encouragement being offered, nor did they do anything to prevent him from seeking help on his own accord.

The court reasoned that the University did not increase Jain's risk of harm, and refused to find that a special relationship existed which gave rise to a duty to notify his parents.

Since the Jain case, several recent high-profile court decisions have caused schools concern that a special relationship and duty to prevent suicide could be extended to postsecondary schools [56]. In *Schieszler v. Ferrum College* [57] student Michael Frentzel committed suicide by hanging. After an argument with his girlfriend, Frentzel sent her a note indicating that he would hang himself. She shared the note with the resident assistant (RA) and campus police, who responded to Frentzel's room. Frentzel had bruises on his head, which he admitted were self-inflicted. The Dean of Students was advised, and asked Frentzel to sign a statement that he would not harm himself. Although there appeared to be an imminent probability that Frentzel would harm himself, neither the RA nor the dean referred Frentzel for counseling or assessment. Days later, Frentzel wrote additional notes telling his former girlfriend he loved her and stating "only God can save me now". She reported this to the Dean and RA, who prevented her from going to Frentzel's room. They did not take any affirmative steps to ensure Frentzel's immediate safety. When the Dean and RA ultimately went to Frentzel's room, he had already committed suicide.

The family of Michael Frentzel sued Ferrum, alleging that the school knew or should have known that Frentzel was likely to harm himself if not properly supervised, and negligently failed to take adequate precautions to insure that he did not hurt himself. In refusing to dismiss the case as a matter of law, and allowing it to proceed to trial, the Virginia federal court found that a special relationship may exist because of the particular circumstances of the case. Specifically, the court was persuaded that the school's failure to take steps to aid Frentzel – by ensuring he was supervised or by contacting his guardian, while preventing his girlfriend from returning to his room – *may* have been a proximate cause of injury. It acknowledged that "[w]hile it is unlikely that Virginia would conclude that a special relationship exists as a matter of law between colleges and universities and their students", a jury might find that a special relationship existed on the particular facts alleged in this case.

It is significant that *the court did not find as a matter of law that there was a special relationship between schools and students. Nor did the court find that the school was liable*. Rather, the court found that, based on the record before it, it could not say that Frentzel's suicide was not foreseeable or the school's conduct was not a proximate cause, and therefore allowed the case to proceed to trial. Thereafter, the case was settled.

Three years later, the reasoning of *Ferrum* was followed by the Massachusetts Superior Court in *Shin v. MIT* [58]. In that case, student Elizabeth Shin had a history of mental health problems and suicidal ideation for which she received treatment from the school counselor. Despite treatment, she continued to experience suicidal ideation. The dorm housemaster received numerous reports of Shin's self-injurious behavior, which she reported to the Dean. The Dean also met with Shin several times to discuss her mental health and received reports from professors and graduate resident tutors of concerns for Shin's safety. On April 8, 2000, in response to a suicide threat, campus police brought Shin to the mental health center, where she spoke with an on-call psychiatrist who determined that she was not acutely suicidal.

On April 10, 2000, other students related to the housemaster that Shin had made suicide threats, which she relayed to the Dean. Later that day, the Dean attended a multidisciplinary group including deans and mental health treatment providers in which they discussed Shin's case. Following the meeting, one of the psychiatrists made an appointment for Shin for an outpatient program the following day, and notified Shin of the appointment and his availability. However, neither the housemaster nor the Dean made any effort to have Shin evaluated by a mental health professional to determine if she was an imminent risk of injury or to otherwise supervise her or notify her family. Shin died that night either as the result of an accident or suicide.

Shin's family sued for failure to prevent her suicide. The Superior Court dismissed all claims against the institution, as well as some of the claims against individual administrators and staff members. However, in refusing to dismiss claims against the Dean and house-master, the court found that they had a "special relationship" and a duty to exercise reasonable care to protect Shin from harm because they were aware of her mental health problems, and could reasonably foresee that she would hurt herself without proper supervision. Accordingly, the court found that they, "failed to secure [her] short term safety in response to her suicide plan in the morning hours of April 10, 2000. By not formulating and enacting an immediate plan to respond to [her] escalating threats to commit suicide", there was a genuine issue of fact as to whether the administrators were negligent ([58] at *14). The court did not find that MIT was liable. In fact, the Court refused to find as a matter of law that the administrators owed Shin a duty. Instead, the Court ruled that there existed a genuine issue of material fact whether the administrators were grossly negligent and whether their negligence was the proximate cause of Shin's death. As such, the case against the administrators was not dismissed and was allowed to proceed toward trial. The case settled shortly thereafter.

Significantly, in both *Ferrum* and *Shin*, in the wake of a suicide threat, the school administrative personnel did not take adequate preventive measures to refer the students for evaluation, to otherwise supervise the students, or to notify family members.

In the most recent reported case involving potential liability for failure to prevent suicide, *Mahoney v. Allegheny College* [59], the PA state court rejected the reasoning of *Ferrum* and *Shin* and declined to find liability. Charles Mahoney had a history of depression for which he received counseling and medication. He had frequent suicidal ideation and resisted the school counselor's requests to contact his parents. On February 11, 2005 he expressed his suicidal thoughts to a counselor who assessed his safety and determined that he was not an immediate threat. She considered contacting his parents, but did not feel that doing so would be beneficial. Later that day, he killed himself.

Mahoney's family sued, claiming that Allegheny College breached a duty to prevent his suicide and breached a duty to notify his parents. In deciding that there was no special relationship and no duty had been breached, the Mahoney court found the *Jain* case factually and legally persuasive. The Mahoney court specifically rejected the decisions in *Shin* and *Ferrum* as "neither precedential, nor persuasive" and factually distinctive. The court reasoned that any finding of a special relationship "is subjective in nature . . . and is in effect an attenuated and unarticulated form of *in loco parentis*:"

> Clearly the increasing incidence of suicide on campuses throughout the United States is cause for grave concern. . . .However, incurring or creating a new duty of care in such cases is not the answer. Nevertheless, "failure" to create a duty is not an invitation to avoid action. We believe the "University" has a responsibility to adopt prevention programs and protocols regarding students self-inflicted injury and suicide that address risk management from a humanistic and therapeutic as compared to just a liability or risk avoiding perspective. In our view, the likelihood of a liability determination (even where a duty is established) is remote, when the issue of proximate causation (to be liable the university's act/omissions would have to be shown to be substantial) is considered. By way of illustration, even as to the issues of the lesser duty of notification of parents/others, there is always the possibility that such may make matters worse and increase the pressure on the student to commit the act. Rather than create an ill-defined duty of due care the University and mental health community have a more realistic duty to make strides towards prevention. In that regard, the University must not do less than it ought, unless it does all that it can ([59]. at 25).

The Mahoney court's opinion cautions against finding a special relationship and corresponding duty to prevent suicide, and instead encourages suicide prevention, referral and assessment. In addition, the court's reasoning suggests that schools that implement suicide prevention best practices are unlikely to be found liable for failure to prevent suicide.

As the court cautions, fear of liability should not overshadow logic, confidentiality principles, and sound clinical judgment. Yet, unfortunately, schools have acknowledged that fear of liability may color their reactions to students with mental illness such that administrators take actions that are not in the best interest of students and that conflict with the judgment of the student's treating mental-health professionals. For example, administrators may second-guess the judgment of mental-health experts and substitute their own judgment, by forcing "students who appear to be at risk to be hospitalized or to withdraw from the university, even though such steps may be contrary to, and disrupt or terminate altogether, any treatment the student may be have been receiving" [60]. In addition, schools say they may be less likely to admit students with potential mental health problems (a form of unlawful discrimination), and may be more inclined to dismiss students who threaten suicide, even if such separation would disrupt the student's treatment or make it more difficult for the student to receive treatment and thereby increase the risk of suicide. Id. Fear, stereotypes and prejudice about individuals with mental illness, and fear of liability have prompted some schools to take punitive actions against students who express self-injury or exhibit serious mental illness in violation of antidiscrimination laws – even when these students appropriately seek out help (see [4,61]). Such actions on the part of universities constitute discrimination and are illegal under the Americans with Disabilities Act [62].

Recommendations

- Schools that implement responsible suicide prevention best practices are unlikely to be found liable for failure to prevent suicide.

- The best interests of the student and sound clinical judgment, not fear of liability, should govern school policies and practices.

- School personnel should have adequate suicide prevention training and access to consultation with mental health experts.

7.3.3 Discrimination

The Americans with Disabilities Act ("ADA") and Section 504 of the Rehabilitation Act of 1973 both prohibit discrimination against individuals with disabilities by colleges and universities. Section 504 provides that "no otherwise qualified individual with a disability in the United States. . . shall, solely by reason of his handicap, be excluded from participation in, be denied the benefits of, or be subjected to discrimination under any program or activity receiving Federal financial assistance" [63].

Title II of the ADA extends the prohibition of discrimination to services of all state and local government entities, including state colleges and universities, whether or not they receive federal financial assistance. Title II can be found at 42 USC §§ 12131–34 (1990). It provides that "no qualified individual with a disability shall, by reason of such disability, be excluded from participation in or be denied the benefits of the services, programs or activities of a public entity or be subjected to discrimination by any such entity". Title III of the ADA similarly prohibits discrimination "on the basis of a disability in the full and equal enjoyment of the goods, services, facilities, privileges, advantages, or accommodations of any place of public accommodation," such as private schools and colleges. 42 USC. §12182(a). Title III can be found in the United States Code at 42 USC. §§ 12181–12189. In all relevant respects, the ADA and Section 504 impose identical requirements [64].

In the educational setting, the prohibition on discrimination extends to academics, research, occupational training, housing, health insurance, counseling, financial aid, physical education, athletics, recreation, transportation, other extracurricular or post secondary aid, benefits or services [65]. Other federal or state anti-discrimination laws may provide further protections. For example, the Fair Housing Act prohibits discrimination in the terms, conditions, or privileges of housing and the provision of services or facilities in connection with such housing because of disability.

These anti-discrimination laws broadly prohibit the denial of participation, the provision of unequal benefits, and the use of criteria or methods of administration that discriminate and actions that have the effect of excluding people with disabilities [66]. Section 504 requires reasonable accommodations when an "otherwise qualified" disabled student "would otherwise be denied meaningful access to a university" [67]. Similarly, the ADA specifically includes as discrimination the failure to make reasonable modifications in policies, practices, or procedures to accommodate a disabled individual, unless the school can demonstrate that making such modifications would fundamentally alter the nature of the services [68]. Reasonable accommodations are discussed in more detail below.

Section 504 also requires that all schools that receive federal funds designate a compliance officer and "adopt grievance procedures that incorporate appropriate due process standards and that provide for the prompt and equitable resolution of complaints" [69].

The United States Department of Justice is the agency charged with interpreting the portions of the ADA relevant to education, and has issued implementing regulations, which can be found in the United States Code of Federal Regulations at 28 CFR Parts 35 and 36 (for Titles II and III respectively). The Office for Civil Rights (OCR) of the US Department of Education ("DOE") enforces both Title II of the ADA and Section 504 with respect to the rights of college students. DOE also issued implementing regulations for Section 504 which can be found at 34 CFR. Part 104.

Who is a Person with a Disability?

The ADA was intended to have broad coverage [70]. Consistent with this intent, the ADA defines "disability" as: (1) a physical or mental impairment that substantially limits one or more of the major life activities of such individual; (2) a history or record of such an impairment; or (3) being regarded as having such an impairment. A person can meet the last requirement by showing that he or she was subjected to an action prohibited by the ADA based on an actual or perceived impairment, whether or not it limits or is perceived to limit a major life activity [71].

Major life activities include functions such as "caring for oneself, performing manual tasks, seeing, hearing, eating, sleeping, walking, standing, lifting, bending, speaking, breathing, learning, reading, concentrating, thinking, communicating and working" [71]. "Major life activities" also include the "operation of major bodily functions", such as functions of the "immune system, normal cell growth, digestive, bowel, bladder, neurological, brain, respiratory, circulatory, endocrine and reproductive functions" [71].

The ADA makes clear that, "the question of whether an individual's impairment is a disability under the ADA should not demand extensive analysis" [70], and a determination of whether an impairment is substantially limiting must be consistent with the findings and purposes of the ADA [72]. The test is not a demanding standard but rather one that ensures "appropriately broad coverage under this Act" [72], and specifically rejects a requirement that the impairment "prevents or severely restricts the individual from doing activities that are of central importance to most people's daily lives" [73]. Impairments that are episodic or in remission meet the definition of disability if they would be substantially limiting when active [74]. Finally, the ADA requires that the determination of whether an individual has a disability is to be made without taking into account the ameliorative effects on an individual's impairment of any reasonable accommodations or mitigating measures such as medication, medical equipment, supplies, or appliances [75]. Mental or psychological impairments such as emotional or mental illness are protected impairments [76].

In general, students who have a mental illness that substantially limits one or more major life activities such as sleeping, working, learning, speaking, caring for themselves, reading, or concentrating, or who have a history of such a problem, will be protected by the ADA even if their symptoms are controlled by medications or some other form of treatment.

When is a Student Qualified?

The ADA protects "qualified" individuals with disabilities from discrimination. A "qualified individual" under the ADA is "an individual with a disability who, with or without reasonable modifications to rules, policies or practices... meets the essential eligibility requirements for... participation in programs or activities provided by a public entity" [77]. The Department of Education implementing regulations define a "qualified" handicapped person, as one who "meets the academic and technical standards requisite to admission or participation in the recipient's education program or activity" [78].

In the education context, a student is qualified if he or she meets the essential eligibility requirements for admission to a school. Thus, as long as a student meets the academic and technical criteria for admission to the university, and for continued matriculation as a student, the student is qualified. The technical standards include essential provisions, such as paying tuition. There is some debate regarding whether a school can consider a student with a disability not qualified if he or she poses a "direct threat" to his or her own health or safety. Under Titles II and III, a "direct threat" is defined as "a significant risk to the health or safety of others..." [79]. See also *Hargrave v. Vermont* [80] and *Celano v. Marriott Intern., Inc.* [81].

To rise to the level of a direct threat, there must be a significant risk to health or safety that entails a high probability of substantial harm, not just a slightly increased, speculative, or remote risk. In determining whether a student presents a direct threat, a school must make an individualized and objective assessment of the student's ability to participate safely in the school's program, based on the best available evidence. The assessment must consider the duration of the risk, the nature and severity of the potential harm, the probability that the potential harm will actually occur, the imminence of potential harm, and whether reasonable modifications to policies, practices, or procedures will sufficiently mitigate the risk to an acceptable level [82–84]. A student may not be denied participation based upon fear, speculation and stereotype about his perceived disability [85].

7.4 Application

7.4.1 Dismissals/involuntary leaves of absence

Schools hope to create a caring supportive campus community that enables students to remain in school and succeed. However, whether out of misunderstanding about the correlation between mental illness and dangerousness, fear of people with mental illness, or in response to liability concerns, schools have at times adopted intrusive or harsh leave policies that limit participation or even exclude people with mental illness from campus. These policies tend to isolate students from their community and the supports they need during a time of difficulty or crisis. More broadly, these policies may have the unintended effect of discouraging students from seeking help out of fear that doing so may jeopardize their academic careers.

In two recent cases, students challenged the imposition of involuntary leaves of absence as discriminatory under the ADA and Section 504. In *Doe v. Hunter College* [62], a student with a history of depression voluntarily admitted herself to the hospital after ingesting several Tylenol. A few days later, she was discharged from the hospital and medically cleared to return to school with a follow-up treatment plan in place. Upon arrival at her dorm room, she learned that the locks had been changed pursuant to a school policy that provided that students who attempted to harm themselves would be evicted from the residence hall for at least one semester, and had to be evaluated by the school psychologist prior to returning. Doe was also mandated to receive counseling. Doe sued, challenging the zero tolerance policy – a blanket policy that required every student who was hospitalized or engaged in self-injurious thoughts or actions to take a leave of absence from the residence hall of a predetermined length. The District Court found that the school had not conducted an individualized assessment and Doe may have been able to demonstrate that she could have safely lived in the residence hall (http://www.bazelon.org/pdf/Doe-v-hunter-Order-denying-motion-to-dismiss.pdf p. 22). The case thereafter settled for a significant sum, and Hunter withdrew their automatic eviction policy.

In *Nott v. GWU* [61] student Jordan Nott sought treatment for depression through the university's counseling center. Thereafter, he voluntarily admitted himself to the university hospital for suicidal ideation. Shortly after his admission, he received a letter from the residence hall director stating that he could not return to his dorm room until he had been cleared by the counseling center. The following day, he received a letter from Student Judicial Services charging him with violation of the school code of conduct that prohibited "endangering behavior". He was suspended pending a disciplinary hearing, barred from his dorm room and campus, and threatened with arrest for trespassing if he entered campus. Rather than face disciplinary charges, Nott withdrew and sued alleging violation of the ADA, Section 504, the Fair Housing Act, and other state law claims. Specifically, Nott challenged his placement on involuntary leave and the use of disciplinary procedures to address mental health issues. GWU was widely criticized for its conduct. The case was settled and GWU thereafter adopted new involuntary mental health leave policies.

The US Department of Education OCR has issued letters of decision finding ADA violations in several similar cases: see OCR letter to Marietta College (Complaint # 15-04-2060, 3/18/05); OCR letter to DeSales Univ. (OCR Complaint # 03-04-2041, 2/17/05), OCR letter to Bluffton Univ. (OCR Complaint # 15-04-2042, 12/2/04), and OCR letter to Woodbury Univ. (OCR Complaint # 09-00-2079, 6/29/01), available on the Bazelon Center's web site at http://www.bazelon.org/issues/education/StudentsandMentalHealth.htm#2.

The decisions counsel that an involuntary leave of absence should only be used in those rare situations where it is determined that a student cannot remain safely at school even with accommodations and other supports. A student may be placed on leave (or removed from a dormitory) only if he or she poses a "direct threat" to the health or safety of others (see above discussion on the ADA). In a complaint against DeSales University, involving a student who was evicted from university housing after posting information about suicide on his dorm door and engaged in self-cutting, OCR stated that:

> In a direct threat situation, a college needs to make an individualized determination of the student's ability to safely participate in the college's program, based on reasonable medical judgment relying on the most current medical knowledge or the best available objective evidence (OCR letter to DeSales Univ).

In determining whether a student constitutes a direct threat, the assessment must consider the duration of the risk, the nature and severity of the potential harm, the probability that the potential harm will actually occur, the imminence of potential harm, and whether reasonable modifications to policies, practices, or procedures will sufficiently mitigate the risk to an acceptable level (OCR letter Marietta College; OCR letter to National University (OCR Complaint # 09-99-2014, *3/23/00*)). Schools must consider less restrictive alternatives to leave (such as leave from housing) that would allow a student to safely remain in school before placing a student on involuntary leave of absence.

Numerous OCR decisions hold that a school should provide due process protections before students are placed on leave. Those protections include notifying the student that the school is considering placing the student on involuntary leave and providing the student an opportunity to submit and respond to any evidence. The student should also have an opportunity to appeal an adverse decision (OCR letter to Marietta College, OCR letter to Guilford College (Complaint # M-02-2003, 3/6/03); OCR letter to DeSales Univ).

Provision of such process will help ensure that students with disabilities are not placed on leave on the basis of unfounded fear, prejudice, or stereotypes. In rare cases, where safety is of immediate concern, a college may immediately impose a leave as long as minimal due process (such as notice and an initial opportunity to address the evidence) is provided, and a final decision with full due process (including a hearing and the right to appeal) is promptly offered (OCR letter to DeSales Univ).

If a student does present a direct threat and treatment is necessary to reduce the threat to an acceptable level, a school may require the student to participate in counseling as a condition of remaining in school or returning from leave. However, the student and mental health treatment provider – not administration – should determine the duration of treatment and scope of issues addressed. Requiring treatment to stay in school or as a condition of return to school for students whose conduct does not rise to level of direct threat violates disability law.

OCR decisions state that the same type of individualized assessment required to place a student on leave is required to determine the student's ability to return. If a student was placed on leave because he or she constituted a direct threat, the school can require that the student demonstrate that he or she is no longer a direct threat. Schools can require documentation that a student is taking steps to reduce the threat to an acceptable level (OCR letter to DeSales Univ). A school may not insist on open ended or unlimited access to medical records or treatment providers (OCR letter to Woodbury University (Complaint # 09-00-2079, 6/29/01)).

OCR has also stated that a school cannot require as a condition of return that the illness be cured or that disability-related behavior no longer occur, unless it is a direct threat and cannot be mitigated. Nor can a school require an assurance that a student's direct threat behavior will not recur. The school must make a fair, stereotype-free assessment based on reasonably reliable information from objective sources such as knowledgeable medical professionals (OCR letter to Skagit Valley College (Complaint # 10-92-2080 4/21/93); OCR letter to DeSales Univ).

Leaves of absence, even voluntary leaves, separate the student from structure, friends and social and professional support systems. Unless a student on leave presents a significant risk to the health or safety of others, there is no reason to prohibit the student from maintaining contact with friends and associates on campus or from attending campus events. Restrictions to a student's interactions may be limited only as needed to ensure safety. These individually tailored policies ensure that if students are limited, it will only be due to dangerousness, not discrimination.

For more information on helpful interventions for students in crisis see Chapter 9 and [86,87]

7.4.2 Reasonable accommodations

Reasonable accommodations are modifications to policies, procedures, and rules that are designed to provide students who have disabilities with an equal opportunity to meet academic and technical standards so that they remain and succeed in school. Schools must modify academic and other requirements as necessary to ensure that they do not discriminate or have the effect of discriminating, on the basis of handicap. However, a school need not make changes that would fundamentally alter their operations, alter the essential nature of their program, waive essential academic and technical requirements or standards, or cause them undue financial burden [90].

When a student informs a school that he/she has a disability and requests a reasonable accommodation, the school must engage in an interactive process with the student to determine what accommodations are needed. An accommodation cannot be denied on the grounds that a student did not meet an artificial deadline or did not report to a specific individual. In requesting accommodations, there are no special words that a student must use, or particular form that the request must take (OCR letter to Guilford College). A school may request information regarding the nature of the disability and how it affects the student's ability to participate in and benefit from the academic program and shape the accommodation.

In addition to accommodations such as extended time to take examinations, students may request: reduced course loads; to drop courses; to change roommates or rooms; a private environment or alternate location in which to take exams; that absences be excused; postponement of assignments and exams; classes online or work from home; provision of an aide or helper in the student's room; retroactive withdrawal for students whose disability prevented an earlier request for leave; and pro-rated financial reimbursement. For a list of additional accommodations, see Campus Mental Health: Know Your Rights! available at http://www.bazelon.org/l21/YourMind-YourRights.pdf.

Schools should offer liberal voluntary leave policies for students with disabilities and remove existing barriers to taking a voluntary leave of absence. For example, taking a leave of absence can cause financial hardship; students may have to repay student loans and may not have funds to complete their education. If the need for a leave of absence arises after the drop/add period, taking a leave of absence may adversely effect their grade point average and academic transcript. Many students receive health care through the school and will lose needed health insurance and mental health treatment if they take a leave of absence. Schools might provide tuition reimbursement and tuition insurance. Schools may allow students to withdraw from courses or receive an incomplete rather than a failing grade if they need a leave of absence. Schools can also offer a retroactive withdrawal to students who can demonstrate that academic difficulties were the result of mental disability and that they were unable to request a leave during the term as a consequence of their disability. Schools can work with insurers and community mental health treatment providers to ensure that students who take a leave of absence have access to mental health services, and can provide funds for uncovered treatment or prescriptions.

Students are also concerned with social stigma associated with taking a leave. To combat stigma, schools can raise awareness about mental health issues, support peer-run groups that support students with depression or other mental illnesses, and ensure that their policies promote help-seeking behavior. It is important that schools remove barriers that discourage students from taking needed voluntary leaves of absence. For more information about reducing stigma see [89,90].

7.4.3 Mandatory assessments and treatment

In those rare circumstances where a school reasonably believes that a student may constitute a direct threat, the school may require the student to undergo an assessment by a mental health professional. An assessment from the student's mental health treatment provider should be sufficient (OCR letter to Skagit). It is important that the assessment be objective, and conducted by an individual without a conflict of interest. If assessments are conducted by the counseling center, it presents a potential conflict of interest. It must be clear whether the mental health provider conducting the assessment is serving the student or administration as the client. In addition, if the counseling center is involved in determining whether students will be placed on involuntary leave, students may be discouraged from using campus mental health services. Conversely, it could erode confidence in the campus counseling center if students get the impression that the "tough cases" get sent off campus. Whoever conducts the assessment, it is essential that the assessor keeps the student's best interest as a primary concern.

If a student undergoes a mandatory assessment, the contours of the assessment and information that will be shared with the school should be clear from the outset, and no more than necessary should be shared. If the counseling center conducts the assessment, it should be clear what information will be shared with the student's treatment provider. Students who refuse to undergo a mental health assessment can only be placed on involuntary leave if they meet the direct threat standard discussed above and are provided due process protections.

Some schools have adopted policies that mandate treatment as a condition of continued enrollment, including for students who express suicidal ideation or engage in self-injury. In addition to being an ADA violation if the student is not a "direct threat', this practice raises a myriad of ethical and legal concerns. Legally, a state can mandate inpatient or outpatient treatment only if an individual presents an imminent threat of significant physical harm to themselves or others. Individuals who do not pose an imminent threat can chose whether or not they wish to pursue treatment. State mandated treatment also requires due process protections. Schools that mandate treatment rely on a much lower standard. They do not require that students be an imminent danger to themselves or others or even that students be actively suicidal. Nor do they often afford any due process protections. Such coercive policies will discourage students from seeking help due to the fear that they may lose their autonomy or that they will be suspended or expelled if they continue to experience self-injurious thoughts or behaviors. Moreover, treatment that is involuntary is less likely to be successful as students may not be truthful with their treatment providers, and may not establish an effective therapeutic relationship.

7.4.4 Discipline/safety

Some schools have recently adopted zero-tolerance policies as part of their disciplinary process. These schools interpret prohibitions against endangering behavior to include students who express self-injurious *thoughts* or behaviors. Inevitably, these policies punish students for help-seeking behavior and encourage students to be secretive about their problems. While schools may believe that they are acting in the best interests of the students or the university community, disciplinary action for such thoughts or actions discourages students from seeking help and therefore actually increases the risk of harm [91]. Students overwhelmingly report a feeling of betrayal when schools take disciplinary action against students who have admitted that they have self-injurious thoughts [3,92–95]. Removing the student from a dorm or the school also isolates students from their community and social and professional supports at a time of crisis and increases the amount of stress and distress experienced by students when they are vulnerable.

Under the ADA, disciplinary rules must be non-discriminatory, must be applied in a non-discriminatory manner, and may not be imposed based on unfounded fear, prejudice, or stereotypes. Nonetheless, many schools address mental health issues (suicidal ideation, self- injury, bulimia) by disciplining the student under the theory that the school is not responding based on a diagnosis of mental illness, but based on conduct, regardless of its cause. Such actions violate the ADA. This conduct represents symptoms of depression and overwhelmingly occurs because of mental disability. Disability discrimination includes discrimination based on an impairment itself but also discrimination based on the effects of an impairment, on the person himself or others [96,97].

In recognition of this problem and in the wake of the *Nott v. GWU* case [61], Virginia passed a law requiring all public colleges to implement procedures for identifying and addressing the needs of students exhibiting suicidal tendencies or behavior. The law required that the policies ensure that "no student is penalized or expelled for attempting to commit suicide, or seeking mental health treatment for suicidal thoughts or behaviors" [96].

In general, when disciplinary action is imposed on students, a student's disability should be considered as a mitigating factor in determining whether to impose a penalty as part of providing a reasonable accommodation. This means that a student's psychiatric condition should be weighed as a factor in determining what penalty, if any, should be imposed (and schools can waive disciplinary action altogether). This is especially true when, as a result of treatment or other interventions, the student is likely to comply with the code of conduct in the future (see OCR letter to San Diego Community College (Complaint # 09-98-2154, 12/30/99)). Where a student raises his/her disability in a disciplinary proceeding, and the student's disability is related to the disciplinary infraction, schools can conduct the proceedings in an alternate forum that includes personnel familiar with disability issues and does not include other students on the conduct board to address privacy considerations (see Woodbury, above). The disciplinary process should be flexible enough to integrate new information and mitigating considerations regarding a student's psychological condition.

Disciplinary proceedings should be halted if a student takes a voluntary leave for mental health reasons when the disciplinary breach was a direct result of the student's condition.

Some schools have used behavioral contracts to address mental health issues. Generally, a behavioral contract is a document that lists various conditions with which a student must comply. Often it specifies consequences for violation. Behavioral contracts can take the form of post-hospitalization plans. To the extent that these behavioral contracts impose conditions on students with mental illness not imposed on non-disabled students, they are discriminatory (OCR Complaint 05-04-2094 (University of Southern Indiana, 9/43/04)). Additionally, they pose the same legal and ethical problems presented by mandatory assessment and treatment discussed above.

7.4.5 Student support committees/threat assessment

Many schools have developed behavioral intervention or threat assessment committees. The Department of Education has encouraged schools to have such committees:

> The Department encourages schools to implement a threat assessment program, including the establishment of a threat assessment team that utilizes the expertise of representatives from law enforcement agencies in the community [98].

While school-wide multidisciplinary committees may be helpful in addressing the needs of students with mental illness, threat assessment committees should focus on addressing actual threats of violence, not mental health issues. Using "threat assessment" committees to address mental health issues equates mental illness with violence and stigmatizes those who may come to the attention of the committee for support. It also sends the message that the school is concerned with "how can we protect ourselves from you" instead of "how can we provide support to you".

In contrast, student support committees (and behavioral intervention committees) can be valuable when used to support students who might be exhibiting academic or social difficulty. Such committees may include representatives from student life, residential housing, student judicial services, and disability services. Committees can include treatment providers from the counseling center, however it is important that counselors act as consultants and provide general advice for responding to students in distress. Counselors can receive collateral information about clients but cannot breach student confidences, including acknowledging that a particular student is receiving counseling. Committees can intervene with the student in distress and offer supportive services, refer students to counseling or academic advising, or recommend accommodations before the student fails or requires a leave of absence. Student support committees might meet weekly to share information, and discuss the status of students who might be in distress. A committee that monitors students to impose disciplinary action rather than provide supportive services to help students succeed can create a campus climate where students are discouraged from seeking counseling.

For more information on student support teams see Student Mental Health and the Law, The Jed Foundation, available at http://www.jedfoundation.org/programs/legal-resource.

7.4.6 Parental communication/notification

College students are young adults, and as discussed above, information about them is governed by confidentiality rules. While school administrators can communicate their personal observations to parents, they are not required to do so. Pursuant to FERPA, a school cannot release information from the student's educational record to parents without the student's consent unless the parents claim the student as a dependant for tax purposes, there is a health or safety emergency or, in certain circumstances, where the student violates a law regarding alcohol or substance abuse (see FERPA discussion above). Mental health information enjoys even greater protection.

It is always preferable to obtain consent to a disclosure of information. School administrators and counselors may want to encourage parents and students to communicate with each other. Since release of a student's information to parents may exacerbate situations, school administrators should judge each situation on a case by case basis and may want to consult with school counselors about specific situations. Students may not know that if insurance is used to pay for counseling services, that they have sought counseling will appear on insurance statements or bills related to their care.

7.4.7 Screening

School administrators recently have considered screening students for mental illness. Some have discussed asking potential applicants if they have a mental health history or have suggested monitoring social networking sites like Facebook for indications of self-injurious impulses or behavior. See for example [99,100]. Others are concerned that increased screening and suicide prevention efforts will subject schools to liability if a student later commits suicide.

As an initial matter, screening postsecondary school applicants for mental illness is impermissible. A post secondary institution "may not make preadmission inquiry as to whether an applicant for admission is a handicapped person but, after admission, may make inquiries on a confidential basis as to handicaps that may require accommodation" [100]. Institutions may only invite applicants for admission to indicate whether and to what extent they are handicapped if they clearly state that "the information requested is intended for use solely in connection with [affirmative action efforts to benefit people with disabilities]; and the information is requested on a voluntary basis, that it will be kept confidential, that refusal to provide the information will not subject the applicant to any adverse treatment" [100].

In addition, large scale mandatory screening programs have several specific drawbacks. First, affixing diagnoses without offering treatment is unhelpful and can harm individuals by labeling them. Second, screening programs are time and cost intensive. School's limited resources are better used to provide outreach and actual supports and services to students. Finally, mandatory screening is intrusive and a violation of privacy.

Evaluation and assessment of mental health needs within the context of overall healthcare, in accordance with healthcare privacy protections and informed consent, can serve to inform the student of risk factors and of the array of treatment and support options available to them. Rather than screening large populations for whom immediate service might not even be available, schools would be better served by making outreach and suicide prevention a priority. Students with mental health problems need ready access to counseling and other support systems without long delays and without fear of repercussions. Schools can take actions to encourage students to seek counseling and mental health treatment through campus services or other available avenues.

An interesting approach has been developed by the American Foundation for Suicide Prevention (AFSP). In collaboration with Emory University, in Atlanta, and the University of North Carolina (UNC) Chapel Hill, AFSP has created a web-based interactive screening program that aims to identify high-risk students and encourage them to get treatment. It is voluntary and confidential and provides referral to students who participate. All students are invited to participate. Interested students can anonymously visit a secure web site, and complete the online questionnaire based on the diagnostic criteria from the *Diagnostic and Statistical Manual of Mental Disorders-IV.* A clinician reviews the responses and invites students with more serious problems to come for an in-person evaluation. Students can also have anonymous follow-up conversations with the clinician via a "dialog" feature. Eighty five percent of students who completed the screening questionnaire were experiencing significant psychological problems and were not receiving any form of treatment. The online, anonymous dialogues played a key role in encouraging help-seeking. Students used the dialog to address concerns about confidentiality, costs, parental notification, and possible sanctions for disclosing self-injury. AFSP has reported that students who used the dialog feature "were three times more likely than others to come for an evaluation and to enter treatment" [101,102].

Colleges can also integrate information about mental health issues and services into student orientation and other aspects of campus life. Equally important, schools can provide training so that faculty, staff and students know what supports and services are available, how to make referrals, and how to access those supports and services. Schools can encourage the formation of peer-run groups on campus to support students with depression and other mental illnesses, and can ensure that emergency psychiatric services are available at all times, either on campus or in the community. Schools should embrace the "no wrong door" concept and provide access and referral to students wherever they are. Mental health programs need to reach out to people who demonstrate a need for services to engage them and keep them engaged.

Recommendations

- Case law suggests that schools that implement suicide prevention practices are unlikely to be found liable for failure to prevent suicide. Schools should offer liberal voluntary leave policies for students who feel that they would benefit from time off and remove barriers to taking a voluntary leave of absence.

- While schools may believe that they are acting in the best interests of the students or the university community, use of disciplinary action for self-injurious thoughts or acts discourages students from seeking help and actually increases the risk of harm.

- Rather than screening large populations for whom immediate service might not be available, schools would be better served by making outreach, training and suicide prevention a priority.

- Schools need to encourage student support groups and activity as students are frequently aware of problems well before the administration.

- Universities have an ethical responsibility to make certain that students have adequate access to mental health services through the provision of direct on-campus services, referral to off-campus facilities or clinicians, and/or assuring adequate insurance coverage for the student body. Students and their families should be recruited as partners in this enterprise.

7.5 Conclusion

In this chapter, we have attempted to explicate the law relevant to college mental health in some detail while at the same time being clear and straightforward enough to make these, at times, complex issues accessible to the broadest range of readers. We have also tried to highlight the ethical principles underlying these laws.

In the midst of a clinical crisis or legal debate about these complex issues it is often difficult to remember that colleges and universities are unique communities that are established to facilitate the education, maturation and growth of the young women and men who attend them (and as noted above, students, parents, university administrators and faculty are all working toward the ultimate success of the student). For learning and growth to occur, colleges must strive to establish a balance between safety, predictability, structure and conformity versus personal freedom and experimentation with ideas and values. (This is actually no different from the challenge that every parent confronts in raising a child.) Too much oversight or control can squelch creativity, enthusiasm, and free thought; too little supervision and security can result in chaos and unmanageable anxiety. We have tried to suggest that the trends in legislation and case law applicable to college mental health are mostly attempts to express, put into practice, and ultimately balance these subtle and lofty principles.

With these considerations in mind, we hope that our readers would recognize these laws not as anxiety provoking problems to be dealt with or worked around. Rather, they should be seen as outer boundaries and general signposts for decision-making. In almost all situations, there is ample space within these boundaries for thoughtful common sense and good clinical judgment.

References

1. Warren S., Brandeis L. (1890) The right to privacy. *Harvard Law Review*, Vol. **4**, No. 5, Dec.
2. See, for example Slovenko, R. and Usdin G. (1966) *Psychotherapy, Confidentiality and Privileged Communication*, CC Thomas, Springfield.
3. Arenson, K. (2004) Worried colleges step up efforts over suicide, *New York Times*, 2 December 2004.
4. Appelbaum, P. (2006) Law and psychiatry: "Depressed? Get out": dealing with suicidal students on college campuses. *Psychiatric Services*, **57**: 914–916.
5. Responsibility to Contact Parent of Student at Imminent Risk of Suicide, VA Code Ann. § 23–9.2:3(C).
6. Colorado Higher Education Student Suicide Prevention Act, Colorado Revised Statutes, § 23-20-101, June 2, 2006.
7. *Tarasoff v. Regents of the University of California*, 17 Cal.3d 425 (1976).
8. Herbert, P.B., and Young, K.A. (2002) Tarasoff at twenty-five. *Journal of the American Academy of Psychiatry and Law*, **30**: 275–281. See also, Restatement Third of Torts, section 41 and internal citations for discussion of the duty owed to third parties).
9. Ann. Cal. Civ. Code § 56.10(a) and (c)(1) (West 2007).
10. NY Mental Hygiene Law § 33.13(c) (McKinney 2008).
11. Texas Health and Safety Code § 611.004 (2) and (7).
12. VA Code Ann. § 23-9.2:3(C) (2009).
13. Family Education Rights and Privacy Act 20 USC § 1232g.
14. United States Code of Federal Regulations at 34 CFR Part 99. 20 USC 1232g(a)(1). see also http://www.gpo.gov/nara/cfr/waisidx_00/34cfr99_00.html

15. 20 USC § 1232g(a)(4)(A); 34 CFR § 99.3.
16. 34 CFR § 99.10.
17. 20 USC § 1232g(a)(4)(B).
18. 20 USC 1232g(a)(4)(B)(iv).
19. 20 USC § 1232g(a)(4).
20. Statement of Leroy Rooker regarding disclosure of information from education records to parents of students attending postsecondary institutions, http://www.ed.gov/policy/gen/guid/fpco/hottopics/ht-parents-postsecstudents.html. See also [21].
21. Letter to Montgomery County Public Schools (MD) re: Law Enforcement Unit Records (February 15, 2006) (on file with the Family Educational Rights and Privacy Act Online Library) http://www.ed.gov/policy/gen/guid/fpco/ferpa/library/montcounty0215.html.
22. 34 CFR § 99.3 (2006).
23. 20 USC § 1232g(b)(1). See also [24].
24. 20 USC § 1232g(a)(5)(A).
25. 34 CFR § 99.37 (2006).
26. 20 USC § 1232g(b)(1)(A).
27. Letter from Leroy S. Rooker, Director, Family Policy Compliance Office, to David Cope, Assistant Professor, Mathematics Department, University of North Alabama (Nov. 2, 2004) (on file with the Family Educational Rights and Privacy Act Online Library) http://www.ed.gov/policy/gen/guid/fpco/ferpa/library/copeuna.html.
28. USC § 1232g(b)(1)(I); 34 CFR 99.31(a)(10) and 99.36.
29. 34 CFR § 99.36(a) (December 9, 2008).
30. 34 CFR § 99.36(c).
31. Letter from Leroy S. Rooker, Director, Family Policy Compliance Office, to Melanie Baise, Associate University Counsel, The University of New Mexico (Nov. 29, 2004) (on file with the Family Educational Rights and Privacy Act Online Library) http://www.ed.gov/policy/gen/guid/fpco/ferpa/library/baiseunmslc.html.
32. FPCO Guidance on "Recent Amendments to FERPA Relating to Anti-Terrorism Activities (April 12, 2002).
33. Dear Collegue Letter, http://www.ed.gov/policy/gen/guid/fpco/hottopics/ht12-17-08.html.
34. 20 USC § 1232g(b)(1)(H).
35. USC § 1232g(b)(1)(J).
36. USC § 1232g(b)(1)(B-G).
37. USC § 1232g(i). 99.31(a)(15).
38. USC § 1232g(b)(6).
39. USC § 1232g(b)(4)(B).
40. USC § 1232g(b)(4)(A), 34 CFR § 99.32.
41. 34 CFR § 99.34(a).
42. 34 CFR § 99.32(a)(5).
43. 45 CFR § 164.501.
44. 45 CFR § 160.103.
45. 45 CFR §§ 160.103, 164.501.
46. HIPAA Privacy Rule preamble; 65 Fed. Reg. at 82483.
47. 45 CFR 164.512.
48. 45 CFR § 164.512(j).
49. The Principles of Medical Ethics § 10.01, American Medical Association 2001.
50. Code of Medical Ethics: Current Opinions § E-5.05, American Medical Association 2007.
51. The Principles of Medical Ethics: with annotations especially applicable to psychiatry § 4.2, American Psychiatric Association 2008.
52. Ethical Principles and Code Of Conduct § 4.05, American Psychological Association 2003.

53. National Association of Social Workers § 1.07(e); Ethical Principles and Code Of Conduct [54]§ 4.02, American Psychological Association 2006).

54. *Jain v. State*, 617 N.W.2d 293 (Iowa 2000).

55. Restatement (Second) of Torts § 314, at 116 (1965); where one person depends on others for protection and is deprived of opportunity for self protection (§ 315, 319, 320).

56. Lake, P. and Tribbensee, N. (2002) The emerging crisis of college student suicide: law and policy responses to serious forms of self-inflicted injury. *Stetson Law Review*, **32**(1).

57. *Schieszler v. Ferrum College* 236 F. Supp 2d. 602 (W.D. Va 2002).

58. *Shin v. MIT*, 19 Mass L. Rptr. 570, 2005 WL 1869101 (Mass. Super. June 27, 2005).

59. *Mahoney v. Allegheny College*, No. AD 892-2003 (Pa. Commw. Ct. Dec. 22, 2005).

60. Brief of Amici Curiae Brown University, Cornell University, Dartmouth College, Emory University, Rice University, Stanford University, the University of Chicago, and the University of Southern California in Support of Petition for Relief Under G.L. c. 231, § 118 (first paragraph) by MIT Administrators Arnold Henderson and Nina Davis-Millis.

61. *Nott v The George Washington University et al.)*, Civil Case No 05-8503, Superior Court of the District of Columbia (2005); http://gwired.gwu.edu/dos/merlin-cgi/p/downloadFile/d/18181/n/off/other/1/name/AdministrativeMedicalMentalHealthLeaveofAbse/.

62. *Doe v. Hunter*, 04-CV-6740; (SDNY Sept. 23, 2005).

63. Section 504 of the Rehabilitation Act of 1973 as amended, 29 USC § 794 *et seq*. ("Section 504").

64. *Henrietta D. v. Bloomberg*, 331 F.3d 261, 272 (2d Cir. 2003) ("[U]nless one of the subtle distinctions [between the two acts] is pertinent to a particular case, we treat claims under the two statutes identically".)

65. 34 CFR 104.43.

66. 34 CFR §104.4.

67. 29 USC § 794(a); 34 CFR § 104.12.

68. 42 USC § 12182(b)(2)(A)(ii).

69. 34 CFR §104.7.

70. 42 USC § 12102(4)(A).

71. 42 USC § 12102(2).

72. 42 USC § 12102)(4)(B).

73. 12101(b)(4).

74. 42 § 12102)(4)(D).

75. 42 USC § 12102(4)(E).

76. 29 CFR §1630.2(h) (2001).

77. 42 USC § 12131(2).

78. 34 CFR part 104.3(l).

79. 28 CFR Pt. 35, App. A, § 35.104, 42 USC § 12182(b)(3).

80. *Hargrave v. Vermont* [84] and 340 F.3d 27, 35–36 (2nd Cir 2003).

81. *Celano v. Marriott Intern., Inc.* [85] Slip Copy, 2008 WL 239306 (N.D.Cal., 2008).

82. *School Bd. of Nassau County v. Arline*, 480 US 282 & n.7 (1987).

83. *Hargrave*, 340 F.3d at 36, *quoting Albertson's, Inc. v. Kirkingburg*, 527 US 555, 569 (1999).

84. 29 CFR 1630.2(r).

85. 42 USCA. § 12102(2)(c).

86. *Supporting Students*, A Model Policy for Colleges and Universities, The Judge David L. Bazelon Center for Mental Health Law, available at http://www.bazelon.org/pdf/SupportingStudents.pdf.

87. *Student Mental Health and the Law,* The Jed Foundation, available at http://www.jedfoundation.org/programs/legal-resource; Law and Policy Reports.

88. ADA Title III Technical Assistance Manual § III-4.3600.

89. Active Minds, http://www.activeminds.org/index.php; Community Integration Tools, The College Experience: Tips for Reducing Stress and Getting the Accommodations You Need,

UPenn Collaborative on Community Integration, http://www.upennrrtc.org/var/tool/file/26-CollegeFS.pdf.

90. Bower, K. (2007) How not to respond to Virginia Tech. *Inside Higher Education*, 1 May.
91. Capriccioso, R. (2006) Counseling crisis. *Inside Higher Education*, 13 March. http://www.insidehighered.com/layout/set/dialog/news/2006/03/13/counseling.
92. Kinzie, S. (2006) GWU suit prompts questions of liability. *Washington Post*, 10 March.
93. Di Benedetto, S. (2007) Reliving the past flashback sends student home. *The Daily Eastern News*, 6 October.
94. *Borkowski v. Valley Cent. Sch. Dist.*, 63 F.3d 131, 143 (2d Cir. 1995).
95. *Gambini v. Total Renal Care. Inc.*, 486 F.3d 1087 (9th Cir. 2007).
96. Code of Virginia, Policies addressing suicidal students, § 23-9.2:8 (2007).
97. Federal Register Vol. 73, No. 237/December 9, 2008/Rules and Regulations at 74839. http://www.ed.gov/admins/lead/safety/edpicks.jhtml?src=ln.
98. 34 CFR 104.42 (b)(4) and (c).
99. Reens, N. (2009) Calvin College expels student accused of writing derogatory Facebook message, *The Grand Rapids Times*, 12 February.
100. Hechinger, J. (2008) College applicants, beware: your Facebook page is showing, *Wall Street Journal*, 18 September.
101. American Foundation for Suicide Prevention http://www.afsp.org/index.cfm?page_id=05967029-BC0C-603D-5A32D68043B9D7A8.
102. Garlow, S.J., Rosenberg, J., Moore, J.D.,*et al.* (2008) Depression, desperation, and suicidal ideation in college students: results from the American Foundation for Suicide Prevention College Screening Project at Emory University. *Depression Anxiety*, **25**(6): 482–488.

8 Working with the Campus Community

Lorraine D. Siggins

Mental Health and Counseling Center, Yale University Health Services, New Haven, CT, USA

8.1 Introduction

One of the fascinations of working in the college mental health (CMH) field lies in the variety and breadth of the issues that arise. In addressing the personal concerns of the individual student, the mental health clinician has to understand many other aspects of student life. These involve for example, friends, roommates, family, teammates, coaches, singing groups, faculty members, advisors, career officers, international student deans, academic deans, student affair deans, cultural center deans, tutors, and chaplains. There is a seemingly endless array of people in the college with whom the student may interact who may play an important role in the student's life. One cannot relate to individual students without being aware of the many and varied communities to which they belong. This chapter will focus on the larger university community and the relationship of the college mental health service to this community and to its constituent parts.

8.2 Some Developmental Considerations

The university community is more than an environment in which the student's life is occurring; it is a community with which the student interacts daily, intimately and personally. This community plays a central role in the crucially important phase of personal development that occurs during the college years.

Recent neuroscience research [1–3] has shown that this personal development is neuronal as well as psychological. During these years there are important cerebral structural changes which result in significant improvement in such functions as judgment and impulse control. Thus, for example, 25-year-old students are able to hold more complicated and contradictory views of a situation than 18-year-olds. It is also possible for them to more accurately judge the consequences of actions and to postpone these actions when appropriate to do so.

It seems likely that these cerebral changes are the biological basis for a portion of the psychological developmental change occurring during these years, including the consolidation of the student's personal identity. As this identity formation encompasses more than personal identity (including, as it does, academic or career identity and sexual identity), the various cultural and community ties which the student forms are extremely important.

Mental Health Care in the College Community   Edited by Jerald Kay and Victor Schwartz
© 2010 John Wiley & Sons, Ltd.

Erikson [4] pointed out that in identity development it is important that the student's community perceive him or her as the student does. It is also essential that, while there is an integration and consolidation of this identity, the student retain considerable psychological flexibility (through the multiplicity of identifications, object relations and learned adaptive skills) so as to have access to the many different internalized parts of him or herself as a creative individual. Thus, college is a time of integrating the neurological, psychological, academic, social and community aspects of the student's life.

8.3 The Evolution of the College Mental Health Service Mission

The mission of the college mental health service, in working with the student on this developmental task, coincides with the university's larger academic and educational mission. The success of the university's educational mission depends on students having as few emotional barriers as possible impeding their capacity to take advantage of the educational opportunities the university offers.

This has been part of the role of the college mental health service from its very beginning. As Paul Barreira points out in Chapter 2, the college mental health movement grew out of the mental hygiene movement early in the twentieth century. The mental hygiene movement was begun by Clifford Beers, a Yale college graduate, who himself suffered from manic–depressive illness, and who turned his attention to exploring the possibilities of working with high school and college students with the aim of preventing the development of mental illness [5]. Thus, from the very beginning, the college mental health services, or "mental hygiene departments" as they were then called, were rooted in a preventative and community framework. When President Angell of Yale, for example, in 1925 appointed the first psychiatrist to the college health service, he stated ([6], p. 3), "with this appointment, Yale begins the development of a highly important contribution of medical education to the welfare of the student body and the hygiene interests of New Haven". Professor George Pierson [7] in his history of Yale College stated (p. 516) "A psychological approach on the broadest front had to be increasingly emphasized by the President, and practiced by the University. Among the new currents flowing through Yale life, none was more significant, he (President [8]) said in 1930, than "the rediscovery of personality as a basic and indispensable element in education"". In this charge, it was implicit that the Mental Hygiene Department would be an integral part of the university community. In fact, Dr. Clements Fry, the chief psychiatrist actually resided on campus in an apartment in one of the student residential colleges. He and his staff were called upon not just to work with individual students in a clinical capacity, but also to be a resource for faculty and administration in dealing with both university policy and community development where it had important psychological ramifications for the student body.

Thus, as at Yale, other college mental health services were already operating in the role of a "community mental health center" in the 1920s, 1930s, 1940s and 1950s, well before the national development of the community mental health movement in the 1960s. Yet, as Dr. Barreira indicates in Chapter 2, the model of the community mental health center (CMHC) best fits the college mental health service, even though the university community, and work within the university community, is significantly different from the public sector community mental health movement and poses different challenges.

With the passage of the Community Mental Health Centers Construction Act in 1963, a new system of care was developed. This care focused on community based service and public health concepts. The CMHCC Act ([9], p. 1537) "required centers to provide five basic services:

- Inpatient treatment

- Emergency services

- Partial hospitalization

- Outpatient services

- Consultation and education".

Thus, the community joined the partnership with the clinician and the patient. "Community based service" was the basis of the core system and thus the CMHC became part of the public health enterprise.

In this context, Jacobs et al. ([10], p. 107) describe how the CMHC model placed great emphasis on prevention. "Prevention science represents a further elaboration and alternative to the public health model of primary, secondary, and tertiary prevention. Prevention science identifies three types of primary prevention activities: universal, selective and indicated [11,12]. *Universal* interventions target the general public or entire population groups regardless of risk status. *Selective* interventions target individuals or population subgroups, whose risk of developing a disorder are higher than average due to individual or environmental factors. *Indicated* interventions target high risk individuals with detectable signs of disorder, but who do not meet criteria for a psychiatric diagnosis [12]. Risk reduction and the enhancement of protective factors are the primary emphases of interventions in prevention science [12,13]". All the above preventative elements are clearly identifiable in college mental health services which also focus their preventative activities on risk reduction.

The President's New Freedom Commission (2006) and in Transforming Mental Health Care in America (2006) reported that ([10] p. 156) "in order for the progress in mental health care to continue the following fundamental issues had to be addressed.

- Ensuring the delivery of high quality, culturally competent behavioral healthcare that is directed toward the identification and elimination of health disparity;

- Ensuring the adequacy and stability of funding for services and supports;

- Supporting excellence in preparation of the behavioral work force;

- Promoting person-centered, consumer-driven care that supports consumer efforts to obtain a better education, paid employment or participation in volunteer activities and safe and stable housing;

- Supporting psychoeducation for families of people with serious mental illness;

- Improving safety for consumers and for the communities in which they live".

Again, with very little modification, it can be seen that these fundamental issues are essential to the delivery of mental health care on college campuses. Obviously, such issues as psychoeducation for families would extend in a campus community to psychoeducation for all members of the community as well as for students and their families.

8.4 The College Mental Health Service and the University Community

To extend the concept of the community mental health movement, and current public health concepts of prevention, the whole university community must be responsible for the provision of care to the student. If this is to be effective, it must involve the education of the entire university community in promoting the welfare, well being, psychological development, and health of each of its students. It is in the context of such a positive, university-wide effort that the academic enterprise can thrive. The organization of the many aspects of university life should be developed with the vision of the student's developmental process in mind. A major role of the professional staff of the student mental health service therefore is to embrace the mission of educating the entire university faculty and staff in this respect.

In practice, this would involve presentations to, and interactions with, as many campus groups and academic departments as possible. This includes faculty groups, department chairs, individual academic departments, residential staff, extracurricular organizations, cultural houses, international student office, coaches and team captains, chaplains, student leaders, office staff and tutors. These many and disparate groups constitute the fabric of the university community. The aim of the presentations to these groups would be to:

- educate the members of a particular group about developmental issues

- alert them to the signs of student difficulty so that they would be able to intervene

- refer students for professional mental health care, when appropriate.

Different universities develop different strategies in educating the university community. In recognizing the impossibility of interacting with the entire university community, most college mental health services first focus on the groups they judge to have most contact with students (the so-called "gate keepers"). The scope of this effort obviously depends on the resources committed to the college mental health service including the number of available staff.

Two models are commonly employed for accomplishing this educational outreach. One relies on the clinicians in the student mental health service to provide education as well. Thus, it might be that an individual full-time clinician would devote 60% of his or her time to doing clinical work and 35% to educational outreach. Another organizational model separates the clinical wing of the service from the educational outreach wing. In some universities, for example, the educational outreach is done by a totally separate department from the college mental health service. It may be part of the health education department or of a wellness center. There are advantages and disadvantages to each model. The choice often depends on the university's history and organizational structure.

One university, for example, assigns liaisons to all academic departments, and all the offices with student contact. The mental health service then assigns several of these departments to each clinician, who then arrange an educational outreach program every year or two. Obviously, this would require a large staff and not be appropriate for smaller colleges.

To develop and present these programs, certain staff members may need some special training. Role playing can be a very useful way to present information during these presentations. For instance, a scenario might show how best to talk with a student who is depressed or who has an eating disorder. Using this tool, the mental health clinician can give staff or faculty ways to frame the situation and examples of words and phrases they might usefully employ to engage the student. For this kind of educational outreach to be successful, collegial relationships with participating university faculty and staff must be established. This will encourage them to consult the clinician about difficult student situations they may encounter in the future. It cannot be over-emphasized how important these individual relationships are.

8.5 Outreach Educational and Consultative Services to Students

Student mental health services can effectively operate only through developing relationships of trust with faculty, administration and students. The students must trust the student mental health service to provide outstanding service and to be approachable and easy to access. Twenty-four hour on-call service is essential because it signals to the student that the mental health service is approachable and available if an urgent situation arises. Students must have complete trust in the confidentiality of any interaction they have with a clinician. In sum, it is important that the service be seen as helpful, accessible, approachable and confidential.

Trust can frequently be promoted by outreach activity directed to students themselves. A critical student group in this effort is the student residential advisors. These are usually upperclassmen living in the dormitories with the freshmen or sophomores. Knowing the students extremely well, they are often the first to observe concerning behavioral patterns. They also know about the students' families and friends and the occurrence of stressful life events. Resident advisors are a valuable resource in detecting students in trouble and referring them to the student mental health service. An effective residential advisor program must include a well organized training program for student advisors.

The attitude toward mental health care by students in leadership positions is very important in trying to reduce the stigma associated with emotional difficulties. Thus, developing positive relationships with student leadership groups is essential. The important student groups will vary from campus to campus, but would usually include some student government groups and the captains of the athletic teams. For instance, outreach programs to athletes might address eating concerns, nutrition and athletic performance, or group dynamics and team leadership. Often a specially trained sports psychologist to work with student athletes is invaluable. There may be one such person who works clinically with athletes as they come to the service and another person who is very active working with the athletic department, perhaps spending 2–4 hours every week in the athletic department, holding informal open office hours to be available for "on the spot" consultation with coaches and teams. In working with athletes, it is important to frame the interaction in terms of enhancing their performance in "their sport". Approached in this way, student athletes are much more open to working with mental health clinicians.

Generalizing from this example, it is important to look at a specific student organization to identify its particular needs, and to understand its particular culture. Both the developmental issues, such as autonomy, and student problems must be framed in a way that is acceptable to that specific group. Student government leaders, editors of student newspapers and publications, fraternity leaders, peer health educators, student peer mental health educational groups, and peer counseling groups will have different needs. As several of these student groups may need faculty advisors, it is optimal if a member of the clinical staff of the CMH service is such an advisor. The dean who oversees student groups may appreciate the help. In working with student groups, the CMH staff needs to be sensitive to overstepping appropriate boundaries. If the group already has a faculty advisor, the CMH staff needs to work with that person rather than approach the student group directly.

Because of student turnover, programs and training will need to be repeated each year. The same may be true of the work with faculty and deans as they often move after 3–6 years. In any case, it is important to both review these issues often and keep personal relationships with these important people active and fresh.

8.6 Relationship of College Mental Health Service to the Faculty, University Administration and Deans of Student Life

As indicated earlier, the community mental health center model is the one (with modification) most appropriate in defining the roles of the college mental health service. This model implies the importance of working with the university administration, particularly in regard to the formation of university policies. As well, it would suggest that it is advantageous to have a member of the CMH staff as a member of various college committees, particularly those involved in student life and the development of various leave and re-admission policies. This facilitates the education of the committee members in regard to student development and helps them formulate policies that promote this development. Working as part of one of these committees is also important in increasing the number of people in university leadership roles who would then see the mental health clinician as a colleague, thus increasing the likelihood that they would refer students to the college mental health service. This collegial relationship would be an asset to the college mental health service just as the CMH clinician would be an asset to the committee determining policy.

8.6.1 Relationship to Faculty

The relationship between the CMH service and faculty is also a very important one and one that can be enhanced if some members of the CMH staff have a teaching role or faculty appointment in an academic department. This again nurtures the collegial nature of the clinician-faculty relationship as well as providing opportunities for academic collaboration. There are many opportunities for such interactions. For instance, many colleges have a system of college seminars given by non-ladder faculty or mini courses given during a winter month break between semesters. Probably the most common faculty relationship that CMH service staff has is either a clinical appointment in the medical school or as a supervisor of postdoctoral fellows in the psychology department. In universities that have professional schools, CMH clinicians often have obtained lectureships, for example, in the law school or the school of public health.

8.6.2 Relationship with Campus Security Department

Since the Virginia Tech shooting in 2007 concern about violence on campus has become a prominent issue. Many campuses have set up new committees and developed new policies to try to minimize the possibility of violence on campus. One of the outcomes of the study of both the Virginia Tech incident, as well as other incidents of campus violence that have occurred since that time has been the recognition that there was a lack of communication between campus departments, each of which had some information and each of which had concerns about the student involved. It has been supposed that had information been shared there might have been an organized intervention which may have averted the tragedy. Obviously, the campus mental health service must be a key player in making these assessments and planning possible intervention.

In response to these concerns many colleges have established two committees (or groups) to try to address the issue of violence on campus. The first group has had different titles on different campuses, but has most commonly been called a "students of concern" committee. The second group deals with actual threat assessment as required by particular situations or students. Some colleges have combined both functions in one group, though most colleges have separated these functions.

For the "students of concern" committee, the constituents vary from campus to campus, but usually include the dean of students, the chair of the disciplinary committee, the chief of security, the director of the mental health service, legal counsel, and the dean of residential life. Other people who might be part of such a committee from time to time, or in some colleges may be included regularly, would be the vice president to whom the dean of students and security report, chaplains, and the head of the international office. In these committees, any member of the committee may bring to the attention of the group either a student or a situation about which they are concerned, particularly those where there seems to be a potential for violence. Obviously, in these situations the director of the college mental health service would not divulge any information that he or she had from clinical sources. The director's role would be to participate in the discussion of possible interventions and ways of understanding and thinking about the particular situation. The intent then of such a committee is to provide a vehicle by means of which people from different parts of the university can pool information, thus providing an overall picture that is of more value than the view of any individual participant. Obviously this is a difficult task requiring that the members of the committee be very respectful of one another and that they use good judgment in neither overreacting or under-reacting to the problem.

When a particular situation has risen to a higher level of concern, the college may want a more standardized "threat assessment". It is now generally understood that it is impossible to accurately predict who will undertake a violent action. However, an attempt can be made to estimate the probability as high, medium or low. Some campuses have decided to use forensic psychiatrists to make these assessments, but more often they are made by the security department where increasingly sophisticated computer programs, using detailed information, can make the probability ratings. It is also important to involve general counsel of the college to make sure that, in any situation attention is being carefully paid to both the safety of the community and the rights of individual students.

In regard to this issue it is clear that it is vital that the CMH service director have a well established, collegial relationship with the head of security. It is essential that security and the CMH service have delineated areas of responsibility. They need to have developed protocols as to how to handle such problems as intoxicated students, suicidal students, disruptive students, and violent students, many of whom will have emotional issues. Security and CMH service may have developed different approaches to different situations and these differences need to be sorted out ahead of time. The head of security usually welcomes outreach from the CMH service and is open to a discussion as to how to handle particular problems. As a relationship of trust develops, a fruitful working relationship can then be relied upon. As part of developing that relationship, it is essential that the CMH service show security that they appreciate and respect the work of the security department. It is important that the chief of campus security be included in decision making groups, routinely through the year, and that they can rely on having a "seat at the table". When they are present in these discussions, there can be greater confidence in a coordinated and well-considered approach. This kind of approach is not possible when security is brought in at the last moment to handle a particular crisis that is already out of hand. If there are not already situations where the CMH service director is interacting with the chief of security, it would be important to set up a regular meeting with the person each semester. Sometimes, out of this interaction, advice can be given or shared about the kind of training it would be useful for security to have regarding student development, the student environment, or the handling of difficult and disruptive students.

8.6.3 Responding to Campus Crises

The importance of the relationships within the campus community that have been built up over the years, is seen very clearly when an immediate response is needed to an on-campus crisis. This area is addressed in detail in Chapter 9. It is enough here to emphasize that if there is a mental health liaison person assigned to individual housing units, academic departments, or schools, it means that an immediate and appropriate response can occur as the CMH clinician is already known and trusted by the campus deans, staff and students.

8.6.4 Relationship to other Resources on Campus

There are other student oriented offices on campus with which it is important to develop solid relationships. The international student office, the cultural centers and career services (and the deans and directors who supervise them) are important campus resources. The support, education, and mentoring that occurs in these centers plays an essential role in assisting the student in defining and consolidating his or her identity. The student's nationality and ethnic background, of course, is an essential part of this identity consolidation. To facilitate this process, it is helpful that the CMH service has an ethnically diverse staff, both for clinical work and for consultation.

In addition to providing and directing worship services, chaplains are also important personal and spiritual advisors to students. With the many faiths represented in the student body today, it is essential that the CMH service understand and appreciate different religious points of view. On some campuses an attitude of mutual suspicion between the chaplain's office and the CMH service has developed, resulting in the chaplain's office feeling that the CMH service will not respect the student's religious faith. Continuing dialog is critical, especially in situations where misunderstandings have arisen. As the chaplains and CMH clinicians are frequently brought together in handling the campus-wide response to a crisis situation, as in the case of a student death, respectful collaboration is essential. It is a good idea, for example, to have the chaplains make presentations to the CMH staff regarding their particular faith and the issues they see facing the students on campus. This both helps the CMH staff to become more culturally and religiously competent, and also provides an opportunity for respectful interaction and referral between the two offices. It also makes it more likely that the chaplains will make CMH referrals as needed.

There are two other important offices with which the CMH service interacts, even though these offices have less direct interaction with students. The first is the *university press office*. Again, this is a situation where it is important to develop a relationship with the chief press officer before a crisis occurs as he or she can be extremely helpful within and outside the campus community. For instance, in the situation of a student death or suicide, they can be helpful in working with the student campus newspaper to report the death accurately, but not sensationally. They can also assist in working with campus and off campus media to optimize accurate reporting, and demonstrating how to maintain good relationships with the press.

Finally, *the legal office* is an extremely important resource in addressing the extraordinary number of legal issues and regulations that arise in the course of the CMH service's day to day work. With detailed knowledge of federal and state laws, this office clarifies ambiguities and contradictions in law. They can be extremely helpful where the law is ambiguous, or where two laws are contradictory, in helping to sort out an appropriate course of action. The legal office is likely to be aware of possible legal ramifications of policies or decisions relevant to the CMH service that may not have been appreciated. A good legal office will support the CMH service in providing good clinical care.

8.7 Confidentiality

Since the CMH service must relate to so many campus entities, students may be concerned about the confidentiality and the relationship of clinicians to faculty and deans. This is an important issue, as, without the students' trust in the confidential nature of the interactions with the clinicians, a college mental health service is ineffective. Some larger universities with many mental health clinicians have addressed this problem by designating one staff member, usually the director, to handle most of the relationships outside of the service. This would mean that when the director speaks with various university people, he or she would not have particular information about specific students. Such college mental health services would then have someone more like an associate director handle the day to day clinic operation, though the director would continue to oversee the entire enterprise. This obviously may not be possible for schools with smaller mental health staffs, as the director would be needed to do a substantial part of the clinical work. In these situations, even though it would be possible to establish some of the recommended campus relationships it may not be possible to establish all of them in order to make sure that there is the perception as well as the reality of confidentiality among the student body.

8.8 Conclusion

This chapter has stressed the necessity of conceptualizing the college mental health service as an integral part of the larger college community. It describes the numerous faculty, student and staff constituencies that must be the focus of collaboration. It highlights the central role of the defining and maintaining the confidentiality between student and the student mental health service clinicians.

8.9 Appendix A: A Model "At Risk/Student Support Program" in a Small Residential Campus[1]

The program described below is currently in operation at a small urban university campus. There are approximately 1200 students on campus of whom 70% live in residence halls and another 15–20% live in private apartments within several blocks of the campus. The students are primarily undergraduates but there are also several small graduate programs.

There are several basic features to this program. First, the primary goal of this program is to identify students who may be having any kind of educational, psychological, social or personal difficulty as efficiently as possible and take all prudent steps to support the students' continuation in school to the greatest extent possible. The primary focus of this program is to support student success, not to avoid liability. This program is based on the overlapping and interlocking activities of two groups.

8.9.1 Student Services Component

The Director of Housing and Residence Life (DHRL) manages the student services component (SSC) of the program. Depending on time of year, this sub-committee meets on a weekly or bi-weekly basis. The DHRL maintains a list of any student who has been identified as potentially having a problem. Students may be identified by:

1. an RA-RAs receive training during orientation and throughout the academic year from the director of counseling and the director of housing

2. a parent-any call by a parent expressing concern regarding their child's functioning would result in a student being placed on the "at risk" list

3. dean, administrator, athletic coach or faculty.

These meetings are run by the DHRL and are attended by University Dean of Students Affairs (essentially the director of student services for the university), Director of Counseling Center, Disabilities Counselor, Director of Learning Support, Assistant Director of Housing, Dean for Student Discipline, campus Chaplain. A list is maintained of all students who have been brought to the committee. Problems may include students who appear depressed, who have had a significant conflict with someone on campus, have manifested deterioration in self care or functioning or have manifested change in social interaction. Each student situation is reviewed and an action plan is established. Director of Counseling and Disabilities Officer play a consulting role at the meeting and do not share information they may have about a particular student unless there is agreement that the problem presented may be acutely dangerous in some way.

This plan may include:

1. further observation by RA-RAs are not provided with detailed or specific information as to the nature of the concern (of course they are often the source of the information in the first place)

---

[1] We would like to thank Mr. Jonathan Mantell, Director of Housing and Residence Life at the Wilf Campus, Yeshiva University.

2. a call from the Housing and Residence Life office inviting the student for a conversation/ check in

3. a referral to academic advising, disabilities office or counseling

4. further conversation with parent to see whether problem has improved-it is important to remember that there are no constraints to listening to parents' concerns. Ultimately, when indicated, there may be attempts to engage the student and family in open conversation with deans or clinicians-typically with full agreement of the student (unless there is an acute and serious emergency in which case, in consultation with committee members, a decision might be made to involve a parent without assent of student).

If the problem does not appear to be significant[2], the student will in all likelihood be briefly followed by the RA and then dropped from the active list.

In determining the plan, special attention is given to particularly challenging periods in the school year such as exams, long weekends and breaks and holidays. It is important to note that RAs play a central role in this program so ongoing training and consultation with them is essential. When a discipline or security issue emerges, DHRL consults with Dean for Campus Discipline and Security department (along with other committee members) to arrive at a plan of action. Campus discipline is not directly handled by this committee. If a disciplinary action is needed the Dean for Campus Discipline will pursue this. The SSC may reach out to the student simultaneously to provide other support services as indicated. Planning is dynamic and the progress of each situation is reviewed at each meeting until the situation is no longer felt to be a problem.

8.9.2 Academic Component

At middle of each semester and soon after finals, the Assistant Deans who oversee student progress and directors of student academic advising meet with the student services team noted above. Prior to the mid-semester meeting, the deans reach out to faculty to ask for information regarding any student around whom they may have a concern (either academic, social or personal). The committee meets to review the status of these students and again determine an action plan. Frequently, the plan will involve a call from the academic advising department leading to a conversation about how the student is handling his academic program and whether there are any issues that might be interfering with his success. Academic advisors work closely with student services staff and attempt to remain vigilant toward psychological or personal issues which might be interfering with students' progress. They are quick to refer to disabilities or counseling offices and since these offices attend the committee meetings, they will already have some familiarity with these students.

After the close of the semester, again this large committee meets and reviews students whose GPAs place them on probation and also students whose GPAs have fluctuated significantly (a student who typically scores a 3.4 who suddenly drops to 2.8 may be experiencing some sort of problem). Some follow up plan is again set and the academic deans track the plan and outcomes.

---

[2] An example of this might be a student whose parent calls Housing Dept. because the student has been out of touch for some time. When RA checks in on student they are informed that the student's phone has been broken and they have just obtained a new phone and have now been in touch with family.

8.9.3 Conclusions

1. These interlocking committees function with a primary focus on student support and success.

2. There is emphasis placed on getting as much information into the system from as many different sources as possible (remember administrators or others are not constrained from sharing behavioral observations and anyone can always listen to a concerned parent or faculty member).

3. Having the student services support staff (such as disabilities and counseling) participate in the academic at risk meetings allows them to share their expertise as consultants and experts in disability issues and mental health. At the same time, these professionals become aware of students who are likely to present at their services (or to gain collateral information regarding students who may already be receiving support through their services).

4. Interventions are typically done from the "bottom up". In almost all cases, the first contact with a student who is having some difficulty will be from someone they know-the student's RA or academic adviser- and the intervention will only become more intense if the problem cannot be handled at this level. This, as much as possible, prevents the student from feeling intruded upon.

5. Making the campus community aware of these programs helps faculty, administrators, parents and students to be aware of the problem solvers and supporters on campus. It helps to clarify whom someone who has a problem or is concerned about someone else can turn to.

References

1. Arnett, J.J. (2006) *Emerging Adulthood: the Winding Road from the Late Teens through the Twenties*, Oxford University Press, New York.
2. Sowell, E.R., Thompson, P.M., Holmes, C.H.J. *et al.* (1999) *In vivo* evidence for post-adolescence from post-adolescent brain maturation in frontal and streatal regions. *Nature Neuroscience*, **2**, 859–861.
3. Sowell, E.R., Thompson, P.M., Tessner, K.D. and Toga, A.W. (2001) Mapping continued brain growth and gray matter development in dorsal frontal cortex: Inverse relationship during post-adolescence brain maturation. *The Journal of Neuroscience*, **21**, 8819–8829.
4. Erikson, E. (1968) *Identity: Youth and Crisis*, Norton, New York.
5. Beers, C. (1907/ 1917) *A Mind that Found Itself*, Longmans, Green & Co., New York.
6. Fry, C. (1951) Retrospect and Prospect: A Special Report on the Twenty-fifth Anniversary of the Student Mental Hygiene Services at Yale.
7. Pierson, G. (1955) *Yale, The University College: 1921–1937*, Yale University Press, New Haven, CT.
8. Angell, J.R. (1930) Report of the president 1929–30, in *Yale, The University College: 1921–1937* (ed. G. Pierson), (1955), Yale University Press, New Haven.
9. Lamb, H.R. (1999) Public psychiatry and prevention, in *American Psychiatric Press Textbook of Psychiatry* (eds R. Hales, S. Yudofsky and J. Talbolt), American Psychiatric Press, Washington, DC, p. 1537.
10. Jacobs, Selby and Griffith, Ezra (eds) (2007) *40 Years of Academic Public Psychiatry*, John Wiley & Sons, Chichester, UK.

11. Gordon, R. (1987) An operational classification of disease prevention, in *Alcohol, Drug Abuse, and Mental Health Administration*, DHHS Publication No. AMD 87-1492 (eds J. Steinberg and M. Silverman), United States Government Printing, Rockville, MD, pp. 20–26.
12. National Institute of Mental Health (1996) A report to the National Advisory Mental Health Council. *NIH Publication* No. 96-4093.
13. Kellams, S.G., Koretz, D. and Moscicki, E.K. (1999) Core elements of developmental epidemiologically-based prevention research. *American Journal of Community Psychology*, **27**, 463–482.

9 Crisis and Crisis Intervention on College Campuses

Morton M. Silverman[1,2,3,4] and Rachel Lipson Glick[5,6]

[1]*The University of Chicago, Chicago, IL, USA*
[2]*The University of Colorado at Denver, Denver, CO, USA*
[3]*The Jed Foundation, New York, NY, USA*
[4]*Suicide Prevention Resource Center, Newton, MA, USA*
[5]*Department of Psychiatry, University of Michigan Medical School, Ann Arbor, MI, USA*
[6]*University of Michigan Health System, Ann Arbor, MI, USA*

9.1 What is a Crisis?

A crisis is the response to an event or series of events that tax a person's usual methods of problem solving. Crises can also occur when stress in a person's life reaches a critical level. When coping strategies fail and a person becomes overwhelmed, hopeless and immobilized, he or she can be thought of as being in crisis [1–3].

A crisis is unique to an individual. Some individuals bear massive loss with little difficulty, while others become overwhelmed with seemingly minor events [4,5]. Some students handle the pressure of college well, while others have difficulty coping. A crisis can occur in a student who is psychologically well, or it can occur in a student who is struggling at baseline. In a student who has been functioning well, an unexpected and overwhelming event may temporarily lead to impairment of coping skills. In the student who is otherwise fragile, seemingly less serious events can lead to similar problems coping. Table 9.1 lists personal and historical factors which pre-dispose one to difficulties coping. One can think of crises as occurring as a result of the unique synergy of intrapsychic, interpersonal, environmental, social, and situational variables.

The spark for the initiation of a crisis may be external (death of a loved one, failure in a course) or may be internal (developmental conflict). Once present, the fuel for a crisis often resides within the individual, in terms of the lack of cognitive skills, coping skills, poor perceptual skills, prior exposure or experience with similar situations, underlying psychiatric disorder, or existing stressful situations. The individual's predisposing personality style often dictates the intensity, duration, and form of his or her response to the crisis [6]. In addition, the individual's appraisal or perception of the event/situation itself, as well as how others may have responded to it, is a critical component of the stress experience and

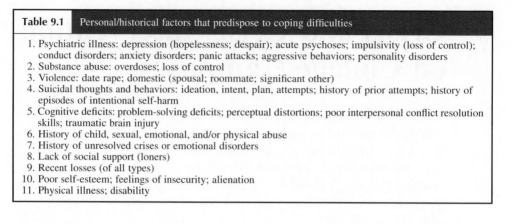

Table 9.1	Personal/historical factors that predispose to coping difficulties

1. Psychiatric illness: depression (hopelessness; despair); acute psychoses; impulsivity (loss of control); conduct disorders; anxiety disorders; panic attacks; aggressive behaviors; personality disorders
2. Substance abuse: overdoses; loss of control
3. Violence: date rape; domestic (spousal; roommate; significant other)
4. Suicidal thoughts and behaviors: ideation, intent, plan, attempts; history of prior attempts; history of episodes of intentional self-harm
5. Cognitive deficits: problem-solving deficits; perceptual distortions; poor interpersonal conflict resolution skills; traumatic brain injury
6. History of child, sexual, emotional, and/or physical abuse
7. History of unresolved crises or emotional disorders
8. Lack of social support (loners)
9. Recent losses (of all types)
10. Poor self-esteem; feelings of insecurity; alienation
11. Physical illness; disability

response. Hence many factors are at work and interact as an individual perceives the crisis, attaches meaning to it, and appraises its effect on their status quo (or abrupt change in their homeostasis).

Sometimes the student first has a visceral or psychological response to an event or stressful situation, and only afterwards seeks understanding of its meaning and relief from the attendant negative response. At other times, students are unable to integrate the event with their own self-perception ("I shouldn't have allowed this to get to me. I always thought that I was stronger than that and knew how to deal with it". Or, "I don't understand why this is happening to me. I never thought it would affect me so much".). Hence there may be both emotional and cognitive failures or misperceptions in response to the crisis itself, and this development and evolution may not be apparent right away ("I don't know why I am still bothered by that event. I thought I handled it well and it is behind me now".)

Problems emerge in students as a consequence of many challenges students commonly face such as transition from home to college, transition from college to the workplace (or graduate school), relationship problems, financial problems, academic performance, developmental delays, psychiatric symptoms, and the use and abuse of alcohol and other drugs. The student in crisis often reports experiencing subjective distress and impaired social, academic, emotional and/or physical functioning. More often than not, the crisis involves a variation on a type of perceived or actual loss: loss of significant other (death, divorce or separation, relational), loss of self-esteem (failing an exam), loss of financial support and/or autonomy, loss of a sense of a future, loss of physical autonomy or well-being, loss of emotional stability, and so on. Table 9.2 lists common crisis situations seen in college students.

Crises can be thought of as occurring in four distinct phases [7,8]. The first phase is the ordinary tension that marks the beginning of a problem-solving response to a potential crisis in an effort to regain homeostasis. The second phase begins when there is lack of success of the usual methods to resolve the crisis and a continuation of the challenging stimulus, which then leads to a stage of "upset and ineffectuality". The individual reports subjective feelings of unease or displeasure (disequilibrium) characterized by anxiety, fear, guilt, or shame. The individual reports feeling helpless in trying to resolve an "insoluble problem". The third phase is characterized by the rise of tension that results from the attempt to mobilize emergency coping skills and other resources, both internal and external, including an appeal to novel methods of problem solving, a linking with neglected social resources and/or

Table 9.2	Common crisis situations in college students

1. Grief reactions to any loss or perceived loss
   -Death of family member or friend
   -Serious illness in family member or friend
   -Death of pet
   -Break-up of relationship
   -Disruptions in friendships
2. Sudden changes in academic status
3. Developmental issues that overwhelm the individual
4. Suicidal or homicidal ideation or behavior
5. Sequelae of drug/alcohol intoxication
6. Acute anxiety, depressive, or psychotic symptoms
7. Personal loss of control or perceived loss of control
8. Problems with impulse control
9. Physical or emotional trauma
   -Date rape
   -Partner violence
   -Natural disasters
   -Sexual assault
   -Physical assault
   -Other traumatic events such as fires, accidents, suicides, crimes

personal capacities, or an active giving up of certain aspects of unattainable goals. The steady state of homeostasis is disrupted. The fourth phase occurs if the problem remains unresolved and the tension reaches a breaking point, resulting in major disorganization of the individual.

Ultimately, just as beauty is in the eye of the beholder, crisis is in the mind of the person in crisis. As noted above, a key determinant in the intensity and duration of a crisis reaction is the individual's appraisal of the threat and the meaning that is attached to it. A crisis is when an individual is unable to manage an important life goal or reduce the stress associated with a life event. For the individual in crisis this challenge is perceived as insurmountable despite the enactment of customary methods of problem solving or coping. They want to feel better and return to normal function. On the other hand, for the clinician a crisis is a brief non-illness response to severe stress that overwhelms the usual coping skills of the person in crisis.

9.2 Crisis Intervention

Crisis intervention has two immediate goals. It aims to reduce the intensity of an individual's emotional, mental, physical and behavioral reactions to a crisis and it aims to help the individual return to their pre-crisis level of functioning. But an additional goal of crisis intervention goes beyond helping the person feel better. Done well, crisis intervention can result in further growth and development for the individual, by teaching new skills and bolstering the individual's ability to confront obstacles and challenges in the future. On college campuses, where a basic goal is to assist students in their learning processes in all realms, the knowledge that experiencing crises and crisis resolution can actually facilitate growth is a key concept; and the importance of learning to deal with crises as normative is paramount.

Students often turn to people they know for help when in crisis. Often it is faculty, student services personnel, coaches, trainers, clergy, other staff, or even friends who first become aware that a student is in distress. These individuals complement the role of the mental health professional. Because these non-mental health professionals are often the first point of contact, they need to be prepared, willing, and able to assist students in distress by inquiring about the circumstances surrounding a crisis presentation, making an initial assessment of relative risk, and presenting mental health services as a viable and trusted intervention. Widespread training in the Question, Persuade, Refer approach (QPR), a model developed by Quinnett to teach non-mental health providers a constructive way to interact with potentially suicidal individuals [9], has been adopted by many campuses to provide first line crisis responders with tools when encountering a student in crisis. Another popular program is Applied Suicide Intervention Skills Training (ASIST), which teaches skills to competently and confidently intervene with individuals at risk [10]. We recommend that every campus provide similar education and training to all staff and faculty.

Once the student gets to the counseling center or other mental health provider, crisis intervention treatment is typically brief and completed within days to several weeks. Interventions should be structured with a clear timeframe in mind and this time frame should be conveyed to the student at the time of the first encounter. This approach is analogous to a brief dynamic psychotherapy.

To be effective, the crisis counselor must remember a few key points. First and foremost, the clinician must recall that the student in crisis is extremely vulnerable. People who are vulnerable are open to hurt as much as to help and no one wants to be hurt or abused when they are defenseless. The goal of crisis counseling is to protect the student from further disruption or traumatization while providing them with immediate assistance in managing themselves and the situation [11].

No one trusts a stranger unless there is hope that that person can help overcome current distress and re-establish a sense of equilibrium. This requires the clinician to be empathic to the student's plight and immediately establish a sense of security, safety, stability and predictability. It is counterproductive to be aloof, dismissive, preoccupied, disdainful, cajoling, or condescending. Crisis counselors must be genuine and caring. They must provide brief, clear and gentle directions and support to distressed individuals. Assisting the individual to gain a sense of control of self and situation is central to effective crisis intervention. Some do's and don'ts of crisis intervention are listed in Table 9.3.

Crisis intervention occurs in eight steps or phases [13]:

1. **Establishing rapport**   On campus, counselors must have experience in connecting and working with young adults and must be aware of the campus "culture" around seeking counseling services. If psychological distress is seen as not acceptable, counseling staff must help the student accept the need for intervention as a first step.

2. **Assuring safety**   Students in crisis may feel or be out of control. The first step in helping them gain control is to keep them safe. For example, if they voice suicidal thoughts, these must be addressed first (see below). If they feel threatened in their living situation, alternative places to stay may have to be arranged before other crisis intervention steps can be taken.

3. **Examining the problem in detail**   The task here is to help the student understand the crisis and their response to it. Establishing a realistic perception of what happened and the path to recovery is the necessary work that needs to be done to resolve the crisis.

Table 9.3	The do's and don'ts of crisis intervention [1,12]

Do's:
1. Provide a safe, secure, and quiet setting to conduct the initial assessment
2. Recognize cultural differences and vary counseling styles accordingly
3. Use an individualized approach that is tailored to the student
4. Speak clearly, in a calm manner at a moderate pace, and maintain good eye contact.
5. Be aware of your body posture and facial expressions
6. Remain calm
7. Be clear and explicit
8. Try to put yourself in their "shoes" and see the traumatic events from their perspective/point of view
9. Listen carefully and compassionately ("I'm so sorry that this has happened".)
10. Emphasize mutual dialog and genuineness whenever possible
11. Be goal directed
12. Provide accessibility and availability of professional support
13. Stabilize the student and the surrounding events as quickly as possible in order to restore a semblance of order and routine
14. Acknowledge that they are in crisis and provide feedback ("I can see that you are really upset and are having difficulty functioning, or thinking clearly, right now".)
15. Provide opportunities for the student to discuss fully (and often) their experiences, feelings and thoughts at their own pace and in their own words ("It is important for or me to hear your story as you experienced it, and in your own words".)
16. Reinforce that their reactions are "normal" or "within a normal range" of responses to the current crisis ("It is natural to be having these difficulties at this time")
17. Explore the specifics of the traumatic event(s) that lead to a crisis reaction, including talking about the person(s) who might have died or been injured
18. Share similar experiences or feelings when appropriate
19. Reassure and be supportive when appropriate ("I would like to be of help to you", or "Together I think that we can work through this", or "Help is available and an improvement in your current state is possible".)
20. Explore previous exposures to crises and their resolution
21. Discuss the role of coping skills and problem solving in addressing crises
22. Inventory the tactics that have been unsuccessful with this current crisis
23. Begin to develop an inventory of coping skills that have worked in the past, especially under similar circumstances
24. Support their identification of healthy and appropriate solutions to the current crisis
25. Encourage self-reliance
26. Identify the student's support network, friends, roommates, and so on
27. Identify others who the student can trust to be available to them as the crisis resolves
28. Stay focused on the "here and now" and what immediately lies ahead
29. Define goals clearly and keep them limited to a manageable plan of action
30. Help students find meaning to their experiences, and facilitate understanding of what has happened, so they can begin to assimilate traumatic events into how they approach the future
31. Support the student when he/she acts on their own behalf for their own resolution to the crisis

Don'ts:
1. Dismiss their sense of being in a crisis as inappropriate or mislabeled ("It's not that bad", or "Crying won't help".)
2. Make premature assumptions or imposing stereotypes about the student's problems or reactions ("Why, if I were you, I would have responded differently".)
3. Argue with the student, especially regarding details and specifics of the traumatic event itself
4. Overwhelm the student with information or ideas
5. Take full responsibility for their emotional state
6. Offer judgments about what might have been done differently or how the student might have responded differently to the event
7. Be chastising or judgmental
8. Make decisions for the student
9. Take sides or assign blame. ("I agree with you that this is all the fault of the university".)
10. Give false assurances. ("There is no need to be upset", or "Everything will be better tomorrow".)
11. Challenge their thinking or emotional feelings ("I'm surprised that you are so upset".)
12. Challenge or agree with mistaken or illogical beliefs ("I can't believe that you think that", or "You are absolutely correct in how you understand what happened".)
13. Be confrontative, authoritative, or controlling
14. Engage in humor
15. Demand, command, or order. It is best to discuss options and elicit the student's opinions and perspectives before making a decision.

4. **Encouraging an exploration of feelings and emotions while providing support**   The clinician must provide the opportunity for the student to vent his/her anger, fear, frustration, and grief. Furthermore, the clinician must sit with, be comfortable with, and validate the emotional reactions of the student.

5. **Assessing past coping skills**   A major focus of crisis intervention is exploring coping strategies. Strategies that the individual previously used but that have not been used to deal with the current crisis may be enhanced or bolstered. Also, new coping skills may be developed. Coping skills may include such things as relaxation techniques, exercise to reduce body tension and stress, and putting thoughts and feelings on paper through journal writing. In addition, options for social support or spending time with people who provide a feeling of comfort and caring should be explored, including parents, guardians, or other authority figures. Encouraging the student to communicate their distress level to his/her parents may lead to the initiation of a new level of communication, understanding, and support.

6. **Generating specific solutions**   Another central focus of crisis intervention is problem solving. This process involves thoroughly understanding the problem and the desired changes, considering alternative methods for solving the problem, discussing the pros and cons of alternative solutions, selecting a solution and developing a plan and, then, evaluating the outcome. Cognitive behavioral therapy, which is based on the notion that thoughts influence feelings and behavior, is effective in crisis intervention.

7. **Restoring cognitive functioning through implementation of an action plan**   In this phase of crisis intervention, the clinician reviews changes the individual has made/can make to point out that it is possible to cope with difficult life events. Continued use of the effective coping strategies that reduced distress is encouraged. Also, assistance is provided in making realistic plans for the future, particularly in terms of dealing with potential future crises. Information is provided about resources for additional help should the need arise.

8. **Providing appropriate and timely follow-up**   A telephone follow-up may be arranged at some agreed-upon time or a determined number of follow-up sessions can be scheduled to resolve any unaddressed or unresolved issues.

9.3 Common Crises and Suggested Responses

Although crises can be divided into some major categories, there is often overlap between and among these artificially defined categories [14]. Furthermore, one type of crisis can promulgate, initiate, or precipitate another type of crises. On campus, most crises can be thought of as either developmental, or situational, or both, as demonstrated by the following examples.

Case 1

Jonathan, an 18-year-old freshman from a suburban high school from which he graduated first in his class of 1500, has enrolled in a small very competitive liberal arts college where he takes several seminar type classes. He feels "dumb" because other students seem to know so much more than he does. He also feels uncomfortable with his roommates who know each other from high school and seem more accomplished and more comfortable with girls than he does. He misses his family, and feels lonely much of the time. His resident advisor has noticed that Jonathan seems sad, and has walked him to the counseling center after explaining to Jonathan that a lot of students need help adjusting to how different their lives are at college, and assuring Jonathan that there is nothing wrong with talking to a counselor once or twice to help get adjusted.

Case 2

Phyllis is a 20-year-old junior in a premed program at a large state university. Both of her parents are physicians and she "has always just assumed I'd be a doctor too". Although her grades are good, she doesn't enjoy her science courses which require long hours of study to achieve B+ to A− grades. She has found that she enjoys reading and writing, and has no difficulty getting excellent grades in her English classes. She questions her career choice, and has developed symptoms of depression, including difficulty sleeping, weight loss, lack of energy, and anhedonia.

Case 3

Derek is a 21-year-old senior who is graduating in several weeks and is still unsure what he is going to do after finishing school. He has been having difficulty sleeping because he cannot stop thinking about his future and worrying about why he feels so immobilized and unsure.

These three cases are examples of developmental crises that can occur during transitions from one stage of life to another or one familiar environment or location to a novel one. In the context of a college environment, developmental crises are often seen as students initially adjust to campus life, and when they approach graduation and are faced with the prospect of leaving a supportive, friendly, safe, and predictable environment for one that is unknown or one that has fewer assurances associated with it.

A developmental crisis may occur when the individual first arrives on campus, having left behind at home familiar turf and relationships, as Jonathan has in Case 1. Jonathan is no longer the outstanding high school student and valedictorian. He now has a number of developmental challenges to master including:

- establishing new relationships with peers

- realistically assessing his academic skills and talents

- developing relationships with professors

- establishing his academic and social identities on campus

- adjusting to group living arrangements

- being exposed to new cultures and different lifestyles

- adjusting to new rules and regulations

- solidifying gender and sexual identities

- learning to take risks (new courses; trying out for the sports teams; engaging in romantic relationships).

Here the clinician must assist the student in identifying prominent issues and reviewing prior successes and failures in mastering previous life challenges and relationships. The counselor provides guidance, support and encouragement in facilitating the student's adjustment to college.

Phyllis (Case 2) is in the process of firming up her identity. The process of consolidating, re-examining, experimenting, and critically evaluating one's beliefs, values, ethics, and morals can cause internal conflict and be perceived as a crisis – especially when these "positions" are not held by others or are challenged in such a way that the individual is left shaken, confused, and defenseless. Phyllis has always believed she will be a doctor. When she finds that her interests and skills may lie elsewhere, she struggles to reconcile this discrepancy, and she worries that her parents will not understand. Although the crisis clinician can re-assure Phyllis that her struggles are normative and part of "growing-up and finding one's own identity", Phyllis' crisis is causing her to have symptoms of a depressive episode that must be acknowledged and may require treatment. This case illustrates that while developmental crises can be normative, they may precipitate psychiatric illness and consequently require a different mode of treatment.

For many, such as Derek (Case 3), graduation signifies the successful mastery of their formal educational career, Leaving such "friendly quarters" often is experienced with trepidation, uncertainty, and insecurity. The fear of the unknown can be immobilizing. Here the role of the clinician is to remind the individual that they have already experienced these transitions as they moved from high school to college or from college to graduate school. It is an opportunity to review and muster coping skills and abilities as the individual faces new situations and locations. This is an opportunity to explore the individual's sense of self-worth, resiliency, and resourcefulness, while reflecting on accomplishments and failures to date, experiences and acquired skills of independence and autonomy. It is also an opportunity to catalog the fears of the future – whether real or imagined – and explore their likelihood of occurrence while preparing for such events or challenges.

Case 4

Hillary is a 19-year-old sophomore who comes to the counseling center in tears 5 days after her grandmother died. She explains that she was very close to her grandmother and knew that her grandmother was quite ill, but had not expected to feel this overwhelmed by her grandmother's death.

Case 5

Robert is an 18-year-old freshman who just learned that he failed his first economics exam. He has found the adjustment to college difficult in that he misses his friends from home and still feels out of place, but when he got the failing grade he became very upset, went to talk to his professor and started to cry, saying he might as well just quit school since if he failed the class he would lose his scholarship anyway. His professor tried to reassure him by pointing out that the exam would not determine his grade, but Robert said this didn't matter. At the professor's encouragement, Robert came to the counseling services to talk about dropping out of school before taking any action.

Cases 4 and 5 are situational crises. These result from some event that may cause immediate distress and inability to function. These may include deaths, injuries, failures, or financial problems, to name a few. Situational crises call upon the clinician to best understand the "who, what, when, where, why and how" the individual became engaged in the situation. Often these types of crises stimulate the re-emergence of reactions to prior incidents or situations that the individual never fully mastered or resolved. These crises are often perceived as direct threats to the individual's sense of integrity, identity, and self-reliance.

A situational crisis can develop in the setting of a developmental crisis, as illustrated in Robert's story (Case 5). If Robert had not been struggling with the adjustment to college, failure of a single test may not have lead to a crisis. Alternatively, if he had not failed the test, his adjustment to college may not have risen to the level of a developmental crisis.

9.3.1 Response to Traumatic Events

Case 6

Cheryl is a 20-year-old junior referred to the counseling center after being attacked and raped by a stranger on campus. Her first appointment with the counselor was just 2 days after the event, and she describes feeling frightened, easily startled, with difficulty falling and staying asleep because of nightmares.

Some situational crises follow events that are so unexpected, and are, or can be, perceived as so frightening and life-threatening, that they deserve special attention. Victims of crime, such as Cheryl (Case 6) benefit from immediate supportive intervention. Under these circumstances, immediate crisis intervention involves establishing a rapport with the victim, gathering information for short-term assessment and service delivery, and averting a potential state of crisis.

An assessment begins with the exploration of what happened and the individual's responses to it. Intense, painful reactions are a common response, and Cheryl is already describing some typical symptoms. An individual's reaction to trauma (see Table 9.4) can include emotional reactions (fear, anger, guilt, grief), cognitive reactions (difficulty concentrating, disorientation, confusion), physical reactions (headaches, dizziness, fatigue, stomach problems), and behavioral reactions (sleep and appetite problems, isolation, restlessness). With a trauma victim, the educational component to crisis intervention is provided through assurances that the individual is experiencing a normal reaction to an abnormal situation. The student should be told that the intense immediate responses are usually time-limited. Although there is not a specific time that a person can expect to recover from a trauma, a clinician can help the victim by:

- Listening and encouraging the person to talk about their reactions when they feel ready.

- Validating the emotional reactions of the person. Intense, painful reactions are common responses to a traumatic event.

- De-emphasizing clinical, diagnostic, and pathological language.

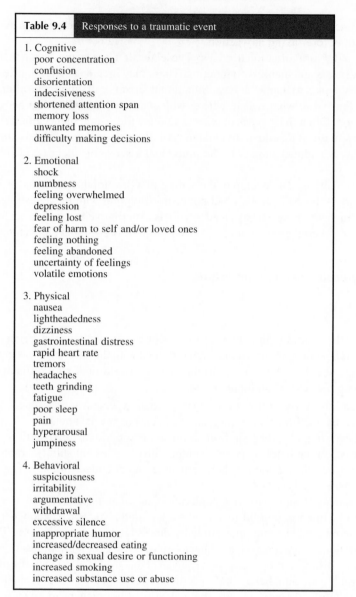

Table 9.4	Responses to a traumatic event

1. Cognitive
   poor concentration
   confusion
   disorientation
   indecisiveness
   shortened attention span
   memory loss
   unwanted memories
   difficulty making decisions

2. Emotional
   shock
   numbness
   feeling overwhelmed
   depression
   feeling lost
   fear of harm to self and/or loved ones
   feeling nothing
   feeling abandoned
   uncertainty of feelings
   volatile emotions

3. Physical
   nausea
   lightheadedness
   dizziness
   gastrointestinal distress
   rapid heart rate
   tremors
   headaches
   teeth grinding
   fatigue
   poor sleep
   pain
   hyperarousal
   jumpiness

4. Behavioral
   suspiciousness
   irritability
   argumentative
   withdrawal
   excessive silence
   inappropriate humor
   increased/decreased eating
   change in sexual desire or functioning
   increased smoking
   increased substance use or abuse

- Communicating, person to person rather than "expert" to "victim", using straightforward terms.

- Identifying specific concerns and attempting to help. Traumatized persons are often preoccupied with focused issues (e.g. "How do I know if my friends made it to the hospital?").

- Based on a review of the person's coping skills and strengths suggesting some or all of the following: keep to a usual routine, identify ways to relax, face situations, people and places that remind them of the traumatic event – and not to shy away, take the time to resolve day-to-day conflicts so they do not build up and add to their stress, identify sources of support including family and friends, and encourage talking about their experiences and feelings with friends, family, or other support networks (e.g. clergy and community centers).

Students who are victims of crime or who suffer injuries of any kind may develop post-traumatic stress disorder (PTSD). One goal of crisis intervention is to avoid the onset of a traumatic stress disorder which will be discussed later in this chapter.

9.3.2 The Suicidal Student

The emergence of suicidal thoughts and actions is a potentially life-threatening event, and therefore is categorized more as a psychological emergency than a crisis. However, a psychological emergency can arise in the context of a life crisis. So, it is incumbent upon the clinician helping the student in crisis to determine whether suicidal thinking or behavior is present and what crisis intervention tools and techniques need to be utilized to reduce the risk of ongoing suicidal thoughts and behavior.

Suicidal impulses and behaviors are largely temporal, transient, and situation-specific, except when the student has a history of being chronically suicidal [15]. Suicide intent is state-dependent and tends to wax and wane. Most people who die by suicide have given some prior warning or communicated their intent to others. Hence, the crisis clinician is in a pivotal, potentially life-saving, position. Fortunately, the symptoms of agitation, dysphoria, and the associated sense of urgency to act in a self-destructive and potentially life-ending manner usually subside with adequate time and protective intervention.

Crisis intervention and management approaches to the suicidal patient are designed to ensure the patient's safety and protect life until the precipitant crisis situation can be resolved with a return to precrisis equilibrium. The steps of crisis intervention might include [15]:

1. restricting access to lethal means

2. decreasing personal isolation

3. decreasing agitation, anxiety, or insomnia

4. increasing accessibility and frequency of contact with a health provider

5. establishing a collaborative, problem-solving focus to treatment fostering the patient's problem-solving skills

6. removal from stressful or toxic environments

7. system interventions to shift immediate dynamics contributing to the crisis

8. negotiating safety considerations and developing contingency plans

9. using hospitalization in cases of clear and imminent suicidal risk.

Unfortunately, many suicidal students present with underlying skill deficits in emotion regulation, distress intolerance, interpersonal dysfunction, impulsivity, problem-solving, and related cognitive distortion and rigidity which typically do not remit spontaneously even with crisis care. These issues and interpersonal deficits usually require appropriate clinical intervention and longer-term care [16], but getting the student through the crisis is the first step.

Table 9.5	General guidelines for working with suicidal students

Do's

1. Fully explore the presence of suicidal ideation. If you suspect that the student is potentially suicidal, don't take an initial "No" as evidence of not having suicidal thoughts or intent, because suicidal ideation and intent can fluctuate over time.
2. Discuss suicide and suicidal behaviors in a calm, self-assured manner
3. Acknowledge that the student may be ambivalent about dying and that they may be in a great deal of psychological pain and distress
4. Talk specifically about suicide, contemplating self-injury, death, and dying
5. Address the sense of hopelessness and despair often associated with suicidal thoughts and behaviors
6. Ask about prior episodes of suicidal ideation, intent or planning.
7. Determine if there is a history of prior suicidal attempts or self-harm
8. If there is a positive history of prior self-injurious behavior, fully explore each and every event, by exploring the "who, what, when, where, why, and how" of that episode, paying especially close attention to the circumstances, the events that precipitated the behavior, the degree of lethality involved, and the resolution ("Were you satisfied with the outcome?" "What did you learn from that experience?" "Are things better for you as a result of the incident?" "Are you sorry that you did not die as a result?" "What would you do differently if you were to attempt again?")
9. Determine whether the current situation is similar to, or different from, prior episodes
10. Explore the level of suicidal ideation, intent and planning (including writing or posting suicide notes on the internet)
11. Assess whether the student can implement the plan (e.g. has access to lethal means of suicide)
12. Determine whether there is an exacerbation of a psychiatric disorder or the onset of a psychiatric disorder
13. Determine whether the student is under the influence of a drug or alcohol
14. Remove or decrease agitation, anxiety, and sleep loss
15. Conduct an "environmental scan" – where does the student live, with whom does he/she live, who is in the support network
16. Assess for the safety of the student and for others involved with the student
17. Restrict access to means of death
18. Decrease the student's interpersonal isolation. Access the student's support network (with the student's permission)
19. Consult with colleagues about the best way to proceed
20. Determine whether the student is intoxicated or under the influence of a drug (including a potential overdose of prescribed medications)
21. Negotiate the establishment of a safety net, contingency plan, and/or safety protocol
22. Discuss available resources and options to consider, including temporary hospitalization until the clear and imminent suicide risk and crisis passes
23. Offer hope and collaboratively generate a course of action

Don'ts

1. Fail to identify the precipitating event in order to identify the context of, and specific triggers for, the suicidal behaviors.
2. Be passive. The clinician needs to be active, engaging, focused, and structured in eliciting the needed information upon which to determine a treatment plan.
3. Avoid an in-depth assessment of suicidal intent. ("It is what's underneath all this that is making you suicidal today, so let's talk about that instead".)
4. Minimize the seriousness of the situation (e.g. "Don't be upset, I'm sure that you'll feel better tomorrow".)
5. Provide superficial reassurance. A tendency to emphasize the positive aspects of a situation risks alienating the student in distress, implicitly rejects and contradicts a communication of anguish or hopelessness, and deepens feelings of isolation. ("But you have so much to live for". "Things can't possibly be all that bad".)
6. Criticize or demean the student for considering suicide as an option ("Most people wouldn't turn to suicide as a way of dealing with that problem".)
7. Argue with the student, especially regarding the decision to engage in suicidal activity
8. Engage in philosophical discussions about the meaning of life or the right to die. Acknowledging that the student always retains the right to die will often facilitate the consideration of other alternatives.
9. Engage in a "no-suicide contract".
10. Avoid the expression of painful affect. A retreat into intellectualization or premature advice-giving simultaneously avoids empathic understanding and models the containment of strong emotions. ("The best way to deal with this situation is to put you on medication".)
11. Be defensive about your own competence, ability to understand, and/or degree of caring. Suicidal students in crisis may be angry, outwardly hostile, distrustful, provocative, and help-rejecting. ("Well, no, I've never been suicidal myself, but I can still be of help to you".)
12. Promise that you will keep all information or discussions secret or confidential.
13. Leave the student alone until you are absolutely sure that the student is no longer actively or imminently suicidal.

The bottom line of crisis intervention with suicidal individuals involves assessing the prospect of "clear and imminent" danger. As discussed elsewhere [17], what exactly constitutes "clear and imminent" is both cloudy and time-indeterminate. Furthermore, Simon has presented an argument that "imminent" is a legal term but not a clinical term, and hence there is no agreed-upon definition of imminent risk [18]. Hence, clinicians must call upon their clinical judgment about the potential for physical danger within a short time frame. This is never easy or straight-forward. There is only one goal of crisis intervention when dealing with a suicidal individual: namely, to keep that individual physically safe and alive until the crisis situation has resolved.

Working with depressed and suicidal students can be frightening and difficult. Indeed, the assessment, treatment, and general management of an acute suicidal crisis are perhaps among the most difficult challenges faced by a mental health professional [15]. Often feelings of anxiety and helplessness can be evoked as the counselor addresses the student's desperation. The capacity to tolerate such intense affect and not overreact is in itself mutative.

There are some helpful guidelines in emergency interventions with suicidal students [19–21] and these are summarized in Table 9.5. They are based on the fundamental goal of keeping the student physically safe (and, of course, alive) until the crisis situation has resolved and the student is no longer actively suicidal [22]. If the suicidal crisis cannot be resolved in the counseling center, referral to a psychiatric emergency setting or an acute hospitalization may be required.

9.4 When Does a Crisis Become a Psychiatric Emergency?

A psychiatric emergency is defined as any unusual behavior, mood, or thought, which, if not rapidly attended to, may result in harm to the patient or to others [23]. In other words, an emergency is a life-threatening situation that demands an immediate response that is life-preserving. A crisis is not necessarily the same as an emergency, although by definition, if a crisis leads to a life threatening situation, it becomes an emergency. The challenge for the clinician is determining whether the response or reaction to the traumatic event or stress (the crisis) falls within the range of "expected" or "anticipated" responses for which the crisis intervention strategies outlined in this chapter are appropriate. If and when the level of pathology reaches a point where a new psychiatric disorder is diagnosed, the disorder must be treated (Table 9.6). If the crisis reaches the point of becoming a true life-threatening emergency, appropriate referrals must be made.

A common example to illustrate these points might be the student who has experienced the break-up of a romantic relationship. When he first comes to the counseling center, the day after the break-up, he is trying to cope with the loss of his girlfriend. His distress can be normalized and crisis intervention techniques employed. When he returns several weeks later and he is still not sleeping, has little appetite, has no interest in pleasurable activities, has no energy, and has failed a mid-term because of his inability to concentrate, a diagnosis of depression is made. He should be referred to a psychiatrist for assessment and probable antidepressant therapy. When he is seen again several weeks after starting an antidepressant, is still quite depressed and is now thinking constantly about suicide, stating he has no reason to go on, and admitting he stood on a highway

Table 9.6	Risk factors for long-term impairment following traumatic event

1. Proximity to the event. Closer exposure to actual event leads to greater risk (dose- response phenomenon)
2. Multiple stressors. More stress or an accumulation of stressors may create more difficulty
3. History of trauma (incest, and/or child physical, sexual or emotional abuse, interpersonal violence)
4. Meaning of the event in relation to past stressors. A traumatic event may activate unresolved fears or frightening memories
5. Chronic medical illnesses
6. Pre-existing psychological disorders
7. Family history of depression, psychosis, suicide, abuse (of all types), substance abuse
8. Instability of relationships at home or on campus

bridge for 15 minutes the night before trying to see what it might feel like to jump, he requires referral to an emergency service.

Although psychiatric emergencies often arise in the context of chronic psychiatric illness, they may also occur secondary to a medical condition, as a result of an adverse drug reaction or intoxication or drug-drug interaction, or as the result of being a victim of severe physical or emotional trauma. Some crises also develop in the context of a psychiatric emergency, for example a student who experiences new onset of psychotic symptoms may present in crisis because they have no mechanism to cope with the cognitive dysfunction. These individuals need psychiatric treatment as well as crisis intervention. Often the latter cannot proceed until psychotic thinking is resolved.

Glick and Schwartz [24] reviewed common reasons for college students to require psychiatric emergency care. These included:

- suicidal thoughts or behaviors

- depression and anxiety leading to acute symptoms requiring urgent treatment

- substance use/abuse issues

- psychosis

- adjustment issues accompanied by intense anxiety and dysphoria (crises as described in this chapter) occurring in settings or at times when no other mental health providers are available

- abnormal behavior that is overtly or perceived as threatening to others (stalking, verbal or physical threats).

Referral for emergency psychiatric care requires campus personnel to contact the psychiatric facility to assure coordination of services. This can be challenging because of privacy regulations, but also because of complicated bureaucratic structures on both campus and in the mental health system. The individual counselor or university administrator who is or becomes aware of the student's visit to the emergency department should work to assure the student that information will only be shared as it needs to be for his or her safety, but should push for this sharing of information. It also behooves the college administration to have processes and procedures in place ahead of a crisis or emergency, and to know the facilities and have contacts within the facilities at which students may be receiving care [25].

9.5 Disasters and Other Crises That Affect Multiple Students

Some events may lead to simultaneous crises in many students. Disasters (fires, attacks, mass shootings, earthquakes, other natural disasters) and events such as violent or unexpected deaths or accidents can all be considered potentially traumatic and may become the stimuli that set the stage for widespread stress and distress [25]. These events are characterized by a sense of horror, helplessness, serious injury, or the threat of serious injury or death. Traumatic events affect survivors, rescue workers, and friends and relatives of victims who have been directly involved, in addition to potentially affecting those who suffer injuries or losses, as well as those who have witnessed the event first-hand or through the media (e.g. television). Stress reactions following exposure to a traumatic event are very common.

The intensity of the impact of a disaster on an individual depends on the: (1) degree of personal loss (including injury to self, injury or death of loved ones, loss of home and/or job); (2) expected duration of the loss (short, long, irreversible); (3) victim's perception and interpretation of the loss; and (4) effects of terrifying and/or horrifying experiences.

Those exposed to traumatic events experience disruptions in reasonable mastery of their environments, in caring attachments to others, and in sustaining a purposeful meaning in life [26–28]. Almost all people who experience severe trauma will develop some symptoms after the event [29]. Common symptoms include:

- hypervigilance

- sleep disturbance

- intrusive recollections of the event

- tendency to withdraw from full participation in daily activities [26,30,31].

When these almost ubiquitous symptoms persist greater than a month in an individual who has experienced a trauma, the diagnosis of PTSD is made [32].

Individuals may be at increased risk for longer lasting reactions to traumatic events. Some factors that contribute to the risk of long-term impairment to traumatic events are listed in Table 9.6 and include: proximity to the event, presence of multiple stressors, history of trauma, activation of unresolved fears or frightening memories, and presence of chronic medical or psychological problems.

Research suggests that about 9% of those exposed to a traumatic event will develop PTSD [33]. Exposure to a traumatic stressor is a necessary, but not sufficient, condition for the development of a potentially disabling posttraumatic reaction. Some people have the ability to experience horrific events with little or no psychological sequelae. Studies of what leads to this resiliency are on-going with the goal of understanding who may be at greatest risk as well as assessing whether interventions can increase resiliency [34].

The challenge in the midst of a crisis is to determine who is at risk for developing a post-traumatic stress disorder and how to appropriately intervene to prevent this outcome. The belief that the traumatized person must relive and come to terms with the trauma emotionally as techniques such as critical incident stress debriefing (CISD) or critical incident stress management (CISM) espouse is now being questioned. Evidence suggests that at best this approach is not helpful, and at worst it may be harmful [35]. Instead "psychological firstaid", (http://www.ncptsd.va.gov/ncmain/ncdocs/manuals/nc_manual_psyfirstaid.html)

has become the recommended approach. This form of crisis intervention focuses not on the person re-living the emotions of the event, but rather on taking care of basic needs, such as shelter and finding whereabouts of loved ones, with a willingness to listen to the person's story if they choose to tell it.

Although there is no one single model for the provision of crisis intervention in disaster situations [36], many subscribe to general principles that alleviate the acute distress of individuals, restore independent functioning, and prevent or mitigate the aftermath of psychological trauma or development of PTSD [26,28]. Advice to traumatized individuals might include:

1. identifying specific worries and needs and resolving them

2. keeping to a usual routine

3. helping identify ways to relax

4. facing situations, people and places that remind them of the traumatic event and not to avoid or shy away from confronting or engaging

5. taking the time to resolve day-to-day conflicts so that they do not build up and add to their existing stress levels

6. identifying sources of support, including friends, family, and clergy, and encouraging talking about their experiences and feelings with them.

9.5.1 Counseling Center Role in Crisis Response

Mental health clinicians will be asked to play a crucial role in the event of a disaster or an event that impacts more than one student on campus. Just as no two disasters or traumatic events are exactly the same, no two campuses have the same student body, history, values, and resources. However, some basic roles and functions that mental health professionals and counseling centers may play during campus-wide crises will be delineated.

Often clinicians must deal with upset students who are in various stages of grief and bereavement: shock, denial, dismay, anger, and so on. What is often not openly addressed is that counseling personnel are called in because the administrators, faculty and staff are ill-equipped to handle the students and/or are themselves having similar reactions as the students and also need support.

The first order of business is to identify who are the clients and what are their needs – and the list may well go beyond the students themselves. The second task is to mobilize and organize a response. This often takes the form of making multiple therapists available on short notice to accommodate requests for interventions. It is often better for at least one mental health specialist to go to the "scene", and stay there as long as possible. In most circumstances, students prefer to be supported in their familiar environments – classrooms, dormitories, apartments, fraternity houses, and even at sports team meetings.

The mental health professional must operate on at least two conceptual levels. The first is not to be "clinical" or play the role of a therapist. The first order of business is to identify those exposed to the event and provide them with good crisis intervention. Table 9.7 outlines a basic approach to helping the student who is traumatized. The goal is to accept individuals wherever they may be in their response to the event, acknowledge their reactions, and

Table 9.7	Response to incidents affecting multiple students

1. When you arrive in the scene of a crisis or emergency situation (man-made, natural, or otherwise), you need to take charge if you are the designated professional. You need to be directive, but calm and reassuring
2. Remain calm, clear, and decisive
3. Assess if related parties also need assistance and respond to them
4. Speak clearly, at a moderate pace, in a normal tone, with appropriate eye contact.
5. Try to develop and establish trust with the affected individuals
6. Be prepared to make decisions for the "victims" and to serve as a role model
7. Don't offer false assurances or theories or best guesses (you can't guarantee that you have all the answers or that you can predict the future)
8. Identify and reinforce the student's prior successful coping strategies
9. Work on collaborative problem-solving, not on analysis or therapy
10. Work towards the student regaining and retaining "power" or "control" over his/her setting and self
11. Don't take sides or assign blame
12. Avoid discussions about "ideal situations" or "what might have been"
13. Don't argue if the student is criticizing you, something you said, or the failure of the college or university to protect them from this situation
14. Enter into a dialog about the best way to proceed, being respectful and attentive, although cognizant that your objective perceptive may well be the best way to proceed
15. Define actions, goals, and solutions
16. Ensure that goals are achievable and time-limited
17. Do not say that you will keep information secret or confidential if it potentially affects the health and welfare of the individuals involved
18. Mobilize support from natural support networks

normalize their responses. The second task is to identify those other students (as well as faculty, staff, and administration) who might be adversely affected by the event and reach out to them in a clinical and therapeutic manner. This may take the form of a mental health clinic staff meeting with staff to identify current or past clientele likely to be affected by the event, and reach out to them in a professional manner. It may also take the form of discreetly suggesting to a member of the faculty, staff, or administration that it would benefit them if they engaged in some crisis intervention work themselves.

Mental health professionals may be called by the school newspaper or the local media to provide commentary on the event, how it has changed life on campus, or what is being done to ensure that it won't happen again. Although we all enjoy seeing our names in print or being on television, we caution you about entertaining such public opportunities. Your statements may be taken out of context or shortened to "sound bites" that do not reflect your thoughts or opinions. Most colleges have a public relations officer or a designated administrator who handles press releases. Defer to them whenever you are approached by the media – no matter how innocuous the questions or requests may seem to be, or how engaging or non-threatening are the media representatives.

Another cause for caution in speaking to media about a public or community disaster or traumatic event is the tendency for both speaker and listener to "fill in the blanks", especially as it relates to questions of why someone died by suicide, or speculate why a certain traumatic event occurred. Often these crises become public and may involve police investigations, so you need to think long and hard about sharing theories and hypotheses, for you may be quoted by others based on what they think they heard you say.

The mental health clinician should not take charge of the situation. Unless you are the only official present at the scene of the crisis, it is always better to defer to the designated staff or administrator. Why? Because it is the college that must "own the crisis" and reassure its students and faculty that they are investigating the event and are taking steps to ensure that it won't occur again. Rarely do campus clinicians have the authority or responsibility to speak on behalf of the college. Often crises require the coordination and intervention of many different components of the university, and only a designated official should be making those decisions. Furthermore, students and others affected will be watching to see who and how things are being handled, and so it is always preferable for an administrator or senior staff member to be in charge.

Timing is crucial. The best way to assure that a mental health response will be rapid is to have it planned out ahead of time. University officials must be educated about the role crisis intervention can play in responding to emergencies and in preventing long term psychological impact. Mental health providers must have a seat at the table as pre-disaster planning occurs. This allows development of working relationships with other important offices on the campus that may be called upon to assist when a disaster does occur. It also helps assure that if an event does occur, rapid mobilization of mental health personnel can occur in an organized way.

9.6 Working with Campus Leadership to Prevent Crisis and Improve Mental Health

In 2006, The Jed Foundation, a foundation dedicated to improving college student mental health and preventing college student suicides, published a "Framework for Developing Institutional Protocols for the Acutely Distressed or Suicidal College Student" to assist colleges and universities in developing and revising protocols suitable for their unique campus environment [37].

The Framework document does not prescribe policies, protocols, processes, or procedures, but rather outlines a list of issues to consider when drafting or revising protocols relating to the management of the student in acute distress or at risk for suicide. By developing protocols in a methodical manner prior to crisis situations, it is hoped that the need for *ad hoc* decision-making during a crisis is greatly minimized. Furthermore, these protocols should remain broad enough to cover many potential crisis situations while at the same time allowing flexibility for application to individual cases. Furthermore the protocols emphasize how decisions are made and by whom. The three areas that the document addresses are: (1) developing a safety protocol; (2) developing an emergency contact notification protocol; and (3) developing a leave of absence and re-entry protocol.

Mental health professionals need to be involved in these matters, if for no other reason than to provide their expertise as consultants and advisors (if not as integral members of the response teams themselves). Often it is the campus mental health professionals who appropriately are lobbying for the establishment of such working groups and development of applicable protocols to address emergencies on campus.

The Jed Foundation emphasizes that suicidal and acutely distressed students are not only a clinical issue, but also a public health (or environmental) issue. Hence this necessitates a shift from prevention and treatment at the individual level to prevention and treatment at the community level. Prevention of self-injurious behaviors and situations that may induce crises are the responsibility of mental health professionals and the entire campus community. A comprehensive effort to confront the problems of suicide and distressed and distressing students should include three parts – prevention, intervention, and postvention. The "Framework" uses the following example to illustrate how planning around one component impacts the planning (and effectiveness) of the other two components. "For example, programming that targets the friends of a student who had died by suicide could both identify someone at heightened risk for suicide (intervention) and encourage

Table 9.8	Examples of prevention, intervention, and postvention efforts

Prevention
1. Creating a mental health task force to develop and implement a campus-wide suicide prevention and mental health promotion plan
2. Raising awareness among students, parents, faculty, and staff about the signs and symptoms of mental illness and the risk factors for suicide and other self-injurious behaviors
3. Restricting access to lethal means of self-harm
4. Offering programs aimed at strengthening life skills (e.g. outreach programs)
5. Matching the mental health resources on campus to the demand for services

Intervention
1. Establishing a case management committee to monitor students of concern
2. Developing formalized crisis management protocols, including those for emergency contact notification and medical leave and re-entry
3. Providing accessible and effective mental health services

Postvention
1. Promoting responsible reporting by the media
2. Providing outreach programs and mental health resources to those students, staff, faculty, and others affected by a suicide, suicide attempt, or crisis event on campus (e.g. community support meetings)

Adapted and Modified from The Jed Foundation, 2006 [37].

help-seeking in others prior to an emotional crisis (prevention)". (pp. 4–5) Table 9.8 provides some possible efforts associated with each component.

Many common crises could have been avoided if the student had addressed the problem(s) at the time they first appeared. Here we are thinking about failed examinations, lower course grades than expected/anticipated, interpersonal conflicts (roommates, significant others, teammates), financial aid, selecting academic majors, and career choices. For the older graduate school population we can add: marital and relationship difficulties, dysfunctional mentoring relationships, failure of a research endeavor, change of career focus, financial support, lack of jobs after graduation, and dismissal from the graduate program for lack of academic progress or poor grades [38].

There are common problems that exist on many campuses that can potentially aggravate the development, onset, and maintenance of student crises. These include:

- insufficient resources and funds to address the development of crisis protocols

- lack of wellness programs and outreach activities

- inadequate effort to de-stigmatize mental health issues

- absence of ongoing dialog with local community entities who could potentially be involved in caring for a student at risk (e.g. local police, emergency department staff, community mental health providers)

- improper training of staff and faculty in identifying students at risk and providing them with tools and techniques for appropriate referral; of at risk students.

9.7 Conclusion

To paraphrase Shneidman [39], in the last analysis, the prevention of suicide and other crisis situations are everyone's business. If we truly believe this to be so, than this scenario on a college campus might look something like the following:

1. immediate access to emotional support

2. programs "destigmatizing" mental illness and emotional distress

3. education of the campus community about the warning signs and risk factors for self-injurious behaviors

4. education of campus faculty and staff about identification, initial intervention, consultation, and appropriate referral for students at risk

5. development, implementation and distribution of a crisis intervention manual or brochure for faculty, staff, and students with definitions, available resources, websites, telephone numbers, e-mail addresses, and so on

6. access to comprehensive mental health services

7. adequately trained mental health professionals

8. development of a campus-wide student crisis response team that works with a student concerns committee that tracks potentially volatile situations and violent students

9. development and implementation of a crisis response protocol within the counseling center

10. identification of key individuals on campus (e.g. Chief of Police, Dean of Students, etc.) responsible for carrying out a crisis intervention protocol in situations deemed necessary (e.g. natural disaster, man-made disaster, sudden deaths of students, etc.)

11. involvement of students, community leaders, parents, and interested parties in developing protocols and procedures to protect and support students on campus

12. development, implementation, maintainance, enhancement, and celebration of appropriate student and faculty coping and life skills

13. encouragement and enforcement of a culturally-sensitive and civil campus community

14. provision of role models of healthy functioning and problem solving.

References

1. Richardson, V.E. (1995) Crisis intervention in contemporary society: Contributions from critical theory. *Crisis Intervention*, **1**(3), 177–189.
2. Dixon, S. (1987) *Working with People in Crisis*, 2nd edn, Merrill Press, Columbus, OH.
3. Caplan, G. (1961) *An Approach to Community Mental Health*, Grune & Stratton, New York.
4. Gordon, C. (1994) Crisis intervention: A general approach, in *Manual of Psychiatric Emergencies*, 3rd edn (eds S.E. Hyman and G.E. Tesar), Little, Brown and Company, Boston, MA, pp. 12–18.
5. Lindemann, E. (1944) Symptomology and management of acute grief. *American Journal of Psychiatry*, **101**, 141–148.
6. Horowitz, M.J. (1976) *Stress Response Syndromes*. Jason Aaronson, New York.
7. Bloom, M. and Klein, W.C. (1995) Crisis prevention and crisis treatment. *Crisis Intervention*, **1**(3), 167–176.

8. Caplan, G. (1964) *Principles of Preventive Psychiatry*, Basic Books, New York.

9. Quinnett, P. (2006) The QPR Theory Paper, http://www.qprinstitute.com/.

10. LivingWorks (2009) ASIST Program. Accessed at: www.livingworks.net.

11. Doherty, G.W. and O'Dochartaigh Associates (2000) Crisis intervention training for disaster workers. Accessed at: www.angeklfire.com/biz2/dmhs/crisis.html.

12. University of Wisconsin Oshkosh (2008) *How to Help a Student in Crisis*, Counseling Center, Oshkosh, WI.

13. Roberts, A.R. (1991) Conceptualizing crisis theory and the crisis intervention model, in *Contemporary Perspectives on Crisis Intervention and Prevention*, (ed. A. R. Roberts), Prentice-Hall, Englewood Cliffs, NJ, pp. 3–17.

14. Callahan, J. (1998) Crisis theory and crisis intervention in emergencies, in *Emergencies in Mental Health Practice: Evaluation and Management* (ed. P.M. Kleespies), The Guilford Press, New York, pp. 22–40, Chapter 2.

15. Berman, A.L., Jobes, D.A., and Silverman, M.M. (2006) *Adolescent Suicide: Assessment and Intervention*, 2nd edn, American Psychological Association Press, Washington, DC.

16. Rudd, M.D. (1998) An integrative, conceptual, and organizational framework for treating suicidal behavior. *Psychotherapy: Theory, Research, Practice, Training*, **35**, 346–360.

17. Jobes, D.A. and Maltsberger, J.T. (1995) The hazards of treating suicidal patients, in *A Perilous Calling: The Hazards of Psychotherapy Practice* (ed. M.B. Sussman), Wiley, New York.

18. Simon, R.I. (2006) Imminent suicide: The illusion of short-term prediction. *Suicide and Life-Threatening Behavior*, **36**(3), 296–301.

19. Cimbolic, P. and Jobes, D.A. (1990) *Youth Suicide: Assessment, Intervention, and Issues*, Charles C. Thomas, Springfield, IL.

20. Jobes, D.A. and Berman, A.L. (1993) Suicide and malpractice liability: Assessing and revising policies, procedures, and practice in outpatient settings. *Professional Psychology: Research and Practice*, **24**, 91–99.

21. Niemeyer, R.A. and Pfeffer, A.M. (1994) Evaluation of suicide intervention effectiveness. *Death Studies*, **18**, 131–166.

22. Maris, R.W., Berman, A.L. and Silverman, M.M. (2000) *Comprehensive Textbook of Suicidology*, The Guilford Press, New York.

23. Fauman, B.J. (2000) Other psychiatric emergencies, in *Kaplan & Sadock's Comprehensive Textbook of Psychiatry*, 7th edn, vol. **2** (eds B.J. Sadock and V.A. Sadock), Lippincott Williams & Wilkins, New York, pp. 2040–2042, Chapter 29.2.

24. Glick, R.L. and Schwartz, V. (2007) Collegiate mental health: Assessment and management: Special considerations for college students in psychiatric crisis. *Psychiatric Issues in Emergency Care Settings*, **6**(4), 7–13.

25. Flannery, R.B. Jr and Everly, G.S. Jr (2000) Crisis intervention: A review. *International Journal of Emergency Mental Health*, **2**(2), 119–125.

26. Flannery, R.B. Jr (1994) *Post-Traumatic Stress Disorder: The Victim's Guide to Healing and Recovery*, Crossroad Press, New York.

27. Raphael, B. (1986) *When Disaster Strikes: A Handbook for the Caring Professions*, Hutchison, London.

28. Wollman, D. (1993) Critical Incident Stress Debriefing and crisis groups: A review of the literature. *Group*, **17**, 70–83.

29. Connor, K.M., Foa, E.B., and Davidson, J.R.T. (2006) Practical assessment and evaluation of mental health problems following a mass disaster. *Journal of Clinical Psychiatry*, **67**(suppl 2), 26–33.

30. Flannery, R.B. Jr (1995) *Violence in the Workplace*, Crossroad Press, New York.

31. Mitchell, J.T. and Everly, G.S. Jr (1996) *Critical Incident Stress debriefing (CISD): An Operations Manual for the Prevention of Traumatic Stress Among Emergency Services and Disaster Workers*, Chevron, Ellicott City, MD.

32. American Psychiatric Association (2000) *The diagnostic and statistical manual of mental disorders (IV-TR)*, American Psychiatric Press, Washington, DC.
33. US Department of HHS (2000) *Mental Health: A Report of the Surgeon General*, Government Printing Service, Rockville, MD.
34. Connor, K.M. and Davidson, J.R.T. (2003) Development of a new resilience scale: the connor-davidson resilience scale (CD-RISC). *Depression and Anxiety*, **18**, 76–82.
35. Foa, E.B., Cahill, S.P., Boscarino, J.A. *et al.* (2005) Social, psychological, and psychiatric interventions following terrorist attacks: recommendations for practice and research. *Neuropsychpharmacology*, **30**, 1806–1817.
36. Jacobson, G., Strickler, M. and Morley, W. (1998) General and individual approaches to crisis intervention. *American Journal of Public Health*, **58**, 338–343.
37. The Jed Foundation (2006) *Framework for Developing Institutional Protocols for the Acutely Distressed or Suicidal College Student*, The Jed Foundation, New York, NY.
38. The Jed Foundation (2008) *Student Mental Health and the Law: A Resource for Institutions of Higher Education*, The Jed Foundation, New York, NY.
39. Shneidman, E.S. (1985) *Definition of Suicide*, Jason Aronson, Inc., London.

10 Working with Parents and Families of Young Adults

Kristine A. Girard

Massachusetts Institute of Technology, Harvard Medical School, Cambridge, MA, USA

10.1 Introduction

The adjustment to college provides a normal developmental opportunity for young adults in their drive towards autonomy and self-reliance which tests their coping skills and resilience. Psychological and neurological development, generational influences, the style of parental attachment, family system dynamics, temperament as well as parental and societal expectations color the negotiation of this complex transition. Given the demands of adult life, young adults face an exciting yet stressful period at the time of life when serious mental illnesses including schizophrenia, bipolar disorder, major depression and substance use disorders, often first present. According to longitudinal analysis, the suicide rate for young adults rose markedly between the 1950s and 1980s to 12.5/100 000 for the 15–25-year-old age group, remained fairly stable through the 1990s and has declined modestly since then [1–3]. Despite the recent decline, suicide remains the second leading cause of death for college students, accounting for an estimated 1100 deaths per year [4].

The National College Health Association Surveys (NCHA) of college students over the past several years consistently report suicidal ideation in the 9–10% range with a majority of students indicating periods of hopelessness, feeling overwhelmed and depressed mood sufficient to affect their studies. When asked to whom they turn for help, college students rate peers first and parents second with mental health professionals trailing far behind (NCHA). Thus, an effective strategy to minimize health and safety risks for young adults is working effectively with their parents who remain a primary support resource. As university mental health clinicians work with millennial generation students, studies of generational attitudes suggest that clinicians need to please not only the students but also their parents given the very active role that millennial parents have played in their lives [5,6]. Working effectively with parents requires understanding and successful negotiation of the privacy regulations governing the sharing of information within heath care, the Health Information Portability and Accountability Act (HIPAA), and within higher education, the Federal Education Rights and Privacy Act (FERPA). Within this privacy framework and with a community systems consultation liaison approach, mental health clinicians can incorporate evidence based

Mental Health Care in the College Community   Edited by Jerald Kay and Victor Schwartz
© 2010 John Wiley & Sons, Ltd.

education models and prevention strategies to strengthen the care that they provide for students in their educational community. This chapter will provide a summary of pertinent research related to young adult development, generational attitudes, cultural influences, family system dynamics and privacy regulations, using case examples to introduce guidelines on how to work effectively with students and their families in the higher education setting.

10.2 Young Adult Development

Cognitive, social, and emotional development continues during the college years as evidenced by both psychological and neurological changes. Eric Erikson introduced the psychosocial perspective in his 1959 seminal work, *Identity and the Life Cycle* [7], and further elucidated his theories in his 1985 *Childhood and Society* [8]. Erikson described the life cycle as composed of eight phases of life, each characterized by a central psychological conflict while not confined exclusively to that particular phase of life. According to Erikson, successful negotiation of each of the successive psychological conflicts was essential for the development of a healthy, fully integrated individual. Using Erikson's schema, one would expect young adults to be consolidating the work of adolescence, identity versus role confusion, actively working through the central conflict of young adulthood, intimacy verses isolation, and beginning the work of adulthood, generativity versus self-absorption. While research since Erikson has built on his life stage model, particularly in the areas of moral development [9], cognitive development [10] and key aspects of identity [11,12], the central themes in Erikson's life stage model remain evident in clinical work with young adults.

An exciting area of research is the study of the changes in the brains of pre-adolescents, adolescents and young adults in efforts to better understand both normal development and the neuroscientific correlates to pathophysiology. Magnetic resonance imaging (MRI) studies of brain maturation during the adolescent years have shown increases in total brain volume, particularly in the frontal lobes, correlated with measures of cognitive functioning [13–16]. Studies of the tissue density changes in young adult brains show patterns consistent with findings observed post-mortem with myelination and pruning [17,18]. Review of the neuronal findings along with studies of social behavioral changes reveals a growing convergence of evidence supporting a relationship between brain physiology and the developmental changes in social behavior, the social information processing network [19–29]. Longitudinal studies to assess patterns of development in resiliency from childhood through young adulthood interestingly show the most dramatic changes in measures of adaptation occurring during the period of emerging adulthood [30–34]. Young adults enter college at a uniquely crucial and vulnerable stage of life, coming with variable maturational capacities for encoding and managing an increasingly complex social environment and a range of practical life skills. Thus, university administrators face the dilemma of balancing parental expectations for safety with a level of autonomy to allow for age appropriate personal growth and risk taking at a time of ongoing neurodevelopment and shifting societal and generational influences.

10.3 Generational Effects

Universities are charged with the task of creating a learning environment both conducive to the learning needs of its students and to maintaining the academic integrity of their faculty and institution. Since typically a generation gap exists between academic faculty and students, systems may particularly notice the influence of generational attitudes when a new generational cohort has entered that system such as the millennial generation (born between 1982 and 2005) who have recently entered the higher education system [35]. College environments that have developed operational procedures which smoothly handled the baby boomer generation (born between 1943 and 1960) and generation X (born 1961–1981) may find their systems taxed by this large millennial cohort. Neil Howe and William Strauss, authors of *Millennials Rising: The Next Great Generation* (2000) [36], among other books, describe generations as "among the most powerful forces in history", noting that "tracking their match through time lends order – and even a measure of predictability – to long-term trends". ([36] *Harvard Business Review* p1) Although researchers of generational effects generally agree on each generation's core characteristics, the inclusion year cutoffs vary among researchers by roughly 3–4 years [5,6,38]. It is also important to remember that specific individuals do not fully embody all of the characteristics of their generation. However, for those providing mental health care in a university environment, understanding the generational characteristics of students and their parents helps to inform strategies for outreach, treatment and work with families.

10.4 The Baby Boomers

Generational attitudes are formed as historical events and the national mood affect individuals differently depending upon their stage of life when the events occur [37]. For example, baby boomers born between 1943 and 1960, now approximately age 49–65 and 78 million strong, represent the largest proportion of academic faculty and parents of current college students. As children working through Erikson's childhood stages of life focused on building *trust, autonomy, initiative and industry*, the boomers were raised largely in traditional families during a time of post-War optimism. Historic events such as the invention of the television and man traveling to the moon reinforced their belief in the possible through initiative and hard work. Baby boomers tend to be optimistic, political, respect experience, live to work and want recognition for their efforts [5]. During adolescence while working to develop a cohesive sense of identity, they encountered McCarthyism, civil rights unrest, the assassination of John F. Kennedy and the beginning of the Vietnam War, which fueled their sense of selves as political advocates and reformers. As college students, the baby boomers staged protests, expected to be heard by the university leadership, demanded expanded freedoms and saw themselves as accountable only to themselves. This baby boomer generation no longer accepted the then prevailing *in loco parentis* doctrine which legally viewed the university as a substitute family for the young adults in their charge. As adults, baby boomers have used their initiative and hard work to advocate, designating themselves as arbiters of the nation's values within a breadth of fields [37] including issues related to the health, education and safety of children. The *Wall Street Journal* observed in a 1990 piece, "It is college presidents, deans, and faculties – not students – who are the zealots and chief enforcers of Political Correctness". As parents, they have developed close relationships with their children, maintain more frequent communication as compared to previous generations, in part related to advances in telecommunications, and tend to be more present and involved with the lives of their young adults in college than previous generations. For baby boomers, their children represent a central aspect of their life's work, one to which they have invested emotion, time, aspirational hopes and resources – a cause worth advocating for potentially to the point of hovering.

10.5 Generation X

Generation X including those born 1961–1981, now aged approximately 27–47, are a relatively smaller group at 47 million and include graduate students, junior faculty and a small portion of undergraduate parents. As children, this group grew up during an economic decline with mothers who entered the workplace before child care was widely available and in an era of failing schools and marriages [37]. The more pessimistic historic climate influenced this generation of children, as they worked through Erikson's childhood issues (trust, autonomy, initiative and industry), to distrust institutions including families, corporations and politicians. As adolescents, they lived with the impact of divorce and the sexual revolution, negotiating the consolidation of their identities in a world with higher crime, increased teen pregnancy and acquired immune deficiency syndrome (AIDS). Not surprisingly, generation X incorporated cynicism, pragmatism and self-reliance into their sense of identity [5]. While higher education institutions may have been bothered by the cynical attitude of generation X, administrators likely also noticed their self-reliance, limited expectations for caretaking and relatively uninvolved parents. Following the shift away from the *in loco parentis* doctrine during the 1960s, the self-reliant attitude of generation X put little pressure on institutions to deviate from the status quo that had worked for the baby boomer collegiate. As adults, generation X value freedom and time, preferring free agency over corporate loyalty. Many of them have begun to develop the strong families that they longed for in childhood [37]. One can begin to see that the cycle of generational attitudes is far from random, but rather a macro-model of family systems dynamics that mental health clinicians routinely encounter. The historic events and climate which affect generational groups during key developmental stages cause large scale shifts in work place attitudes, life approach, sources of meaning and parenting which in turn influences the next generation.

10.6 The Millennial Generation

The millennial generation includes those born 1982–2005, now aged 3–26. They are largest generational group at 80 million strong, the most culturally diverse cohort and make up the majority of the student body at universities currently [6]. As children, they have grown up during a technological boom with protective baby boomer parents and affirming teachers, kept busy in scheduled activities by parents involved with their lives [5,6]. Recalling the Eriksonian tasks of childhood, the millennials have learned to trust grown-ups and institutions, and to socialize and work in groups. Coming of age in a post 9/11 era at a time of economic crisis, the millennial generation identity has incorporated concerns about safety, civic mindedness and risk management. They value loyalty, work-life balance, technology and team work [5,37]. In contrast to generation X, millennial college students trust rather than feel cynicism for large institutions and expect institutions to provide clear expectations, community standards and care-taking. University systems designed to work well for the baby boomers who demanded freedom and autonomy or for the pragmatic and self reliant generation X work less well for millennials who expect university administrators and faculty to provide clear goals, affirming support and ongoing, involved interaction. As the millennial generation has moved into the workplace, they have been viewed as trusting and teachable, but also more pampered, risk averse, and dependent [35]. It is ironic that it is the same baby boomer generation who railed against the *in loco parentis* doctrine in the 1960s who now expect greater institutional caretaking for their legally emancipated young

Table 10.1	Generational profiles			
	Veterans **1922–1945** **55 Million**	**Baby boomers** **1946–1964** **78 million**	**Generation X** **1965–1980** **47 million**	**Millennium** **1981–2000** **80 million**
Style	traditional	personal satisfaction	self-reliant	modern traditional
Size	rapidly declining	dominant	small group	large
Ethic	respect, loyalty	ambitious, political	progressive, cynical	loyal, conservative
Gender Role	classic gender roles	mixing gender roles	unclear	gone
Work	respect for system work for security	respect experience likes to work	respect expertise work to live	work to live
Heroes	strong heroes	some heroes	no heroes	anti-heroes
Seminal Events	Depression, WWII	Vietnam, BCP	weak USA	9–11
Upbringing	traditional family	traditional family	absenteeism parents	protective parents
Reward	a job well done	money, title, recognition	freedom, time	work

Data source: Zemke R *et al. Generations at Work.* American Management Association, New York, 2000 [5].

adult children. The generational attitudes of both millennial students and their baby boomer parents are aligned such that university administrators and clinicians should expect greater family involvement which puts pressure on universities to develop an institutional understanding of FERPA and procedures to negotiate family involvement when serious behavioral, psychological, disciplinary and/or academic concerns present (Table 10.1).

10.7 Privacy Standards in Higher Education

Universities struggle with developing procedures that both respect the privacy of students while appropriately involving parents as part of the students' support network. The Family Education Rights and Privacy Act (FERPA) applies to university employees and restricts disclosure of student educational records to parents. However, there is an explicit exception to allow for "disclosure reasonably directed toward avoiding harm to the student or others". In December 2008, the Department of Education published its Family Education Rights and Privacy Final Rule to further clarify the FERPA rules and regulations. In this report, the health and safety exception was further amended to include a provision stating, "if an educational agency or institution determines that there is an articulable and significant threat to the health or safety of a student or other individual, it may disclose the information to any person, including parents, whose knowledge of the information is necessary to protect the health or safety of the student or other individuals". Clinicians are generally expected to follow strict patient confidentially as outlined in the Health Insurance Portability and Accountability Act (HIPAA) if their facility collects fees or electronically submit insurance claims, or similarly restrictive state privacy statues and codes of ethics for clinical disciplines. Many university health services do not bill or electronically submit insurance claims, and are therefore not regulated under HIPAA. University administrators not only may notify parents under FERPA when there are circumstances that significantly threaten the health and welfare of their college students, but according to the added FERPA provision are given further latitude and encouragement to do so. Procedures to allow for coordination of care around high risk students and guidelines for notification of parents can help to ease anxiety when crisis situations present.

A June 2007 report from the Family Policy Compliance Office (FPCO) provided additional reassurance to higher education personnel who share information with parents.

As an office within the Department of Education, the mission of the FPCO is to meet the needs of learners of all ages by effectively implementing two laws that seek to ensure student and parental rights in education: FERPA and the Protection of Pupil Rights Amendment (PPRA), (Department of Education FPCO web site 2007 [39]). The FPCO report noted, "Nothing in FERPA prohibits a teacher or other official from letting a parent know of their concern about their son or daughter that is based on their personal knowledge or observation". Recalling that FERPA pertains only to educational records, sharing by university personnel of their personal observations about concerning behavior or inter-personal interactions, with support personnel including mental health clinicians promotes early case finding and treatment, important in crisis prevention. The December 2008 FERPA Final Rule further clarified sharing in relation to behavior including records held by university disciplinary departments noting, "Investigative reports and other reports created by an institution's law enforcement unit are excluded from the definition of education records under § 99.3 and, therefore, are not subject to FERPA requirements". Development of FERPA training and procedures for university employees are essential to dispel myths and decrease barriers for appropriate sharing with parents, student support personnel and university health services. Use of social support networks, training, community leadership endorsement and policies/procedures to promote coordinated risk management planning have been shown to decrease self and other directed violence [40–42]. See also Tables 10.2 and 10.3.

Table 10.2	Family Education Rights and Privacy Act (FERPA): exceptions when disclosing allowed without consent
School officials with legitimate educational interest Other schools to which student is transferring Specialized officials for audit or evaluation purposes Grades on peer-graded papers before they are collected and recorded by a teacher High schools and postsecondary institutions with dually-enrolled students Appropriate parties in connection with financial aid to a student Information returned to the party identified as its source Directory information not including social security numbers Organizations conducting certain studies for or on behalf of the school Accrediting organizations To comply with a judicial order or lawfully issued subpoena Appropriate officials in cases of health and safety emergencies State and local authorities, within a juvenile justice system, pursuant to a specific law	

Data source: http://www.ed.gov/policy/gen/guid/fpco/ferpa/index.html; Office of Planning, Evaluation, and Policy Development, Department of Education. (Dec 2008) Rules and Regulations. *Federal Register*, 73(237): 74806–74855 [54].

Table 10.3	Material excluded from educational record and not protected under FERPA
Personally identifiable information related sole to a student's activities as an alumnus of an institution Education record for student who is claimed as a dependant for Federal income tax purposes by either parent Personal observations of university personnel Information from law enforcement unit records to anyone, including local police and other law enforcement authorities Information concerning registered sex offenders provided to the educational agency or institution under state and Federal guidelines Student medical and psychological treatment records made, maintained, and used only in connection with treatment	

10.8 Influence of Case Law on Privacy

Societal change in the medical–legal climate with increased litigiousness and generational influences contribute to the complexity of decision making for higher education administrators. Recent cases challenge the traditional expectations about who assumes the risk of college life [43]. Are students responsible for adverse consequences of impulsive, immature, or even illegal choices? Or is the college institution responsible for an adverse outcome by virtue of creating a campus environment that allows for an impulsive, immature, or illegal choice to occur? Higher education cases involving Ferrum College 2002 [44], Massachusetts Institute of Technology 2005 [45], Allegheny College 2006 and Clark University 2007, reviewed more comprehensively in Chapter 7 on law and ethics, bring into question whether non-clinicians such as administrative deans and campus residence staff legally have a special relationship that charges them with a duty to protect students with whom they live or work. The plaintiffs in these cases attempted to expand the legal duty to warn and protect which has heretofore been reserved for clinicians in their work with patients when knowledge exists regarding an imminent risk for harm to a specific party. The 2006 Allegheny College jury ruling that no "special relationship" existed for the university administrators and the 2007 Massachusetts court dismissal of a wrongful death case involving the death of a student by heroin overdose at Clark University denying the existence of a duty to protect students from illegal drug use provide some reassurance for college administrators that courts seem to be limiting the expansion of the duty to protect.

10.9 Privacy Meets Generational Attitudes

As previously discussed, generational attitudes influence today's parents as they have increased expectation for the university to ensure the safety of their young adult sons or daughters which stretches the more traditional expectation for institutions of higher learning. As college students, the baby boomer generation highly valued their autonomy, protested intrusions from authority figures such as university administrators and demanded to be treated as legal adults. Their attitudes around independence and free choice contributed to erosion of the *in loco parentis* doctrine during the 1960s. As the baby boomers came of age, societal beliefs around individual responsibility equally supported the view of college students as legal adults where young adults were expected to manage the stresses associated with the transition to college, even if that burden of stress was high [43]. As adults, baby boomers continue to view themselves as arbiters of the nation's values within a breadth of fields [37], now advocating for increased legal protections and assurances related to the safety of their young adult children.

Compared to previous generations, these parents expect more caretaking of their college student including clinging to the false hope for a guarantee of safety. Rather than experiencing involvement of authority figures as intrusive, the societal perspective has shifted such that authority figures are now expected to provide a variety of systems including education, health care, national defense and social security. Thus, the safety of young adults leads baby boomer parents and higher education administrators to re-examine the balance between young adult autonomy. Parents expect universities to maintain tighter control and have greater expectation for involvement of faculty, administrators and clinicians. And millennial students described as risk averse and dependent [37] may experience involvement by authority figures as familiar and in keeping with the clear guidelines with which they have been raised. While university clinicians are encouraged to routinely explore to what extent each particular case reflects the generational attitudes, the dimensional characteristics of millennial students and their baby boomer parents will tend to promote greater collaboration with parents and consultation-liaison to university personnel.

10.10 Privacy in the Transition from Secondary Schools to Higher Education

Understanding FERPA regulations around the transfer of educational records between schools provides an additional opportunity for the university health service to enhance optimal coordination and continuity of care. Understandably, young adults and their families are reluctant to disclose information about the mental health history during the admission process. The December 2008 FERPA Final Rule clarifies:

> medical and psychological treatment records of eligible students are excluded from the definition of education records if they are made, maintained, and used only in connection with treatment, including treatment providers at the student's new school.

In practical terms, this means that "after a student has already enrolled in a new school, the student's former school may disclose any records or information, *including health records and information about disciplinary proceedings*". Thus, any medical information that has been included on the primary or secondary school forms is excluded from FERPA protection and may be shared with a new school to which the student is transferring. In addition to the medical and disciplinary information disclosed from the secondary school to colleges, parents and young adults may provide the university health service more comprehensive medical and behavioral information to aid health promotion. Parents and incoming students benefit from accurate information from the university health service to reassure them about the separateness of protected medical information from the admission process.

Typically the medical record kept by the pediatrician of the incoming student is considerably more comprehensive than the information which has been released to the secondary school. As the university health service requests health and immunization records, the incoming student and their family may feel more comfortable providing honest and complete health information including mental health history when reassured that the more restrictive HIPAA or applicable state laws regarding confidentiality protect their personal health information from the wider university community protected under FERPA. The university health service is essentially a HIPAA or clinical island within a FERPA sea (Figure 10.1). HIPAA, state laws around confidentiality and ethical codes for clinical disciplines also include provisions to allow for communication of protected health information (PHI) during a health emergency, necessary for treatment or referral; anonymous report of sexual assault to local police in compliance with the Clery Act, and mandated reporting for suspicion of neglect/abuse of minors or dependent elders. It is useful to review the limits of confidentiality in campus educational materials and at the beginning of treatment.

Particularly for incoming students who are already engaged in mental health treatment, complete disclosure of the medical treatment history helps the university clinicians to coordinate care with their current clinicians, to anticipate challenges, to promote

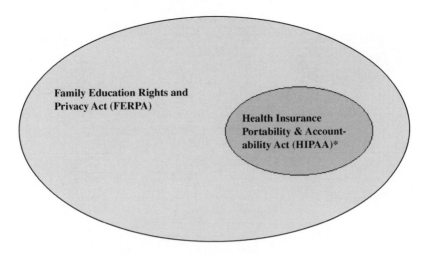

Family Education Rights and Privacy Act (FERPA)

Health Insurance Portability & Accountability Act (HIPAA)*

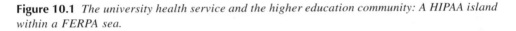

*HIPAA and/or state statutes plus codes of ethics for clinical disciplines

Figure 10.1 *The university health service and the higher education community: A HIPAA island within a FERPA sea.*

continuity of care and to reduce the risk for relapse. As young adults work through identity issues, some may wish to make a fresh start in college, leaving their previous mental health problems behind. Some may decide to discontinue their medications, which puts them at increased risk for relapse. For these as well, complete and accurate health records assist university clinicians as they liaison with the educational community, to promptly and therapeutically respond to the personal observation comments that are brought to their attention.

10.11 The Risk Management Team

Should concerning behavioral observations be brought forward, the formation of a crisis or risk management committee such as the one shown in Figure 10.2 serves as a useful vehicle to allow for regular communication between various community stakeholders. While membership of such a committee might include those represented in this figure, it is likely that the specific representatives will vary according to the decision-making hierarchy of the particular institution. The director of the medical and/or mental health service participates primarily as a clinically informed listener but may provide guidance to the committee as a liaison. Under FERPA, university personnel have significantly more latitude than clinicians for sharing information outside of the academic record. Not only may university personnel share information reasonably directed toward avoiding harm to the student or others in a health or safety emergency, they are unrestricted in sharing personal behavioral observations. Thus, as individual students of concern are discussed in this format, timely decisions may be made weighing the best interests of each student with the needs of the community. Considerations may include understanding the benefits and risks of informing parents, reviewing the student's functioning in the residence, discussing incidents that have involved the campus police, assessing the extent of effort to engage the student and understanding barriers for help seeking.

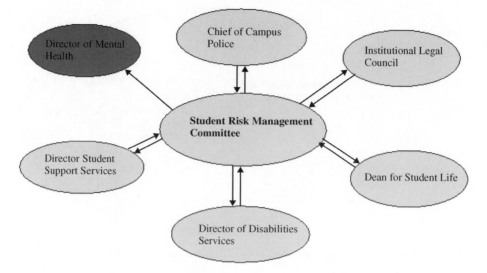

Figure 10.2 *Post-secondary risk management community.*

10.12 Health Insurance

One barrier to help seeking affecting some students may be health insurance. While many undergraduates are eligible for health insurance coverage as dependents under their parents' insurance, an estimated 80% of universities offer some direct health care [46] which can vary from basic medical and urgent care to multi-specialty medical clinics including mental health services. Usually these services are provided to students free of charge or with nominal co-pays, and are financially supported through students' fees. Most graduate students exceed the age typically allowed for dependents, and young adults are believed to be the largest group of uninsured in the United States [47].

Although incoming students and their families are encouraged to acquire/maintain supplemental health insurance coverage for visits, treatments or procedures not available or not covered under the basic student plan, only an estimated 40% of schools require students to provide proof of insurance [46]. Thus, it is relatively easy for students to enroll without having adequate health care coverage. Some students lack supplemental health insurance entirely. Others are covered as dependents on their parents plan, but managed care restrictions allow only life saving treatment or in-network providers – not particularly helpful for a university student in Massachusetts when the network providers are in California.

For young adults unaccustomed to negotiating their own health care and already reluctant to seek mental health care, inadequate health care coverage may feel like an insurmountable hurdle. The recent passage of mental health parity intensifies the need for parents to work closely with their college bound son or daughter, the home pediatrician and the university mental health service to develop transitional mental health care plans. Families are often reluctant to purchase the universities' supplemental health insurance because of cost, misunderstandings about the limitations of their insurance plan or hopes that their student will not need it. Unfortunately, as noted in the introduction, serious mental illnesses such as bipolar disorder, major depression and schizophrenia often first present during late adolescence and early adulthood. Family physicians, university clinicians and administrators play a central role in educating parents about health care options, helping them to understand the importance of fully appreciating the limitations of their current health plan and knowing when there is a need for the university supplemental insurance. Particularly for incoming students, who have benefited from mental health treatment prior to coming to college, perhaps relying on medications as a significant contributor to their high functioning, parents should be strongly encouraged to obtain to the university supplemental health insurance. Supplemental insurances are typically contracted by the university with third-party insurance companies and cover most, but not all, additional medical expenses that students may encounter [46].

10.13 Family Therapy in the University Health Service

Case 1

Melissa is a 17-year-old first-generation Asian-American freshman from out of state who comes to the mental health service early in her first semester accompanied by concerned friends who share that Melissa has been frequently crying and cutting herself. Melissa admits that this has been the longest that she has ever been away from home and feels completely overwhelmed. Schoolwork had always come easily to her, and she feels devastated by getting only average scores on her assignments. She has been telling her parents that everything is fine. She knows how much they have sacrificed to allow her to attend college, doesn't want to admit failure to them and fears bringing shame to her family.

The adjustment to college provides a normal developmental opportunity to foster the young adult's drive towards autonomy and self-reliance, which tests their coping skills and resilience. Cross-cultural factors, family system dynamics, generational influences and the style of parental attachment all color the negotiation of this complex transition. At this transitional time, students are especially sensitive to their ability to maintain academic success. Increasingly, college is viewed as a necessity rather then an option in order to succeed in life for young adults coming of age during a global economic recession and a technological era. Students and their families have worked hard to craft resumes for college admission boards knowing of the keen competition for this largest of American generations. Admission to college can then be viewed by students and their families as validation of their efforts and reinforcement of the young adult's core identity as cognitively competent but also sets up expectations for thriving in college to make good on the family investment.

10.13.1 The Imposter Phenomenon

As young adults transition to the university environment, they take risks which challenge their core identity of a cognitively competent self. Even those students who have excelled typically face cognitive challenges that evoke self doubt. Dimensional characteristics such as degree of perfectionism, familial inter-dependence, parenting style and sociability all influence both resiliency and psychological risk. For Melissa, adaptive aspects of perfectionism include her self-imposed drive towards excellence and familial imposed value placed on academics prior to college. While familial obligation attitudes contribute to greater academic motivation among youth from immigrant as compared with US-born families, greater behavioral demands imposed on Asian American, Hispanic and Afro-Caribbean immigrant youth detracts from their achievement [48,49]. Maladaptive aspects of perfectionism, parent driven perfectionism and extreme self imposed perfectionism are associated with depressive symptoms and complicate the transition to college, presenting a heightened cultural vulnerability for Asian-American students [49]. Perfectionism has also been studied in pre-professional students where stronger associations were found between current psychological distress with perfectionism and imposter feelings than with demographic variables known to be associated with psychological distress [50]. When self and/or other imposed perfectionism becomes exaggerated, the normally expected, transient self doubt that most college students face can become an imposter syndrome such that students feel like imposters at risk for exposure as frauds at any moment.

In the case of Melissa, the university mental health clinician is an unique position to commend her for coming to the service, to offer positive reinforcement to the peers who showed enough concern for her to persuade her to come and to establish initial clinical rapport. During early sessions, Melissa is able to talk about her close family ties. Although not outwardly demonstrative, Melissa knows that her parents love her and are proud of her. Melissa is aware that her parents faced challenges as immigrants to the United States, feel proud of their daughter's academic success and want her to have the top tier university education that they were not able to have. Melissa experiences her parents as both academically demanding and protective. Melissa feels torn about not being truthful with her parents, misses the sense of cohesion with them and longs for their guidance, yet fears disappointing them. With the support of the therapist, Melissa agrees to include the parents in a series of family sessions, first via a conference call and then in person.

As Melissa expects, her parents are concerned and alarmed to learn that she is not having the smooth adjustment to college for which they had hoped. The clinician is able to provide normalizing information about young adult development and the use of mental health services. As the parents more fully understand her level of distress, Melissa is relieved that they respond in a supportive, concerned manner rather than leading with the criticism and disappointment that she had feared. While she is not earning the straight As that she had in grade school, the therapist is able to reframe Melissa's B average by placing it within a university community and developmental context. This allows Melissa and her parents to look at the adaptive and maladaptive aspects of their perfectionism. A safety plan is able to be developed which includes both the therapist and the parents as contacts should Melissa have self injurious impulses. Melissa also agrees to continue individual therapy, to begin a stress management-mood regulation group and to outline what she anticipates would be most helpful in weekly check-in calls with parents.

Perception of familial support, parenting style and sense of familial cohesiveness have all been shown to affect coping efficacy during emerging adulthood [48,51–57]. While adolescents raised by authoritative or permissive parents tend to show stronger feelings of homesickness as compared with those raised by authoritarian or uninvolved parents, it is the group raised by authoritarian or uninvolved parents who show more internalizing and externalizing problems in reaction to their homesickness. Melissa's family represents a highly cohesive, authoritarian system with protective and involved parents. The family constellation along with a cultural vulnerability to maladaptive aspects of perfectionism increase her risk for feeling overwhelmed, using less effective coping mechanisms and experiencing perceived barriers to help seeking. Brief family therapy serves as an opportunity to provide psycho-education, to reframe expectations and to use the protective strengths of family cohesiveness.

10.14 Required Medical Withdrawal

Case 2

Vanessa is an 18-year-old freshman who developed anorexia nervosa during high school. She has always done well academically and is pleased to get accepted at her first choice university. Vanessa's pediatrician completes the required health assessment form, cautiously endorsing Vanessa's enrollment while noting some concern about her current body mass index of 16 and loss of menstruation. Both Vanessa and her parents are aware of the pediatrician's concern but are unwilling to accept an eating disorder diagnosis, preferring to believe that Vanessa is naturally slender and losing weight because of her preference for only healthy foods like vegetables. After arriving on campus, the university health service contacts Vanessa to confirm receipt of her health assessment form and invite her in for an appointment to meet her new primary care provider (PCP). During the initial meeting with her PCP, Vanessa adamantly rejects the possibility that she may have an eating disorder, agrees that she is "a little on the thin side" but says she feels fully capable of managing her weight without the PCP or the nutritionist and therapist that the PCP recommends. Vanessa indicates that she understands the expectation to gain weight, affirms that she can do this on her own and reluctantly agrees to meet with the PCP before the end of the semester. Just prior to winter break, Vanessa returns to meet with the PCP explaining that her 5 pound weight loss is due to her new vegan diet, again rejecting the possibility of having an eating disorder. She reluctantly agrees to have a mental health consultation when she returns to campus since she was not able to prove that she was able to gain weight on her own. Parents are alarmed when they see how thin Vanessa looks when she comes home for winter break and contact the PCP. The parents indicate that Vanessa will be returning to campus in a week. They do not want Vanessa to know that they have been in touch but want the PCP to make sure that Vanessa eats enough protein and does not exercise.

Students with eating disorders present particular clinical and administrative challenges for the higher education community. Despite their precarious nutritional status, students with eating disorders are often doing well academically, have ritualized patterns around eating which are difficult to change and are highly ambivalent about treatment. These students attempt to use their control of food as a method of managing underlying negative psychological states. Interactions with clinicians, family members and others may feel equally controlled. Families concerned about the college student's nutritional status may feel powerless to change things while other families may not acknowledge the problem. Family system dynamics including parental attachment, degree of engagement, and negotiation of control all influence the vulnerability for eating issues and use of less effective coping strategies.

10.14.1 The Eating Disorders Team

Particularly for students who have limited insight about their eating disorder, effective interventions typically rely upon use of a collaborative, team approach. In a university community, the eating disorders team might include a PCP, nutritionist, individual therapist, group therapist, athletics staff and a clinician administrator who serves as a liaison with other university administrators and support personnel. Eating disorder teams find themselves struggling to define minimum nutritional expectations, protocols for engaging reluctant students, and procedures for how to involve parents and administrative support personnel in keeping with FERPA and HIPAA standards.

Universities typically have procedures to require withdrawal for students failing to meet minimum academic standards but may not have developed analogous processes for required medical withdrawals. FERPA allows for *communication to appropriate officials in cases of health and safety emergencies*, and HIPAA (and/or state statutes plus clinical disciplinary codes governing privacy) allows for *communication for treatment, health care operations, safe transfer and in cases of threat to public health or safety*. The presence of significant numbers of students with eating disorders on campus together with shifting generational attitudes will increase pressure on administrations to define campus standards and communication protocols. Millennial students expect clear codes of conduct, involved baby boomer parents expect greater caretaking from institutions, and clinicians are faced with the dilemma of providing guidance to higher education administrators on policy decisions related to the health and safety of its students.

The eating disorder team serves as an effective body to define medical parameters to guide administrations, particularly useful in cases such as Vanessa's where the student refuses to participate in treatment yet remains in good standing academically. In response to the weight loss during the fall semester, the team is able to notify Vanessa in writing of their expectation for her to discontinue exercise, to actively engage in treatment including weekly individual and group therapies, nutritional counseling and PCP monitoring including weight checks in order for the team to medically support her ongoing enrollment. Acceptable minimal goal weight and lab parameters are identified. Vanessa is also informed that her athletic facilities privileges have been revoked through medical request to the Dean for Student Life. During the mental health consultation, Vanessa acknowledges having received the letter from the eating disorder team but denies having any mental health concerns and flatly denies considering an eating disorder. With annoyance, she attributes her inability to gain weight and amenorrhea during the fall semester to following a more strictly vegan diet and exercise. She is aware that her parents are concerned about her health given their comments over winter break, wants to do her academic work and reluctantly agrees to stop exercising and keep appointments. Within a week, Vanessa has made multiple attempts to use her invalidated card to access athletic facilities and lost another half a pound. The PCP makes a recommendation for a medical withdrawal and an inpatient eating disorder program which Vanessa refuses.

10.14.2 The Students at Risk Committee in Action

As universities develop procedures and protocols to assist in the management of vulnerable students at risk for health or safety concerns related to themselves or others, many have formed small, inter-disciplinary bodies to routinely review students known to be of concern. This body is typically composed of a small number of the institutions' decision makers which may include those representing the areas of mental health, student life, disabilities services, discipline and legal counsel. When a severely malnourished student such as Vanessa fails to maintain minimum health standards despite the eating disorder treatment plan and remains a substantial health risk, HIPAA standards allow the eating disorder team to notify the vulnerable student committee who is in turn allowed by FERPA to contact the student's family and empowered to require a medical withdrawal. In practice, the need for required medical withdrawal is extremely rare. Much more frequently, students and their families are able to be persuaded by the medical circumstances and discussions with administrative deans to voluntarily accept the need for a medical withdrawal to allow medically necessary treatment. Should the need for a required withdrawal arise, clear lines of authority, established protocols including appeal processes, and careful medical documentation are essential.

In the case of Vanessa, the Dean for Student Life is able contact her parents who are initially ambivalent about the idea of a medical withdrawal although not surprised to learn that she has been found to be severely malnourished. Family meetings with the dean provide an opportunity to share information about the medical withdrawal and re-admission process and to the address concerns that the family has about costs of the treatment, stigma associated with taking a leave, tuition and housing costs and impact on financial aid. Through use of concerned persuasion and building a shared rapport focused on the best interests of the young adult, the parents and Vanessa are able to agree to a medical withdrawal, understand the expectation for an intensive eating disorder program and are reassured to learn that many students have successfully returned to the university after taking a medical withdrawal to regain their health and optimal functioning.

10.14.3 Health Insurance Revisited

Young adult health care coverage varies between insurances and among universities. According to higher education surveys, only 40% require health insurance [46]. Even for those institutions which require attestation to a minimal level of health care coverage in order to waive the student insurance, many accept the waiver without actually confirming the insurance coverage. In choosing a school, it is important for families to carefully consider the physical and emotional health needs for their young adult. Particularly for students who are applying from out-of-state who have an existing mental health history prior to college, addition of the university's supplemental insurance may provide coverage for local inpatient or day treatment programs which may be excluded by an out-of-state insurer. Health and learning concerns that presented prior to college do not disappear with college matriculation despite conscious and/or unconscious wishes that they might.

Understanding of the temperament as well as the unique health and learning needs of the young adult will help families to carefully investigate and make informed choices about the young adult's fit with each university's environment and support resources. For millennial students who have grown up protected and kept busy by involved adults, this generation of students is likely to need assistance from the pediatrician, family, and university clinicians to foster continuity of care, to build understanding about when and how to access health care, and to help to frame expectations. As the Vanessa case illustrates, early alerts from pediatricians or family members are helpful to allow more proactive treatment planning and crisis prevention. University clinicians welcome concerned input from outside sources and are able to listen whether or not they have the young adult's consent to share information. Understandably, families may feel fearful about sharing health or disability information to clinicians employed by the university and may need clarification about the HIPAA confidentiality standard and its separation from the university admissions process (Table 10.4).

Table 10.4	Tips for parents of young adults

Maintain lines of communication
Make informed choices (university fit, insurance)
Learn about support resources on campus
Support and encourage self advocacy
Actively listen
Take a supportive, non-judgmental stance
Encourage the development of life goals without imposing one's own
Engage in self-reflective discussions to build judgment
Key Message– Young adults need space to grow but still need their parents and families for support and guidance.

10.15 Behavioral Problems in the Residential Community

Case 3

Max is a 21-year-old junior who lives in a fraternity. He has an inconsistent academic record and has struggled with anxiety. On Friday afternoon, shortly after returning from summer break, Max calls his campus psychiatrist to request a prescription for clonazepam which he had been using over the summer, adding that he lost the bottle of medication that he had been prescribed by his home psychiatrist. He is given an appointment with his psychiatrist in 3 days and enough medication to last until then. Over the weekend, fraternity brothers call the university health service to report that Max has had some kind of spell and needs to be taken to an emergency room. The computed tomography scan and physical in the emergency room are unremarkable. He is given an appointment the next day with a neurologist and discharged back to the fraternity. The emergency room subsequently calls to inform him that his urine toxicology screen came back positive for multiple recreational drugs in addition to clonazepam. When Max meets with his psychiatrist, he complains of anxiety much of the time, reports use of the prescribed medication as directed with modest benefit and denies any recreational drug abuse, noting that the urine test in the emergency room was in error. He admits that he missed his neurology appointment due to oversleeping, agrees to reschedule, and then misses his next psychiatrist appointment.

Within 2 weeks, multiple brothers have expressed concern to the fraternity president about Max's 'out of control' use of substances. The fraternity house officers and the residential advisor meet and agree that Max will either have to get treatment for his substance use or move out of the fraternity. After Max denies having a problem when confronted by the fraternity council, fraternity brothers contact the dean-on-call to request temporary housing placement from the university for one of their brothers who they reluctantly identify as Max.

Universities vary regarding their policies and procedures for handling substance use and behavioral problems, some with localized judicial boards such as in this example and others with a more centralized disciplinary committee. Whatever the arrangement, established communication protocols and trainings with residential staff on how to handle various emergencies benefit individuals, perhaps reluctant to engage in needed treatment, take advantage of the protective social support network inherent in universities [40,41,58,59] and promote collaborative, considered crisis management. As behavioral concerns are identified within residences, classrooms, academic departments or athletics for example, individual cases can be presented and discussed in the multi-disciplinary student crisis management committee. In the case of Max, his removal from residence, publicly observed spell of unconsciousness, lack of insight and his resistance to treatment referral by the fraternity council in conjunction with the residential advisor represent both a health crisis and a residential crisis.

An established student risk management committee allows for discussion and decision making around the appropriateness of moving the student to a different campus residence, notification of parents, and/or addressing the substance use issues through campus disciplinary channels. Depending upon the individual circumstances of the case, some institutions may view parental notification as justified through the FERPA health and safety exception. The preamble to the December 2008 FERPA Final Rule explicitly supports university administrators and clinicians, noting the intent to provide "greater flexibility and deference to school administrators so they can bring appropriate resources to bear on a circumstance that threatens the health or safety of individuals" (73FR 155574, 15589). Despite significant concern about Max's welfare, some student risk committees may feel that the circumstances fall short of the threshold to constitute a health and safety emergency if using a threshold based upon an imminent harm model.

Whether or not the aspects of the individual case are determined to reach the health and safety emergency threshold for a particular institution, personal observations and concerns may be shared with the parents by residential staff or other university personnel. Parental notification may also be pursued for financially dependent domestic students as students who are claimed by either parent as a dependent for a US Federal income tax return are also viewed as a FERPA exemption [60]. Although this exception would apply to many undergraduates, the Dec 2008 FERPA Final Rule clarifies:

> we expect the disclosure to be made under the dependent student provision (§99.31 (a) [8]), in conjunction with a health or safety emergency (§§99.31 (a) [10] and 99.36), or if a student has committed a disciplinary violation with respect to the use or possession of alcohol or a controlled substance (§99.31 (a) [15]).

As a member of the student risk management committee, the director of the mental health service functions in an administrative medical liaison role, using the information known in the residential and academic communities to inform the discussion without sharing PHI known only to the mental health service. It is possible to share general concepts related to risks related to substance use, typical treatment strategies and challenges in working with patients who do not yet acknowledge the need for treatment.

In the case of Max, the circumstances are felt to meet the criteria for a FERPA health and safety emergency, and a decision is made for the Dean for Student Life to contact the parents in efforts to facilitate a medical withdrawal rather than to pursue the substance issues through disciplinary channels. Having experience in working with many involved, baby boomer parents, the Dean anticipates that the parents are likely to have a multilayered emotional response. The Dean is able to empathize with the parents' initial disbelief and shock, followed by their sadness and sense of personal failure – a narcissistic injury given their perhaps grandiose projection for all of their advocacy and hard work for their offspring. Although skeptical, the parents agree to come to campus for a face-to-face meeting with their son and the Dean where they become more concerned about Max as they learn about the circumstances leading to the emergency room visit and the residential crisis. The discussion underlines how Max's health issues have interfered with his academic and interpersonal functioning, persuading Max and his parents to accept the need for a medical withdrawal. Max acknowledges that he failed his first round of exams and agrees that taking some time off might be a good way to make a fresh start academically. While continuing to minimize the substance use problem, Max understands that he will be expected to engage in treatment in order to be considered for re-admission.

10.16 Mental Health Prevention

Case 4

The parents of Carlos, a 19-year-old Hispanic sophomore, call the mental health service to share concern about their son who has not been responding to their calls or e-mails for the past month. Parents note that Carlos struggled with depression and suicidal thinking during high school and has always been extremely resistant to using mental health services. They fear that Carlos may be suicidal now and want help from the mental health service to engage him in treatment without letting Carlos know that they have called. They have asked Carlos to come to the mental health service many times and worry that he will definitely refuse to come if he knows that they are involved.

The student risk management committee provides an established forum to discuss strategies when some degree of concern exists insufficient to determine the degree of imminent risk. Following the initial committee discussion, an inquiry to the residence staff reveals that Carlos seems solitary and does not participate in the residence hall's social events. The academic advisor indicates that Carlos did well academically prior to this semester but notices marked decline in his academic performance this semester. The advisor received no answer to an e-mail sent to Carlos a couple of weeks before hearing from the dean. After discussion to remind the advisor of the various university support services, she agrees to contact Carlos again expressing concern and an expectation for a meeting with a plan to walk him over to the mental health service.

When Carlos meets with his academic advisor, he feels touched by her concern and is able to admit that he has not been feeling like himself. Carlos agrees to walk over to the mental health service with his advisor after she reassures him about its confidentiality. Carlos acknowledges a possible need for treatment but makes it clear that he does not want his parents to know about it. Whether involved overtly or behind the scenes, parents may be instrumental in identifying developing concerns before a crisis arises. The extensive social networks present in university communities often allow for referral by someone who already has some connection and rapport with the individual of concern. In this way, social support networks are believed to be an important protective factor to explain the substantially reduced suicide rate in college students as compared to their age matched peers [2,58].

Health and safety training programs campus-wide shift ownership of health and safety problems from solely the concern of the university health service and campus police to a shared concern for the entire community. Standardized curriculums may be a practical and useful way to insure that university staff recognize warning signs, know available resources and feel sufficiently skilled in facilitating referrals [61]. As shown in Figure 10.3 the post-secondary community is quite complex and as such has many competing agendas. Endorsement of health and safety as a priority by the senior leadership is crucial for

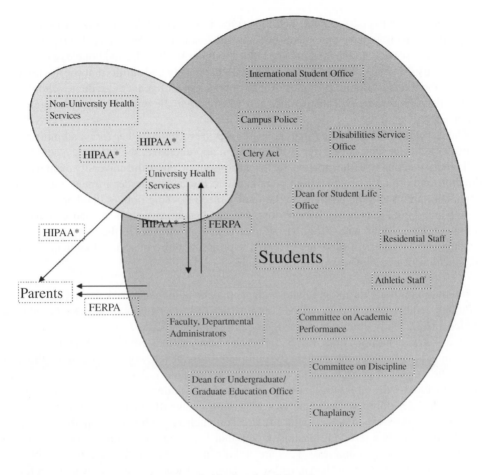

*HIPAA and/or state statutes plus codes of ethics for clinical disciplines

Figure 10.3 *The higher education student resources community with directional flow of information.*

underlining the shared mission. Behaviors and attitudes around help seeking are then able to be transformed as community leaders and trainers value the use of support resources as important, proactive ways to care for oneself and the community [40,41].

10.17 Crisis Management

Case 5

Ying is a 24-year-old graduate student in chemistry from China who takes an overdose of chemicals found in her lab after learning that she has failed her qualifying examinations and will not be allowed to continue in her graduate program. She is transported to a local emergency room after peers find her unconscious. There Ying is able to be medically stabilized. The university mental health service is contacted to authorize a psychiatric hospitalization through her extended student health insurance. Ying had not been previously known to the service. In the hospital she talks about her wish to die and hopelessness, feels burdened by the shame that she has brought upon her family and admits that she has not told parents about her academic struggles over her two and a half years of graduate school. She knows that her parents will disown her and worries that she will be always be seen as a failure.

The director of the university mental health service meets with her for an administrative consultation prior to her discharge. Although a bit apprehensive, she agrees to a conference call family meeting with the inpatient team and consents to allow the university mental health director to coordinate her discharge planning with her academic department, the housing dean, her parents and the hospital. In the family meeting, Ying notices that her parents are disappointed but are also much more concerned and supportive than she had imagined. In follow-up discussions with Ying, her advisor is able to emphasize the work that she has accomplished which will allow her to leave the program with a masters rather than stressing the doctoral degree that was no longer possible.

International students and graduate students may be at increased risk for self harm given their age demographic and the added complexities of life as graduate and/or international students [62]. Many countries have significantly higher suicide rates as compared to the United States including China, Korea, India, and Eastern block countries (WHO database), and China is the only country where the completed suicides of women outnumber those of men. The impact of migration patterns on suicide prevalence deserves more study. Apart from any cross-cultural issues that may exist, graduate students being further along in the young adult development track, are typically more financially independent but also more vulnerable to the vicissitudes of major life stressors such as a failure in the qualifying exams which necessitates a terminal masters. Given that life events which are experienced as a significant failure or embarrassment are a known risk factor for suicide, established protocols for the delivery of "bad news" such as required academic withdrawal, disciplinary sanctions or terminal masters are an important component of a safety plan for an academic community. Routine referrals to the university mental health service in the face of life changing news allows for reaction to and processing of the news in a supportive setting that may prevent hopelessness which accounts for 76% of the association between depression and suicidal intent [63].

Success in college has become the expected path for career development, financial security and prestige for both students and their families. Analogous to the grieving process with the loss of a loved one, a psychiatric hospitalization represents a threatened loss to the idealized trajectory longed and planned for by the student and his/her family. Understandably, many students are initially reluctant to tell their parents that they have had serious enough mental health problems so as to require a hospitalization. Exploration of the family system issues while in the hospital allows a thoughtful determination about the appropriateness of bringing family members into the treatment. In many cases though not all, parents are central to their support system and an important collaborator in the discharge planning. In a liaison role, the university mental health director is able to facilitate a face saving solution with the department, consider the needs of the residential community, mediate discussions with family members, provide psychoeducation and coordinate referrals in conjunction with the inpatient team.

Table 10.5	Tips for college administrators, faculty and clinicians

There is never a constraint to listening to parents' concerns
Develop communication protocols
Use orientation and web site to education students & their families about support resources on campus
Be aware of privacy standards but don't forget to think about safety and use common sense in interpreting the standards
Convey message that it's not only okay but a strength to know oneself and to use appropriate resources to address concerns before they become crises
Actively listen to students, using low threshold for referral to campus resources
Administrators and faculty have a lower threshold for parental contact than clinicians in almost all situations
Administrators, residence staff and faculty may freely share personal observations of behavior with parents and others
Key Message– Treat parents as allies until there is reason to proceed otherwise. Most millennial students maintain close relationships with their parents and see them as a primary resource.

10.18 Conclusion

The adjustment to college provides a normal developmental opportunity for young adults that challenges their coping skills and resilience. Psychological and neurological development, generational influences, the style of parental attachment, family system dynamics, temperament as well as parental and societal expectations color the negotiation of this complex transition (Table 10.5). Young adulthood is also the time of life when serious mental illnesses including schizophrenia, bipolar disorder, major depression and substance use disorders, often first present, and suicide is the second leading cause of death for college students. Media attention to recent campus tragedies highlights underlying fears of parents, clinicians and administrators about campus violence.

As university mental health clinicians and administrators work with millennial generation students, they are likely to notice the need to please not only the students but also their parents given the core generational attitudes. Baby boomer parents tend to maintain close ties with their young adult students, and surveys of college students reveal that when they need help, they rate peers first and parents second. Thus, parents become a natural potential collaborator for clinicians and higher education administrators as they work to balance the needs of individual students with the needs of the educational community. Working effectively with parents requires understanding and successful negotiation of the privacy regulations governing the sharing of information within heath care: HIPAA for universities who submit insurance claims online, state privacy statutes, codes of ethics for clinical disciplines, and within higher education, FERPA. Within this privacy framework and with a community systems consultation liaison approach, mental health clinicians can incorporate evidence based education models and prevention strategies to strengthen the care that they provide for students in their university community. Working effectively with parents who remain a primary support resource for a majority of students becomes an integral component for prevention efforts to minimize health and safety risks for young adults.

Despite challenges, it is possible to work effectively with college students and their families using a community systems approach and common sense. Established communication protocols for university staff with appropriate trainings encourage routine collaboration around emotional and behavioral crises. It is important to remember that FERPA privacy limitations are often not as restrictive as university personnel fear, and university personnel have greater latitude to communicate than clinicians in almost all situations.

Specifically, there are no restrictions on faculty, residence staff, departmental administrators or peers in sharing personal observations with clinicians, other campus support personnel or parents. University communities are in an ideal position to use their natural faculty, departmental and residential life structure to create protective support networks which promote mental health stability, early case finding and effective crisis management.

References

1. Schwartz, A. (1990) The epidemiology of suicide among students at colleges and universities in the United States. *Journal of College Student Psychotherapy*, **3**(4), 25–44.
2. Schwartz, A. Are college students more disturbed today? Stability in the acuity and qualitative character of psychopathology of college counseling center clients 1992-3 through 2001-2. *Journal of American College Health*, **54**(6), 327–47.
3. Centers for Disease Control and Prevention (2003) Web-based Injury Statistics Query and Reporting System (WISQARS). Retrieved April 26, 2009 from www.cdc.gov/injury/wisqars/index.html.
4. National Mental Health Association & The Jed Foundation (2002) *Safeguarding your Students Against Suicide: Expanding the Safety Network*, National Mental Health Association, Alexandria, VA.
5. Zemke, R., Raines, C. and Filipczak, B. (2000) *Generations at Work*, American Management Association, New York, NY.
6. Mangold, K. (2007) Educating a new generation: teaching baby boomer faculty about millennial students. *Nurse Education*, **32**(1), 21–23, Review.
7. Erikson, E.H. (1985) *Childhood and Society*, Norton, New York.
8. Erikson, E.H. (1959) *Identity and the Life Cycle*, Norton, New York.
9. Kohlberg, L. and Gilligan, C. (1972) The adolescent as philosopher: The discovery of the self in a post-conventional world, in *Twelve to Sixteen: Early Adolescence* (eds D.A.J. Kagan and R. Coles), Norton, New York, pp. 144–179.
10. Piaget, J. (1972) Intellectual evolution from adolescence to adulthood. *Human Development*, **15**, 1–12.
11. Taylor, J.M., Gilligan, C. and Sullivan, A.M. (1995) *Between voice and silence: Women and girls, race and relationship*, Harvard University Press, Cambridge, MA.
12. Kegan, R. (1994) *In Over Our Heads: The Mental Demands of Modern Life*, Harvard University Press, Cambridge, MA.
13. Jernigan, T.L., Trauner, D.A., Hesselink, J.R. and Tallal, P.A. (1991) Maturation of human cerebrum observed *in vivo* during adolescence. *Brain*, **114**, 2037–2049
14. Reiss, A.L., Abrams, M.T., Singer, H.S., Ross, J.L. and Denckla, M.B. (1996) Brain development, gender and IQ in children. A volumetric imaging study. *Brain*, **119**, 1763–1774
15. Giedd, J.N., Blumenthal, J., Jeffries, N.O., Castellanos, F.X., Liu, H., Zijdenbos, A., Paus, T., Evans, A.C., and Rapoport, J.L., (1999) Brain development during childhood and adolescence: A longitudinal study, *Nature Neuroscience*, **2**(10), 861–863.
16. Sowell, E.R., Thompson, P.M., Tessner, K.D. and Toga, A.W. (2001) Mapping continued brain growth and gray matter density reduction in dorsal frontal cortex: Inverse relationships during postadolescent brain maturation. *The Journal of Neuroscience*, **21**(22), 8819–8829.
17. Benes, F.M., Turtle, M., Khan, Y., Farol, P. (1994) Myelination of a key relay zone in the hippocampal formation occurs in the human brain during childhood, adolescence, and adulthood, *Arch Gen Psychiatry*, **51**: 477–484.
18. Huttenlocher, P.R. and de Courten, C. (1987) The development of synapses in striate cortex of man. *Human Neurobiology*, **6**, 1–9.

19. Nelson, E.E., Leibenluft, E., McClure, E.B. and Pine, D.S. (2005) *Psychological Medicine*, **35**(2), 163–174.

20. Stevens, M.C., Pearlson, G.D. and Calhoun, V.D. (2009) Changes in the interaction of resting-state neural networks from adolescence to adulthood. *Human Brain Mapping*, [Epub ahead of print].

21. Ernst, M., Romeo, R.D. and Andersen, S.L. (2009) Neurobiology of the development of motivated behaviors in adolescence: A window into a neural systems model. *Pharmacology, Biochemistry, and Behavior*, **93**(3), 199–211.

22. Anderson, S.W., Bechara, A., Damasio, H. *et al.* (1999) Impairment of social and moral behavior related to early damage in human prefrontal cortex. *Nature Neuroscience*, **2**, 1032–1037.

23. Beauregard, M., Levesque, J. and Bourgoin, P.J. (2001) Neural correlates of conscious self-regulation of emotion. *The Journal of Neuroscience*, **21**, 1–6.

24. Gogtay, N., Giedd, J.N., Lusk, L. *et al.* (2004) Dynamic mapping of human cortical development during childhood through early adulthood. *Proceedings of the National Academy of Sciences of the United States of America*, **101**, 8174–8179.

25. Ochsner, K.N., Bunge, S.A., Gross, J.J. and Gabrielli, D. (2002) Rethinking feelings: An FMRI study of the cognitive regulation of emotion. *Journal of Cognitive Neuroscience*, **15**, 1215–1229.

26. Rilling, J.K., Guttman, D.A., Zeh, T.R. *et al.* (2002) A neural basis for social cooperation. *Neuron*, **35**, 395–405.

27. Sowell, E.R., Thompson, P.M., Holmes, C.J. *et al.* (1999) *In vivo* evidence for post-adolescence for post-adolescent brain maturation in frontal and striatal regions. *Nature Neuroscience*, **2**, 859–861.

28. Winslow, J.T. and Insel, T.R. (2004) Neuroendrocrine basis of social recognition. *Current Opinion in Neurobiology*, **14**, 248–253.

29. Winston, J.S., Strange, B.A., O'Doherty, J. and Dolan, R.J. (2002) Automatic and intentional brain responses during evaluation of trustworthiness of faces. *Nature Neuroscience*, **5**, 277–283.

30. Obradović, J., Burt, K.B. and Masten, A.S. (2006) Pathways of adaptation from adolescence to young adulthood. *Annals of the New York Academy of Sciences*, **1094**, 340–344.

31. Masten, A.S., *et al.* (2004). Resources and resilience in the transition to adulthood: continuity and change, *Dev. Psychopath.* **16**, 1071–1094

32. Masten, A.S. *et al.* (2005) Developmental cascades: Linking academic achievement, externalizing and internalizing symptoms over 20 years. *Development and Psychopathology*, **41**, 733–746.

33. Gest, S.D., Reed, M. and Masten, A.S. (1999) Measuring developmental changes in exposure to adversity: A life chart and rating scale approach. *Development and Psychopathology*, **11**, 171–192.

34. Roisman, G.I. *et al.* (2004) Salient and emerging developmental tasks in the transition to adulthood. *Child Development*, **75**, 123–133.

35. Lancaster, L.C. and Stillman, D. (2002) *When Generations Collide*. Harper Collins, New York, NY.

36. Howe, N. and Strauss, W. (2000) *Millennials Rising: The Next Great Generation*. Vintage Books, New York.

37. Howe, N. and Strauss, W. (2007) The next 20 years: How customer and workforce attitudes will evolve. *Harvard Business Review*, **July–August**, 41–52.

38. Borges, N.J., Manuel, R.S., Elam, C.L. and Jones, B.J. (2006) Comparing millennial and generation X medical students at one medical school. *Academic Medicine*, **81**(6), 571–576.

39. Department of Education Part II (2008) Family educational rights and privacy act; Final rule. Federal Register, 20 USC § 1232g; 34 CFR Part 99, 74806–74855. Retrieved March 2, 2009 from http://www.ed.gov/policy/gen/guid/fpco/ferpa/index.html.

40. Knox, K.L., Litts, D.A., Talcott, W.G. *et al.* (2003) Risk of suicide and related adverse outcomes after exposure to a suicide prevention programme in the US Air Force: Cohort study. *British Medical Journal*, **327**(7428), 1376–1378.

41. Knox, K., Conwell, Y. and Caine, E.D. (2004) If suicide is a public health problem, what are we doing to prevent it? *Journal of Public Health*, **94**(1), 37–46.

42. Joffe, P. (2003) An empirically support program to prevent Suicide among a college population. Paper presented at University of Michigan Inaugural National Conference on Depression on College Campuses: Best Practices and Innovative Strategies.

43. Bickel, R. and Lake, P. (1999) *The Rights and Responsibilities of Modern Universities: Who Assumes the Risk of College Life?*, Carolina Academic Press, Durham, NC, pp. 193–213.

44. Schieszler v. *Ferrum College* 236 F Supp 2d 602 No 702CV00131, (WD Va July 15, 2002)

45. Shin v. *MIT*, Middlesex Superior Court, Civil Action No.: 2002-0403A.

46. Brindis, C. and Reyes, P. (1997) At the crossroads: Options for financing college health services in the 21st century. *Journal of American College Health*, **45**(6), 279–288.

47. Molnar, J. (2002) A cross-sectional audit of student health insurance waiver forms: an assessment of reliability and compliance. *Journal of American College Health*, **50**(4), 187–189.

48. Tseng, V. (2004) Family interdependence and academic adjustment in college: Youth from immigrant and US-born families. *Child Development*, **75**(3), 966–983.

49. Yoon, J. and Lau, A.S. (2008) Maladaptive perfectionism and depressive symptoms among Asian American college students: Contributions of interdependence and parental relations. *Cultural Diversity & Ethnic Minority Psychology*, **14**(2), 92–101.

50. Henning, K., Ey, S. and Shaw, D. (1998) Perfectionism, the imposter phenomenon and psychological adjustment in medical, dental, nursing and pharmacy students. *Medical Education*, **32**(5), 456–464.

51. Patock-Peckham, J.A. and Morgan-Lopez, A.A. (2009) Mediational links among parenting styles, perceptions of parental confidence, self-esteem, and depression on alcohol-related problems in emerging adulthood. *Journal of Studies on Alcohol and Drugs*, **70**(2), 215–226.

52. Ying, Y.W., Lee, P.A. and Tsai, J.L. (2007) Predictors of depressive symptoms in Chinese American college students: Parent and peer attachment, college challenges and sense of coherence. *American Journal of Orthopsychiatry*, **77**(2), 316–323.

53. Klink, J.L., Byars-Winston, A. and Bakken, L.L. (2008) Coping efficacy and perceived family support: Potential factors for reducing stress in premedical students. *Medical Education*, **42**(6), 572–579.

54. Nijhof, K.S. and Engels, R.C. (2007) Parenting styles, coping strategies, and the expression of homesickness. *Journal of Adolescence*, **30**(5), 709–720.

55. Neff, K.D., Brabeck, K.M. and Kearney, L.K. (2006) Relationship styles of self-focused autonomy, other-focused connection, and mutuality among Mexican American and European American college students. *The Journal of Social Psychology*, **146**(5), 568–590.

56. Luyckx, K., Soenens, B., Vansteenkiste, M., Goossens, L. and Berzonsky, M.D. (2007) Parental psychology control and dimensions of identity formation in emerging adulthood. *Journal of Family Psychology*, **21**(3), 546–50.

57. Roer-Strier, D. and Rosentahl, M.K. (2001) Socialization in changing cultural contexts: A search for images of the "adaptive adult". *Social Work*, **46**(3), 215–228.

58. Silverman, M., Meyer, P., Sloane, F. *et al.* (1997) The big ten student suicide study. *Suicide and Life Threatening Behavior*, **27**, 285–303.

59. Silverman, M. (2004) College student suicide prevention: Background and blueprint for action. College Mental Health [Special issue]. *Student Health Spectrum*, 13–20.

60. Office of Planning, Evaluation, and Policy Development, Department of Education (2008) Department of Education 34 CFR Part 99 Family Education Rights and Privacy; Privacy Rule. *Federal Register*, **73**(237), 74806–74855.

61. Quinnett, P.G. (2000) *Counseling suicidal people: A therapy of hope*, The QPR Institute, Inc., Spokane, WA.

62. Silber, E. *et al.* (1999) Helping students adapt to graduate school: Making the grade. *Journal of College Student Psychotherapy*, **14**(2), 1–110.

63. Beck, A.T., Steer, R.A., Kovacs M., Garrison B. (1985) Hopelessness and eventual suicide: A 10-year prospective study of the patients hospitalized with suicidal ideation. *The American Journal of Psychiatry*, **142**, 559–563.

11 Psychiatry Residency Training in College Mental Health Services

Jerald Kay[1] and Victor Schwartz[2]

[1]*Department of Psychiatry, Boonshoft School of Medicine, Wright State University, Dayton, OH, USA*
[2]*Yeshiva University, Albert Einstein College of Medicine, New York, NY, USA*

11.1 Introduction

Neither psychiatry nor psychiatric training has historically played a central role in college mental health services. While about half of US college mental health services (CMHSs) employ a staff psychiatrist, many for part-time positions only, most services have not included psychiatric residents among their trainees [1]. By all accounts, this is a missed opportunity for the CMHSs, psychiatric residency training programs and psychiatric residents. As noted in Chapter 1, students are increasingly matriculating having had treatment for psychiatric disorders and therefore are on psychopharmacologic agents prior to college. Many more have their first treatment experience with both psychotherapy and medication once in college [2,3].

11.2 Benefits to Services

Psychiatric resident rotations can provide a number of benefits to CMHSs. One of the challenges for psychiatrists at CMHSs can be the relative professional isolation in which they function. Even in a university that has an affiliated medical school or hospital, CMHS staff are, by and large, geographically and administratively isolated from the medical center. (The staff psychologists and social workers are usually not closely connected to these academic departments or graduate schools either.) Additionally, most CMHSs that employ a staff psychiatrist have only a part-time, or at best, one full-time psychiatric clinician [1] and professional development within the CMHS is quite limited. The lack of collegial relationships within the discipline may have a significant impact on morale and, ultimately, professional recruitment and retention. For example, when the psychiatrist seeks professional consultation or continuing education opportunities, these must occur outside the college service.

Mental Health Care in the College Community   Edited by Jerald Kay and Victor Schwartz
© 2010 John Wiley & Sons, Ltd.

Within all medical specialties, the quality of medical care is improved by services having an academic or teaching program. By virtue of having residents "on service" at the CMHS, supervising psychiatrists are challenged to stay more current in their fund of knowledge. The interaction between residents and staff psychiatrists allows for new information and knowledge sharing among professionals and gives the staff psychiatrist closer contact with the academic department of psychiatry through the residency training program. These factors add to the intellectual and professional vitality and vibrancy of the CMHS for the psychiatrist since teaching, supervising and interacting with other psychiatric colleagues undoubtedly make staff psychiatry positions at a CMHS that much more attractive.

Further, although supervising the work of resident psychiatrists requires the investment of clinical staff time, the addition of these residents can augment the medical coverage at the service. Most CMHSs do not have psychiatric services available during all operating hours yet often students who need immediate attention might require some pharmacologic intervention. Thus, the ability to expand hours of psychiatric coverage on site may obviate the need for an unnecessary emergency room visit for acute medication management. Further, while most CMHSs currently limit their staff psychiatrists' clinical activities to evaluating emergencies, crisis management and psychopharmacology, there are some patients who are best managed by a clinician who can provide combined psychopharmacology and psychotherapy. Psychiatric residents are in an excellent position to provide this combined treatment when indicated. Indeed, one of the chapter authors has argued that combined treatment may be more advantageous in students with significant impairment and severe co-existing chronic medical disorders such as schizophrenia, severe bipolar disorder, treatment resistant depression and a host of medical conditions, such as Crohn's disease, where a student may be on reasonably high levels of glucocorticoids which may cause psychotic and severe mood symptoms [4]. In these situations, effective split treatment, while not impossible, mandates intensive collaboration in a system where time is exceptionally limited.

Psychiatric residents are required to care for patients in hospital psychiatric units, community mental health centers, and psychiatric emergency services in the earlier years of training. Advanced residents, therefore, augment a CMHSs capacity to assess students who may be in the midst of frightening acute crises (psychosis, hallucinogenic or other illicit drug-induced mental disorders, and parasuicidal and suicidal behavior) or who may need to be considered for admission to an inpatient psychiatric service. This can be particularly helpful to CMHSs that do not have clinical staff who are comfortable with or experienced in managing psychiatric crises since it has not been a routine component of their education or training. Residents who are based at the local medical center or community hospital can also serve as liaisons to their local emergency rooms and hospital-based outpatient services for students who may require services beyond the scope of those available at the CMHS. Some departments of psychiatry have specialized clinics for exceptionally challenging patient populations and residents may be in a position to facilitate referrals to these clinics as well as into the hospital system at large. For those services that provide psychiatric training, the connection and communication between the CMHS and the medical centers' departments of psychiatry is generally closer and this brings with it the opportunity for the enhanced sharing of clinical and educational resources. Selected diagnostic procedures that may be indicated for students, but which are rarely available within the CMHS, such as those for sleep studies for obstructive sleep apnea or narcolepsy, can be facilitated by psychiatric residents.

11.3 Benefits to Trainees

The Accrediting Council for Graduate Medical Education (ACGME), the national organization responsible for establishing training requirements, requires a series of psychotherapy competencies for residents (http://www.aadprt.org/training/programs.aspx). Among these competencies are: "brief therapies," "psychodynamic psychotherapies" and "psychotherapy combined with psychopharmacology." Many hospital-based psychiatric outpatient services struggle to attract patients who will provide residents with the full array of psychotherapy experiences expected under these directives since they must often attend to those with severe chronic mental disorders who often function marginally in society. As a result, these patients often struggle with compliance and may not respond robustly to psychotherapeutic intervention. A patient load weighted heavily with severely ill patients often leads residents to an attitude of therapeutic pessimism, or at worst a therapeutic nihilism that psychotherapy is neither efficacious nor helpful. Many residents completing training have never seen a patient with an anxiety or mood disorder respond significantly to psychotherapy as a monotherapy.

The patient population of most CMHSs, on the other hand, provides an excellent and richly varied resource of higher functioning patients more suitable for psychotherapy training. As university students, these patients are often highly appropriate for "talk therapies" and are frequently responsive to brief or focal treatments. They are, moreover, typically motivated for care and interested in understanding themselves. They are often intelligent and relatively psychologically minded. As a function of their youth, many have significant capacity for emotional growth and change during this important developmental phase.

These patients are valuable in helping promote learning of basic therapy skills. Many CMHS patients are struggling with appropriate, but challenging developmental issues, relationship and family problems and, intense life crises with or without other major or incipient clinical concerns. As will be explicated, the trainee faced with assessment and care of these students must be theoretically and clinically flexible and must be cognizant of the importance of prioritizing problems. Treating university students affords the resident the opportunity and challenge of working psychotherapeutically with patients who are often quite similar to themselves; patients with whom they can, and often do, identify. It therefore, provides unique teaching opportunities around issues of idealization and minimization of some types of student concerns. The exploration, for example, of unique countertransference problems is invaluable for the professional development of the young psychotherapist. In some training programs, this opportunity is rarely found in other clinical venues that residents are likely to encounter. As well, working with special college-patient populations (See Chapter 13) such as lesbian–gay–bisexual–transsexual (LGBT) students, student athletes, recently returning veterans, international and minority students, and those with physical disabilities is an attractive option.

Work at the CMHS also provides the resident with the opportunity to consult and manage medications along with other clinicians and to manage medication/psychotherapy cases on her own. Sophisticated split treatment rests upon the development of collaborative skills which are central in the CMHS [5,6]. Since much of residency training is devoted to the care of significantly disturbed patients, many residents do not have extensive opportunity to conduct brief dynamically informed therapy. Residents are required to achieve competency in brief treatment. A resident immersion experience in one of the brief dynamic models, such as those of Mann [7], Luborsky [8], Strupp and Binder [9], or Sifneos [10], to name but a few, is profoundly engaging and rewarding.

College mental health rotations can also afford the resident an opportunity for exposure to general principles of community mental health (see Chapter 2 for further discussion of the interface between community mental health and college mental health) and social psychiatry. An appreciation for the interplay between social, community and personal issues may add to the resident's sophistication; realizing that, for example, students beginning college are often evolving with very different adaptive concerns from those about to graduate can bring the notion of developmental psychology to life for a trainee.

While research is often not treated as central to the role of many CMHSs, some larger and academic programs promote research. This provides another opportunity for psychiatric residents. At times, residents may again act as a conduit between CMHSs and medical school-based departments of psychiatry (which often have better research support). College communities provide an excellent setting in which residents might explore the nexus between psychiatry, prevention strategies and other public health issues. These opportunities will be described in Chapters 14 and 16.

Many CMHSs look for college mental health experience when hiring staff psychiatrists. Residents who rotate through these services are at an advantage in terms of both actual clinical experience and marketability in this setting. It is a priority of the American Psychiatric Association's Committee on College Mental Health to promote the development of a cadre of young psychiatrists who will practice within college mental health. The recently formed Higher Education Mental Health Alliance (HEMHA) has established as one of its goals, the development of comprehensive and best practice-based services for all college and university students (Figure 11.1).

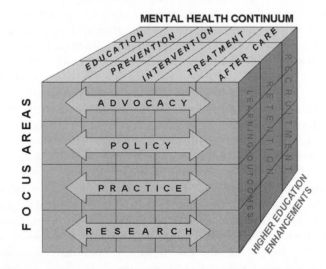

Figure 11.1 *Mission and purpose of HEMHA. American College Health Association. American College Health Association-National College Health Assessment: Reference Group Executive Summary Fall 2007. Baltimore: American College Health Association: 2008.*

11.4 Benefits to Training Programs

For many years, psychiatric residency programs across the United States have offered more positions than can be filled. As such, there is some competition among programs to attract high-quality residents. Providing an opportunity to rotate through CMHSs has typically been an attractive and appealing program component and thus is a positive recruitment tool [11]. The opportunity to collaborate closely with other mental health disciplines outside the traditional hospital in public-sector venues broadens the training experience for many residents and may also make the residency program more attractive to applicants. As noted above, residents can often act as liaison between the CMHS and the local medical center or hospital-based psychiatric outpatient service. This can provide a facilitated conduit between the college service and local hospital service for college student-patients who need longer term or more intensive treatment than can be provided at the CMHS.

11.5 Characteristics of a Rotation

CMHSs are clinically complex and fast-moving services. Most students who present for care are experiencing some degree of personal or psychological crisis. Clinicians working at these services often must respond quickly and nimbly. Further, approximately 50% of CMHSs have a psychiatrist on staff. In other cases, students may be sent to a private consulting psychiatrist or to a nurse practitioner or a general practitioner in the college health service for medication evaluation or management. Given the complexity of the clinical challenges and the often limited options for on-site supervision by psychiatry faculty, residency rotations at CMHSs should be offered to the most senior trainees in a program. Certainly, it is unrealistic to send residents who have not as yet had significant experience conducting outpatient (and especially psychodynamic) psychotherapy. While junior residents (years 1 and 2 of a 4-year program) have the ability to provide an adequate clinical assessment, they are, in all likelihood, unprepared to develop a more sophisticated psychodynamic assessment with any degree of facility. Fourth-year residents general psychiatry or fourth- and fifth-year child fellows (adolescent psychiatry residents) are ideal candidates for work in these clinics. When necessary, talented third-year residents may be able to handle the clinical challenges of these programs when they have access to robust and preferably "on the spot" supervision. Yale University, for example, offers three third-year residents the opportunity to complete their entire outpatient year within the Yale University Health Service (YUHS). This rotation includes two fourth-year, full-time residents as well. Because this program provides care for university students, graduate, and professional students, and often treats patients who may be as old as 60 years of age, there is sufficient patient diversity. Having five full-time residents is possible since the YUHS has eight full time psychiatrists.

While the modal number of visits at CMHSs is one, the average number of visits at most services is approximately five [1]. This means that many patients are seen once but quite a large number are actually seen more than five times. Typical residency rotations, beyond hospital and outpatient settings, are full or half time over 1 to 3 months duration. Ideally, a CMHS residency rotation should allow for a significant number of patients treated by the rotating resident to have a complete course of treatment at the CMHS under one supervising clinician. With this in mind, it is sensible to structure these rotations to last a minimum of 6 months and, whenever possible, it is best if the resident can rotate for a full academic year.

Since the academic residency year begins over the summer and finishes in June and since the typical college academic year (and thus the busy time for most CMHSs) lasts from late August until mid-May, this allows for some flexibility in the duration and timing of resident experiences. If the service has some activity during the summer, it is often helpful to have residents begin a rotation during the summer (or for that matter during January for 6-month rotations) so that residents can become adjusted to this very unique setting while things are not as hectic. They can be assigned some patients during the time that clinical staff has maximal availability to supervise their work carefully.

Given the exigencies of financing residency rotations outside of the traditional medical school or university hospital settings, residency training programs find 6–12 month long, half-time or full assignments impractical. In order for the resident to be properly acculturated to the CMHS experience, for the experience to be educationally useful to the resident, and clinically helpful to the service, the resident must be on site for at least half a day each week. This allows for several hours of clinical time and an hour for supervision and paperwork. As a matter of efficiency and convenience, it is even more helpful if the resident can be on site for a full day each week. This allows enough time for the resident to have a varied array of clinical activities and experiences while at the service. These may include, for example, group therapy for eating disorders, students who self harm, substance abuse, and even stress management.

11.6 Centrality of Supervision

There can be no substitute for in depth supervision of residents assigned to such a novel experience as a CMHS. Although interdisciplinary supervision and case conferences contribute to diversified experiences, all psychiatry residents must receive supervision from a psychiatrist because of significant issues of professionalization as well as accreditation requirements. Residents are not permitted to practice independently. For each rotation, individual or group supervision must be provided so that residents can discuss all of their patients. In the smaller CMHS, minimal supervision may be only 1 hour weekly. However, in complex university settings where residents are responsible for a large assessment and treatment caseload, supervision should approximate the need of the resident. Even in uncomplicated medication management, the wise supervisor insists on familiarity with all of resident cases (see Appendix A for Helpful Hints for Supervisors). Ultimately, the residency training program through its faculty is obligated to:

- Provide phase-appropriate documented clinical experiences

- Ensure that clinical service is balanced with education

- Assess medical knowledge

- Formally evaluate all trainees throughout all didactic and clinical experiences

- Ensure practice-based learning and improvement (e.g. reading, self-directed learning, workshops/conferences, develop lifelong learning habits)

- Stimulate continued interpersonal and communication skill development

- Assess resident professionalism with patients, colleagues, and within clinical systems

- Monitor the number of hours worked by residents

- Develop teaching and administrative skills

- Ensure competence to work within various health care delivery systems (e.g. coordinate patient care within systems, sensitivity to cost containment, advocate for quality patient care).

Types of supervisory experiences vary from one CMHS to another and depend on whether a psychiatrist is employed by the university or college service. The advantage of on-site supervision should not be underestimated. Such an arrangement allows immediate consultation when challenging cases arise, provides opportunity for observed patient encounters, and may permit clinical teaching through shared activities, such as co-leading group treatments. It may also be a vehicle for co-teaching with the supervisor. Group supervision of residents may be required when there is a large number of trainees rotating through the CMHS. One of the authors has six general psychiatry residents and or child adolescent psychiatry residents yearly within two separate universities. Supervision is scheduled for more than 1 hour weekly in each university by on-site psychiatry faculty and lasts until all clinical material is reviewed. Group supervision also promotes resident learning from peers. (See Appendix A for Helpful Hints for Supervisors.)

Off-site supervision is a traditional model in residency training especially regarding psychotherapy. Without a CMHS employed psychiatrist, this is the supervisory model in many residency programs. Although most supervision focuses on clinical experiences, administrative and system issues peculiar to college life arise frequently and are important to discuss. The off-site supervisor, in particular, would be wise to communicate with the CMHS director about the progress of the psychiatry residents and to assist in identifying areas that need special attention. The same is true for the Director of Psychiatry Residency Training in the medical school. It is also often helpful for the resident who is receiving supervision from an off-site faculty member to have regular, brief meetings with a senior clinician at the CMHS to assure that issues specific either to the university setting or the particular institution are being properly addressed and managed.

11.7 Didactic Curriculum

The authors are keen on presentations by residents to their departments of psychiatry grand rounds (continuing medical education attended by faculty, trainees, medical students and community clinicians) as well as conferences within the CMHS. In the case of the former, yearly presentations enforce training program interest in this area, raise potential research or writing opportunities, and expose full-time and volunteer faculty to a growing and challenging mental health care issue of which many are unaware. For those medical school departments that may also have faculty at the college health services, grand rounds presentations with internal medicine and family medicine, for example, often provide an exciting dimension. In large universities, there may be a full-time gynecologist at the student health service, but in most institutions there is likely to be limited on-site service. Issues of sexuality, sexual trauma, infectious disease, to name but a few topics, are often of interest to medical school departments of obstetrics and gynecology. At Wright State University, there is a yearly grand rounds and a conference on college mental health to which clinicians and administrators of all surrounding institutions are invited. The latter provides an opportunity to share program development and address emerging issues. Presentations at CMHS interdisciplinary clinical conferences provide residents with additional teaching opportunities. They also promote greater appreciation for the role of other mental health professionals. These presentations are excellent venues for examining collaborative care issues such as split treatment, conjoint group and individual psychotherapy, campus crisis, legal and ethical dilemmas, and outreach and preventive activities.

The daunting requirements of the psychiatry residency program and the limited time spent by select residents in the CMHS necessitate that, for the most part, didactics occur within the confines of the general residency curriculum. First and foremost, a strong grounding in human development is vital. All training programs teach human development. It is helpful within these courses that when adolescence and young adulthood are discussed, special mention should be made of the college student. Some CMHS psychiatrists urge their residents to read a general introduction to the field, like *College of the Overwhelmed* [12].

Some CMHS psychiatrists have noted that residents are sometimes unfamiliar with the Western concept of adolescence and all of its characteristics. Lectures and readings should address the transitional psychological tasks of early, middle, and late adolescence. These include, but are not limited to:

• Separation from parents and family

• Establishing greater affinity with peer groups

• Consolidation of sense of self

• Increased sexual experimentation

• Emergence of more intimate relationships

• Experimentation with alcohol and drugs for many

• Consideration of the future regarding career and long term relationships [13].

One of the major advances in the study of adult development recently has been the elucidation of late adolescence and early adulthood (18–25 years) as distinct developmental phases; the latter marked by significant exploration, growth, heightened ability to self-focus, possibility of greater variety of social roles, and the emergence of strengths [14,15]. This period has also been called "emerging adulthood" [16].

Although each generation has faced unique challenges, it has been noted [17] that today's early adults are the first generation to:

• Compete in a global economy

• Have instantaneous world-wide communication

• Understand domestic terrorism

• Fear HIV/AIDS throughout their lives

• Experience the destruction of an American city from natural disaster.

11.8 Developmental Psychopathology

Serious psychiatric disorders such as depression, bipolar disorder, panic disorder, eating disorders, substance abuse, self-harm behavior, antisocial behavior and schizophrenia are the illnesses of young people. Residents must appreciate the impact of these disorders on their college patients. They must also be aware that first breaks in severe disorders may not present classically as they do in adults. It is no longer scientifically tenable to think of adolescence as a period of "normal psychosis" or constant emotional upheaval. Symptoms must be taken seriously for most students do not outgrow them.

The vast majority of psychiatric disorders are precipitated by one or more stressors which, while they do not cause an illness, are instrumental in its unfolding. The leading theoretical framework of American psychiatry rests upon interaction between gene and environment. Neither by itself is sufficient to account for most disorders and psychiatry has abandoned the nature versus nurture mythology. However, some common stressors among college students include:

- Separation from family

- Family illness or divorce

- Loss of romantic relationships and friendships

- Emerging gender conflict

- Conflicted sexual experiences with or without sexually transmitted diseases

- Exposure to unanticipated academic competition and academic expectations

- Emergence of a heretofore undiagnosed learning disorder

- Marginal academic performance

- Challenges of living with roommates

- Establishment of new social supports and networks

- Challenges to deeply held religious and other beliefs

- Sexual and physical trauma (e.g., date rape).

Who are the students at greater risk for psychiatric disorders in college? In general, the diagnosis of a disorder earlier in life frequently places the entering student at greater risk for future emotional problems. This includes the student diagnosed with schizophrenia, bipolar disorder, severe personality disorder, sexual disorders, PTSD from sexual trauma, eating disorder, substance abuse disorder, and some anxiety disorders such as panic and obsessive compulsive disorders. Students with significant learning deficits and disorders also constitute an at-risk group. The student with significant physical disabilities, in a college that is insensitive to special needs students, may also be at greater risk for social and academic failure. Larger state universities, in particular, have begun to address some of the unique attributes of returning combat veterans, a group who are entering higher education in increasing numbers. In short, many clinicians working in larger public universities are struck by the similarities to those colleagues currently in the public sector community mental health center. The number of patients is increasing, their acuity is elevated, and the resources to accommodate these shifts have not grown.

Assigned reading on psychopathology might also include national survey data on the incidence, prevalence, and under treatment of mental disorders among college students. The executive summaries of the yearly National Survey of Counseling Center Directors, American College Health Association National College Health Assessment, the National Center on Addiction and Substance Abuse Study [18] and other recent epidemiological investigations [19] are especially recommended. High school studies supporting the vulnerability of some students in the transition period to college are also useful (Jed Foundation Transition Year Project, 2009 [20]).

Protective factors in adolescence and young adulthood are powerful influences against emerging psychopathology. Residents must appreciate that resilience is highly dependent on the development of social support, maturity of defense mechanisms and personality attributes that contribute to the capacity to master stress, and self-understanding [21].

11.9 Psychopharmacology

Beyond required experiences in primary care and neurology, residents initially learn to diagnose and treat psychiatric disorder during early assignments to inpatient mental health services. This is supplemented by rotations in the hospital and clinic providing consultation and liaison to medical and surgical specialties. The art and science of psychopharmacology in treating severely affected hospitalized patients must be complemented with the treatment of outpatients. The CMHS rotation, therefore, is an excellent site for advanced psychopharmacological instruction [22]. Patients within the CMHS may have nearly all of the diagnoses of those requiring hospital-based treatment but with less acuity. This includes anxiety, mood, eating, substance abuse, and personality disorders. Providing an effective medication regimen to college students who cannot be overly sedated because they are required to attend class and study is a central skill. As a group, students may not have the means to afford medication. Learning how to dispense cost-effective medication is a must. Knowledge of generic medications that can be obtained by students for as little as $4.00 monthly enhances treatment compliance. Last, the CMHS provides an excellent introduction to the assessment of learning disorders, and where appropriate, their treatment with medication.

A more complete listing of the traditional goals and objectives of a resident experience in college mental health may be found in Appendix II.

11.10 The Resident's Clinical Theoretical Framework

It goes without saying that the resident who enters a CMHS rotation with a unidimensional view of patients, be that purely biological or psychological, will receive less from a rotation and will undoubtedly give his or her patents less than optimal care. Mention has been made of residents providing psychotherapy during CMHS rotations. The authors feel strongly that residents should not be relegated to prescribing medication only. Although establishing effective collaboration in split treatment is an important skill to attain, rotations must permit treating patients with both medication and psychotherapy. Indeed, most residents may have not treated patients with psychotherapy as a monotherapy in earlier clinical rotations devoted to patients with severe and persistent mental disorders. Skills in brief psychodynamic psychotherapy, cognitive behavioral therapy, interpersonal psychotherapy, and crisis intervention can be consolidated within the CMHS rotation. Some residents may have experiences in or exposure to group therapies. Group treatments, in particular, have received less attention in psychiatry training over the last decade. Most CMHSs offer group treatments for eating disorders, substance use, and self harm behavior. Others can be exposed for the first time to behavioral techniques like relaxation and meditation to name but two. Residents in psychodynamically orientated training programs often have much to share with non-psychiatric trainees coming from a more exclusive cognitive, behavioral, or health psychology orientation.

11.11 Increasing Visibility of Social Media

The age of rapid and increasingly sophisticated electronic communication offers new mechanisms to enhance psychotherapeutic and psychopharmacologic treatment among college and university students. However, these resources and techniques are accompanied by novel ethical and legal issues which are currently being addressed on college campuses throughout the country. It is unlikely that psychiatry residents will receive a more thorough introduction to this topic outside of the CMH service. Because students in higher education are at the forefront of communication technologies such as Facebook.com, the resident will undoubtedly become aware of the advantages and disadvantages of social media. The former includes opportunities for online peer support, reminder mechanisms for medication compliance, and education about mental health resources and services to name but a few. However, the challenges of these new communication venues include many facets of how to use electronic therapeutic interventions while maintaining strict confidentiality and privacy, being careful not to rely on these resources for emergency care as well as the inherent limitations of electronic therapy as a substitute for clinical interaction. Therapist liability issues are also of critical importance. In short, the CMH rotation offers psychiatry residents new learning experiences with technology and outreach efforts.

11.12 Fellowships in CMH

Despite the pressing need for psychiatrists with training experience in College Mental Health (CMH), there are surprisingly few post-residency fellowship programs. Funding such positions appears to be the limiting factor in the creation of these programs. Full-time, year-long experiences can incorporate administrative aspects which are not easily accommodated in fourth-year, part-time rotations. At the University of Chicago, for example, fellows gain experience in mental health disability accommodation policy, consultation to students going on and off medical leave for psychiatric reasons, and consultation for behavioral health issues on campus including working with faculty, staff, and peers about how to deal with troubled students. This may include consulting with student life and student services programs. A fellow also serves as liaison to the department of psychiatry at the medical school around services to students that need more intensive care. Travel support is available to attend national college mental health meetings. A scholarly project is required prior to completion of the fellowship. Providing there is not a complete complement of third and fourth year residents requesting a CMH rotation, Yale University has offered a post-residency fellowship. In another fellowship program at Ohio State University, participation in utilization and quality assurance is encouraged. Last, a fellow could serve as a liaison to a special academic unit, such as the athletic program. Coaches and athletic directors often have unique challenges regarding the welfare and wellbeing of their student athletes.

11.13 Conclusion

Given the recent data supporting the growing prevalence and incidence of mental health disorders among college and university students, as well as the disconcerting studies documenting the need for greater treatment resources, a rotation in the CMHS is exceedingly timely. This type of clinical-educational experience is an example, *par excellence*, of a remarkably beneficial collaboration between psychiatric graduate medical education and a university. Gains to the institution of higher learning, the CMHS, the trainee, and, of course, the patient, are well worth the effort of providing these rich experiences. Hopefully, all college and university mental health services will provide these opportunities in the future.

Appendix A: Helpful Hints for Supervisors

- Encourage flexible listening
  Residents entering rotations at CMHSs have typically worked in hospital-based services with seriously ill patients. As such, their impulse is to listen and assess with their primary attention to "making a diagnosis." While attention to diagnostic concerns is crucial, many students coming for help at their CMHS are not so much concerned with symptomatic complaints as by some more (at least apparently) "real life" problem. If these issues are not acknowledged and discussed, the student will likely feel unheard and not cared for. Residents must learn to listen and respond at multiple levels.

- Help residents to "take a deep breath" and wait a bit before pulling out the prescription pad. As noted above, residents are typically orientated toward making diagnoses and treating. Their training leads them to look for symptoms and treat them, usually with medication. College students (being young adults) can be remarkably changeable and fluid in mood and presentation. Unless symptoms are severe, acute or dangerous, it is often sensible to give things a bit of time. Many presenting symptoms that on their face seem quite disturbing are self-limiting and often improve quickly with supportive care.

- Encourage practical treatment planning
  It is often challenging for residents to balance the demands of assessment, support, symptom management, practical help and psychoeducation all within the limits of what is usually a very short treatment. Patients and residents must be helped to prioritize problems. There should be careful consideration to what therapeutic work can be accomplished in a brief time.

- Familiarize residents with medication costs
  Many students have limited financial resources. Residents should prescribe generic medications and inform students where they may receive the lowest prices. For those patients requiring non-generic medication, residents should be made aware of programs that provide students with these medications at low cost or even without charge.

- Work from the surface down

  In our experience, many student problems are not so much based on neurotic conflict as on lack of information or naiveté about life. It is important to remember that many students are living away from home for the first time while at college. Many life-style issues that their parents may have broadly managed or facilitated (such as when and how much to eat or sleep), may not be obvious to them now that they are living on their own. It is often worth trying to see whether a problem can be resolved through the sharing of a bit of information or by making an environmental adjustment. If this does not solve the problem, then it is likely based on more deeply rooted problems or conflicts.

- Some patients will need a treatment in preparation for treatment

  Many patients presenting at CMHSs have never had prior therapy and have little idea what therapy or psychiatric treatment entails. Others have had treatment as adolescents and often, since this treatment may be imposed on them, the resulting experiences are not positive ones. Thus, it is useful to keep in mind that even patients who need a long-term or fairly intensive treatment, may be uneasy when presented with this recommendation. It is often necessary to do a brief treatment at the CMHS to educate the patient about the therapy process, begin to make them curious about themselves and to prepare them to accept referral for a more definitive treatment.

- It is OK to enjoy treating patients

  As noted earlier, university students are often intelligent and relatively insightful and thoughtful. And although their frequent similarity to their treating resident in background, intelligence and outlook can present treatment challenges, it also often makes them highly enjoyable to treat. While residents need to be monitored in supervision for countertransference issues that may emerge or as a result of identification, it also needs to be communicated that therapeutic work can be fun. Ultimately, this is why most residents find a CMHS rotation so enjoyable.

Appendix B: PGY IV (Postgraduate Year Four) Psychiatric Resident Rotation, Student Mental Health Rotations, Wright State University, University of Dayton

Scope of Program

This program provides PGY IV residents the opportunity to spend one-half day/week to one day/week for 12 months on this service. The goals for PGY IVs are a reinforcement of the skills acquired in the previous years and include psychopharmacological consultations for patients treated in psychotherapy by other clinicians.

Goals and Objectives

Patient care

- Perform a comprehensive initial psychiatric intake interview

- Understand young adults in college within a developmental and biopsychosocial frame of reference

- Appreciate the interaction between personality, temperament, culture, clinical symptoms and the patient's functioning
- Formulate treatment plans within a short-term treatment model
- Treat patients with brief psychotherapy techniques, cognitive-behavioral treatment approaches and crisis intervention
- Integrate pharmacological treatment with psychotherapy modalities.

Medical knowledge

- Build on previously learned *DSM IV* TR diagnostic categories of the major psychiatric syndromes and apply to a population of young adults
- Appreciate the complex interaction between Axis I and Axis II diagnoses
- Complete assigned reading of selected chapters from a textbook on college mental health
- Be familiar with the high prevalence of substance abuse disorders as co-morbid conditions in college students and be able to recognize substance induced clinical symptoms
- Understand the complex etiology and differential diagnosis of academic performance problems
- Perform office screening tests for students with attention deficit complaints
- Know the university/college policy regarding the treatment of students with stimulants.

Interpersonal and communication skills

- Establish rapport with young adults from diverse cultural backgrounds
- Interact effectively with a multidisciplinary staff of psychologists, social workers, care managers, nurse practitioners, psychiatrists and trainees of these respective disciplines
- Educate patients about their conditions and explain the indications for short-term vs. long-term treatment or cognitive-behavioral treatment
- Be aware of the confidentiality policies as outlined in HIPAA (Health Insurance Portability and Accountability Act) and FERPA (Family Educational Rights and Privacy Act)
- Communicate with the student's parents while maintaining confidentiality laws and appropriate treatment boundaries.

Systems-based practice

- Be aware of the different services within the Student Health Center beyond mental health such as primary care, urgent care, women's health, speciality services
- Master the electronic health record, where applicable, and make appropriate referrals within the organization
- Understand the concept of crisis response services and educate the students about these services

- Know about the high prevalence rate of depression and suicidal risk among college students.

Practice-based learning

- Improve clinical skills through case discussion in supervision with a psychiatric attending
- Integrate supervisory feedback and suggestions into the management of cases
- Utilize various electronic databases to search for literature relevant to college mental health
- Seek consultations from staff and supervisors concerning complex cases with eating disorders, substance abuse, trauma, and LGBT issues
- Improve ability for interdisciplinary dialogue by participating in joint case conferences with psychology, social work and counseling trainees.

Professionalism

- Demonstrate respect for patients and staff, regardless of cultural background
- Have a collaborative attitude towards other professional staff within the Student Health Center
- Display an empathic attitude towards patients and their family members
- Conduct yourself in a professional manner and show reliable, responsible and punctual behavior.

Method of evaluation

- Weekly individual supervision by psychiatric attendings with constructive feedback and suggestions for clinical management
- *Ad hoc* case discussions and informal consultations by psychologists and social workers among the staff
- Verbal feedback midway and at the end of the rotation by the attending supervisor
- Written performance evaluation at the end of the rotation as stipulated by the WSU Residency Training program.

Based in part, New York University Goals and Objectives for Psychiatric CMH Rotation.

References

1. Gallagher, R.P. (2008) *National Survey of Counseling Center Directors*, The International Association of Counseling Services, Inc., pp, 1–33. http://www.iacsinc.org/2008%20National%20Survey%20of%20Counseling%20Center%20Directors.pdf.
2. American College Health Association/National College Health Assessment (2007) Summarized Mental Health Data and Trends, Spring 2000, Spring 2007.
3. Eisenberg, D., Golberstein, E. and Gollust, S.E. (2007) Help-seeking and access to mental health care in a university student population. *Medical Care*, **45**(7), 594–601.

4. Kay, J. (2001) Integrated treatment: An overview, in *Integrated Treatment for Psychiatric Disorders: Review of Psychiatry*, vol. 20 (ed. J. Kay), American Psychiatric Press, Washington, DC, pp. 1–29.

5. Kay, J. (2005) Psychotherapy and medication, in *Oxford Textbook of Psychotherapy* (ed. G.O. Gabbard), Oxford University Press, Inc., New York, NY, pp. 463–476.

6. Kay, J. (2008) Combining psychodynamic psychotherapy with medication, in *The Textbook of Psychotherapeutic Treatments* (ed. G.O. Gabbard), American Psychiatric Publishing, Inc., Arlington, VA, pp. 133–161.

7. Mann, J. (1973) *Time-Limited Psychotherapy*, Harvard University Press, Cambridge, MA.

8. Luborsky, L. (1984) *Principles of Psychoanalytic Psychotherapy: A Manual for Supportive–Expressive Treatment*, Basic Books, New York.

9. Strupp, H.H. and Binder, J.L. (1984) *Psychotherapy in a New Key: A Guide to Time-Limited Dynamic Psychotherapy*, Basic Books, New York.

10. Sifnoeos, P.E. (1979) Short-term dynamic psychotherapy: Evaluation and technique. New York: Plenum.

11. Moran, M. (2005) Residents help meet demand for college MH services. *Psychiatric News*, 12; Vol 40:24, 2005 American Psychiatric Association, p. 4.

12. Kadison, R. and DiGeronimo, T.F. (2004) *College of the Overwhelmed*, Jossey-Bass, San Francisco, CA.

13. Towbin, K.E. and Showalter, J.E. (2008) Adolescent development, in *Psychiatry*, vol. 1, 3rd edn (eds A. Tasman, J. Kay, J.A. Lieberman *et al.*), John Wiley & Sons, Ltd, England, pp. 161–180.

14. Beardslee, W.R. and Vaillant, G. (2008) Adult development, in *Psychiatry*, vol. 1, 3rd edn (eds A. Tasman, J. Kay, J.A. Lieberman *et al.*), John Wiley & Sons, Ltd, England, pp. 181–195.

15. Masten, A.S., Burt, K.B., Roisman, G.I. *et al.* (2004) Resources and resilience in the transition to adulthood: Continuity and change. *Development and Psychopathology*, **16**(4), 1071–1094.

16. Arnett, J.J. (2000) Emerging adulthood: A theory of development from the late teens through the twenties. *American Psychologist*, **55**(5), 469–480.

17. National Research Council and Institute of Medicine (2006) *A Study of Interactions: Emerging Issues in the Science of Adolescence*, National Academies Press, Washington, DC.

18. National Center on Addiction and Substance Abuse (CASA) at Columbia University (2007) Wasting the best and the brightest: Substance abuse at America's colleges and universities.

19. Blanco, C., Okuda, M., Wright, C. *et al.* (2008) Mental health of college students and their non–college-attending peers: Results from the National Epidemiologic Study on Alcohol and Related Conditions. *Archives of General Psychiatry*, **65**(12), 1429–1437.

20. Jed Foundation Transition Year Project (2009) http://www.jedfoundation.org/parents/programs/transition-year-project.

21. Beardslee, W.R. (1989) The role of self-understanding in resilient individuals: The development of a perspective. *American Journal of Orthopsychiatry*, **59**(2), 266–278.

22. Schwartz, V. (2006) Medications, in *College Mental Health Practice* (eds P. Grayson and P.W. Meilman), Taylor & Francis Group, New York, NY, pp. 59–78.

12 Psychology and Social Work Training in University Mental Health

David A. Davar

Jewish Theological Seminary, New York, NY, USA

12.1 Introduction

As the sheer number of students grappling with urgent and complex psychiatric difficulties increasingly overwhelms college counseling centers [1], establishing a new training program or maintaining and/or expanding an established training program has many advantages:

- A training program can provide a dramatically increased amount of care, and reduce the clinical burden on professional staff.

- The trainee-staff can be utilized to significantly expand clinical outreach and prevention

- Teaching and supervising trainees can increase the expertise and broaden the experience of professional staff

- A training program can assist in recruitment by helping to guarantee new hires the opportunity to supervise

- A training program may increase the staff's professional and institutional pride.

Though adding a program requires additional funding, additional administration and supervision, and exposes a college to the risks of allowing inexperienced clinicians to provide care, the downsides are more than mitigated by being able to provide care to many more students.

12.2 Administrative Matters

The chief consideration when setting up a new training program is finding the right balance between the primary mission of providing outreach, prevention, and treatment to the university community, and providing trainees with a high level of supervised training and opportunities to gain clinical experience [2].

Mental Health Care in the College Community   Edited by Jerald Kay and Victor Schwartz
© 2010 John Wiley & Sons, Ltd.

By accepting practicum and internship trainees, a training program undertakes the obligation to provide them with a defined clinical caseload and appropriate supervision [3]. Part-time trainees typically provide 6–8 hours of direct care per week, requiring 1.5–2 hours of supervision. Trainees in full-time internships do substantially more direct care hours, and receive approximately 1 hour of face-to-face supervision for every 4 direct care hours provided [3]. Training affiliation agreements typically have clauses outlining the needs and responsibilities of both the academic program and the training site [4]. Individual clauses detail such matters as indemnification and insurance; procedures regarding unethical, incompetent, or inappropriate behavior by a trainee; and compensation, supervision, and evaluation.

Establishing a training program will mark a major change in the way a counseling service operates and affects both the professional and support staff. As such, it is crucial to treat all staff as stakeholders in the new program and involve them in all phases of its planning [5].

In addition to an enthusiastic buy-in from the counseling center staff, gaining support from the university administration is key: a training program cannot operate without cooperation from a college's human resources, legal, and risk management departments [4]. Salary and benefit packages must be coordinated with human resources; training affiliation agreements need to be approved by the legal counsel; and liability/insurance matters must be arranged with the risk management office since psychology and social work trainees are typically insured by their academic programs, which must provide current documentation [4].

Determining the proper size of the program is also essential. While counseling center data on the number of new applications for treatment in prior years is a major factor, not all of them will be suitable for treatment by trainees; a careful assessment of the number of consulting rooms and supervisory hours available will also need to be made before a training director can decide on how many trainees to accept each year.

The senior staff responsible for overseeing the interns must also be knowledgeable about training and supervision and may wish to consider the painstaking – but ultimately rewarding – process of applying for accreditation with the International Association of Counseling Services (IACS) [2].

12.3 Ethical and Legal Considerations

As mentioned, implementing a training program incurs a dual obligation: The counseling service has a primary mission to provide competent and ethical care to university students needing treatment [2]; the training program is obligated to provide trainees with a rich and stimulating training and supervisory experience, exposure to a diverse range of cases, and a caseload sufficient to meet the direct care requirement. But the primary obligation of offering competent care to university students does not exist in perfect alignment with the needs and requirements of the trainees [2]. The accreditation standards of IACS state:

> Counseling centers must provide training, professional development and continuing education experiences for staff and trainees.Training and supervision of others (paraprofessionals, practicum students, pre-doctoral interns, post-doctoral psychology resident/fellows, etc.) are appropriate and desirable responsibilities of counseling services. While training and supervision are legitimate functions, they should not supersede the primary service role of the agency. http://www.iacsinc.org/Accreditation%20Standards.htm

One potential ethical conflict exists within the procedures used to assign cases to therapists in training. The Association of Psychology State Boards recommends that supervisors have direct knowledge of the cases they supervise [3], but this is rarely the case [6]. In fact, in a survey of counseling center supervisors conducted in 1996, Freeman and McHenry found that only 3% of counseling center supervisors had made supervisory client screening part of their practice [7]. To mitigate this, a telephone triage system for entry into care is desirable on many levels [5]. When senior clinicians do the telephone screening, cases that are inappropriate for therapists-in-training can be referred either to professional staff or appropriate resources in the community [5,8].

A good training program will also have thoughtful policies and procedures governing access to supervision. Given the anxiety common among therapists in training and the ubiquity of crises brought to college counseling centers, trainees often need both immediate and after-hours assistance from supervisors [8].

A second ethical conflict exists regarding the assignment of cases too complicated or challenging for an inexperienced therapist-in-training. Ideally, as a trainee grows in experience and clinical competence, the program should also expose him or her to increasingly complex clinical experiences. But assigning a case that is beyond a trainee's ability can have catastrophic consequences for the client and may pose a traumatic setback to a trainee's confidence and professional development. Yet, being too protective of trainees robs them of the opportunities for growth that come through grappling with increasingly challenging clinical realities. This is another reason why senior clinicians should perform a telephone triage of students applying for treatment to ensure that they are assigned to trainees deemed to have sufficient skills, competencies, maturity, and experience to provide adequate care [5].

Training programs have an essential place in the preparation of competent and ethical mental health practitioners because of their critical role in providing real-world experience with supervised clinical practice. However, both purely academic and practical training sites have a duty to protect both the public and the profession by playing a gatekeeping role in identifying and remediating impaired and/or incompetent trainees [9–11]. Lumadue and Duffy caution that legal action can result from a program graduating a clearly incompetent or impaired clinician [11]. The best safeguard against legal jeopardy is to thoroughly document a program's standards and to consistently follow best practices when assigning cases to trainees, diligently supervise their clinical work, and maintain written evaluations of their competence and of any remedial efforts taken to bring a trainee in line with professional standards.

Case 1

Jason had always done well academically. He had gotten into his first choice graduate school with ease. But he sometimes struggled outside the classroom and he knew it. When the practicum supervisors asked who had no previous clinical experience his heart beat wildly. He was excited to finally get to meet his first client but scared he would blow it. Would the client like him. Would he be able to help? How should he handle personal questions? Somehow his thoughts wondered to the night in high school when he forgot his lines on stage and just froze. Then there was the sex thing. Jason was questioning his sexuality and worried he might be gay. His family was very traditional and he knew they would never accept homosexuality. What if his first client was an attractive gay male? Jason took a deep cleansing breath.

12.4 Recruitment and Selection of Trainees

Training programs should devote considerable time and resources to the selection of applicants. A lack of due diligence during the screening process can prove costly if an unprepared or temperamentally inappropriate trainee causes treatments not to go well, increases tension among the trainee cohort, or has unmanageable difficulties with supervision. It is beneficial to have two staff members and a current trainee interview each applicant, then process and discuss the screening interview immediately following its conclusion to determine a rating based on an agreed-upon system. Kay's [12] rating system is useful (Figure 12.1).

The interviewers should place particular emphasis on such foundational capacities and competencies as self-reflection, self-awareness, being open to constructive supervisory feedback, and the ability to relate in an empathic and non-judgmental way [13]. Additional time spent implementing a vigorous screening process is usually well worth the effort in ensuring that only well-qualified trainees are selected.

INTERVIEW RATING FORM

APPLICANT: _____   DATE:

RATER: ___

	Poor	Fair	Average	Good	Out-standing
Past performance and recommendations					
Work and educational history/habits					
Energy and motivation					
Psychological mindedness					
Capacity for mature coping					
Language/communication skills					
Interpersonal relatedness					
Emotional stability, maturity					
Integrity, ethics, professionalism					
Interest in our program					

Estimated Strengths:

Estimated Weaknesses:

Comments (justify any poor or outstanding ratings):

Figure 12.1 *Interview rating form.*

12.5 Running a Successful Training Program

Attracting a large enough pool of talented applicants may require marketing the program. Hunter *et al.* reported in 2009 that more than 90% of large US organizations have dedicated web pages focused on recruitment [14]. To market your program, you will need print materials that include an informative brochure that is also posted on a user-friendly web page. Networking with directors of clinical training is also helpful in getting trainee referrals, as is attendance at events such as psychology/social work training fairs.

Once trainees are accepted, the welcome letter serves an important function in formally welcoming the new trainees, covering such logistics as listing the dates of upcoming mandatory training events, reminding the intern of any days of the week when attendance is expected, and recommending summer readings.

Stressing that trainees will play a critical role in your program and are treated as junior colleagues rather than as slave labor can't be emphasized enough. Once the training cohort is in place, it is helpful to schedule a number of celebrations, such as an end-of-the-year party, where trainees are thanked for their hard work and their important contribution is affirmed. Awards such as books in an area of interest to individual recipients, are an affordable way to recognize distinctive commitment and service [15]. A good training program can also be invigorated by the joint participation of the trainees and supervisors in relevant in-service professional development to which mental health experts are invited to make presentations on topics relevant to college mental health.

Most important to the success of the program will be the qualifications and skills of the supervisors [16]. Supervisors will ideally be capable mentors knowledgeable about university mental health. Kaslow *et al.* recommend the professional development of supervision competencies through activities such as postdoctoral courses on supervising, supervision of supervision, and conducting evaluations of a supervisor's competencies as a supervisor [17].

12.6 From Theory to College Counseling Practice: CAPS Orientation for New Trainees

Orientation is an opportunity for staff and trainees to begin to get to know each other and for supervisors to welcome the trainees, explain their mission, set realistic goals, announce clear expectations, and begin the process of mentoring. An orientation program is an important and exciting opportunity to help trainees acculturate to their role as members of the counseling service and therefore requires careful planning and clear objectives.

A clear explanation of a university's Counseling and Psychological Services (CAPS) policies and procedures is a critical part of a successful orientation. Trainees should be given a handbook that covers the following expectations:

- Record-keeping

- Communicating via e-mail and expectations regarding timely response to students' messages

- Exercising appropriate discretion when leaving messages with a roommate or relative

- Medication referrals and ways to work collaboratively with the CAPS psychiatrist (s)

- Procedures for urgent and after hours supervisory consultation

- Protocol for trainee correspondence with faculty.

- Scheduling logistics: (can trainees see clients in the center after supervisors have left; what are the parameters?)

- Post-termination contact with clients

- Timely reporting of suicidality

- Reporting of suspected child abuse

- Process for evaluation of trainee's competency during her placement at CAPS

- Referrals to off-campus community resources

- Professional demeanor and dress code.

While the majority of trainees may not need any instruction regarding standards of professional dress and behavior, a few trainees seem inclined to come to work attired in ways likely to elicit unhelpful reactions from clients. In one large East Coast counseling center training program, for example, a male trainee wore shorts and sandals to work, a female trainee wore attire more suitable to nightclubbing, and a psychiatry resident insisted on wearing his white laboratory coat even in the university counseling center. So that it not appear as arbitrary and rigid rule-setting, discussion of the dress code can be contextualized as an element of the client-therapist interaction; unnecessarily provocative attire is assigned meaning by student-clients, and introduces unneeded complexity to the therapeutic encounter [15]. Other practical issues that should be covered during orientation include the assigning of supervisors and consulting rooms and the importance of gathering and dealing with the insurance paperwork required by the program.

12.6.1 Orientation: Knowing the History, Mission, Setting, and Population

An introduction to the history and mission of college counseling in general as well as knowing the specific counseling center's setting and the population it serves will also help ground the trainees and contextualize their work and training.

12.6.2 Knowing the History and Sociocultural Shifts

The primary purpose of counseling centers has shifted from academic advising to the evaluation and treatment of mild, moderate, and severe psychopathology [18]. Sociocultural shifts in the perceptions of hierarchy and authority have implications for the therapeutic encounter. These shifts have made the clinical exchange far more egalitarian than previously, in ways that have implications for both client and trainee in the consulting room. In today's more horizontal, less formal social settings, many students and their parents have an attitude of entitlement and an expectation of immediate gratification. A student's definition of what constitutes a mental health emergency might include getting a "B" on an exam and he or she may demand to be seen immediately to somehow treat the "problem". Moreover, the increasingly common phenomenon of "helicopter parents" – that is always hovering – who expect to speak to their son or daughter's therapist or threaten to complain to the dean of students or call an attorney when a situation doesn't turn out exactly as expected, can raise confidentiality issues and adversely affect the therapeutic atmosphere in the consulting room.

Case 2

Pat approached her internship year with confidence. She was annoyed when she didn't get her top choices but put it down to the inability of the selection committees to identify real clinical talent. For her OCD, Pat had been through years of various therapists and considered herself a seasoned pro by now. She respected the older supervisors but secretly thought little of the newly minted fresh-out-of-graduate school ones. She knew their flaws and in fact had had a couple of newly minted just-out-of –graduate school therapists herself. They were a total waste of time. Pat was pleased to be assigned to two wise and seasoned older supervisors. She knew she could learn from them. She was sure she was going to have a bad experience with the third supervisor, a newly hired young psychologist.

12.6.3 Knowing the Mission: The Importance of Outreach and Prevention

Trainees are eager to try out their skills in the consulting room and are far less enthusiastic about learning skills in outreach and prevention. Trainees need to understand that the early identification and referral of at-risk students is a core part of the CAPS role, and should not be viewed as secondary to treatment [1]. Given the historical shifts in the role of CAPS, the primary function of clinicians at counseling centers now revolve around:

- Crisis intervention

- Setting realistic goals for and providing short-term care and referrals for ongoing care

- Re-entry evaluations for students returning from psychiatric leaves of absence

- Suicide and dangerousness assessments

- Evaluation and treatment or referral of other high risk phenomena including severe eating disorders, cutting, alcohol, prescription medication, and other drug abuse, and so on

- Evaluation and treatment or referral of students lacking in the capacity to delay gratification and/or the work habits critical to progressing academically in college.

12.6.4 Knowing the Setting and the Population

Trainees need to be reminded of the irregular rhythms of campus life, in which the ideal of regular treatment and assessment is interrupted by exams, extended holiday periods, and semester breaks. The college campus is by nature a community. As a result, a trainee's encountering such confidentiality and treatment issues as running into clients in public areas of the campus; knowing or having to deal with a client's roommate(s) or other friends; and knowing or working with a client's professors or other authority figures will be much more frequent than in a less confined community.

Trainees must be aware of and sensitive to the subcultures peculiar to universities – international students, students from diverse ethnic backgrounds, athletes, fraternities, and so on. For the CAPS clinician, it is critical to be familiar with national survey data on drug and alcohol use; sleep deprivation; addictive behaviors, suicidal ideation; and so on, within the college student demographic.

Orientation should cover the basics of the therapeutic encounter in the college setting, including intake, crisis intervention, and forging a working alliance with students. Trainees also need to learn CAPS policy regarding confidentiality, session limits, cancellations, and so on. Some useful concepts to cover are self-disclosure and recommendations for handling what both trainee and client may experience as awkward silences.

For trainees who have no prior consulting room experience, it is important to clarify that psychotherapy is a unique and peculiar conversation between two people. New trainees tend to feel pressure to immediately answer any question put to them by their student-clients, but the quick response expected in everyday conversation is not necessarily useful in a clinical setting. It is far more important for trainees to feel free to take the time necessary to formulate a clinically useful therapeutic response. It will come as a relief to trainees to be empowered *not to know* everything a client might bring up and to understand that they can respond to a client's question with a candid – and guilt-free – "*I don't know*".

12.7 From Theory to College Counseling Practice

12.7.1 The Seminar and Case Conference

In *The Successful Internship* [19] Sweitzer and King note that the word "seminar" is derived from the Italian *seminare* or "to sow". The CAPS psychotherapy seminar is a didactic course offered in a practical training site and must bridge the gap between abstract theory and real world practice [4,16,19]. It is here where the trainee can reflect on the applicability of her book learning to the practice of college counseling and begin to digest and metabolize abstract theory in an applied clinical setting; it is therefore critically important that the seminar and case conference be used to demystify psychotherapy theory and to teach practical consulting room skills.

Textbook Therapy versus Real Therapy

The student or trainee . . . often finds himself forced to hide aspects of his actual behavior with patients from his supervisor because he feels these behaviors do not meet the standards of this ideal model therapist. One standard that this approach typically consecrates is the stance of perfect technical neutrality. But when confronted with the reality of treatment, this ideal can actually lead to extremely malignant results: Trainees may develop a false professional self. If a trainee is brave enough, this false self only appears in his interactions with the supervisor, while in his work with the patient he continues to bring his humane self into the relationship. If he is not so courageous, this false self takes over and becomes his permanent professional self. Tragically, this is manifested in his interactions with patients and in his relationships with his supervisors and finally, even in his own self-perception.
From *Dare to be Human*, Michael Shoshani Rosenbaum [20]

12.7.2 Seminar Dynamics and Motivations

It is useful to understand the dynamics and motivations common to trainees participating in a CAPS seminar or case conference. Kahn in 2003 [21] listed four types of internship seminars (Figure 12.2).

- In *"The free for all"*, interns one-up each other, trying to impress supervisors and gain their attention and approval

- In *"The beauty contest"*, each intern shows off his or her own wonderful ideas but, instead of listening to peers, tries to think up the next wonderful idea.

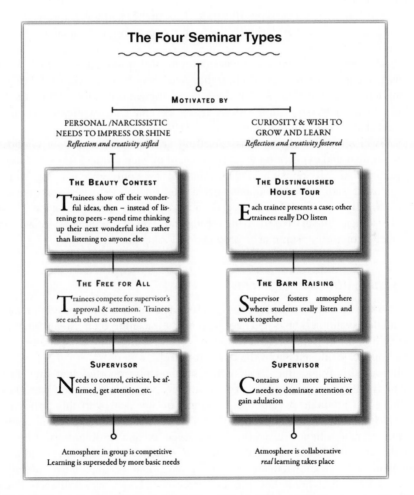

Figure 12.2 *Different Seminar Types, adapted from Michael Kahn,* The Seminar, *and Sweitzer and King,* The Successful Internship.

More desirable are:

- *"The distinguished house tour"*, in which each trainee presents a case or theory and his or her peers actually do listen, and

- *"The barn raising"*, at which interns both listen and learn from one another while working together to gain clinical and theoretical skill, sophistication and wisdom.

Kahn's typology focuses on trainee behavior in the seminar; the typology is important, but does not go far enough. Trainees get less out of the seminar experience if they are motivated mostly by the need to compete, impress, or gain approval. Supervisors, being human, may also find themselves succumbing to a narcissistic desire for attention or admiration, or try to gain affirmation of their personal clinical theory or style by criticizing or devaluing trainees.

The chart of Kahn's seminar types illustrates how higher and lower motivations in both trainees and supervisors can seriously impact the pedagogical value of the seminar experience.

Supervisors need to promote a seminar environment that mitigates interns' understandable need for attention, approval, and admiration and helps them grapple with the struggle to attain confidence as a clinician. But the optimal experience is one where both trainees *and* supervisors have their baser motivations in check and can collaborate openly in an environment that allows real learning to occur [19].

Finally, Sweitzer and King emphasize setting ground rules regarding confidentiality within the seminar and explicating what is expected of each trainee. It is advisable for the supervisor to periodically revisit how the seminar or case conference is going, whether it is functioning well and to make adjustments as necessary [19]. The seminar and case conference usually meet for 90 minutes each and are typically held once a week. Although topics and readings will vary based on the setting and level of training, a suggested syllabus for the college counseling seminar is provided as Appendix A.

12.7.3 Sexual Attraction to Clients

In their 2006 survey, Pope and colleagues [22] found that 95% of male psychotherapists and 76% of female psychotherapists had been sexually attracted to their clients on at least one occasion. While the vast majority never act out such feelings, most psychotherapists feel guilty, anxious, or confused about the attraction [22].

The authors also found that 91% of the respondents reported that they had either received no training on the matter or, if they had received training, that it was inadequate. Noting that most graduate psychology programs do not deal with this important topic, Pope *et al.* emphasize that if seasoned therapists feel anxious, guilty, and confused by sexual attraction to clients, it will pose an even greater problem for trainees [22]. Arguing that the taboo must be lifted, Pope *et al.* conclude that therapists and therapists-in-training must be acknowledged as fully human, that is, capable of feeling sexual attraction to those to whom they provide professional services, and recommend that education on this topic be a part of clinical course work and training [22].

Given the sexually charged atmosphere of many college campuses and the normal sexual experimentation common among college students, it is particularly important that trainees at college counseling centers be able to cope with the feelings of sexual attraction they are likely to experience towards their student-clients. The internship seminar is an appropriate forum for such training. With very limited exceptions not applicable to the CAPS setting (such as, "do you and your patient address each other on a first name basis"), Epstein and Simon's *Exploitation Index* [15,23] is a powerful teaching tool which should be used in the seminar module dealing with sexual feelings and thoughts in the consulting room.

Seminar Topics for Sexual Misconduct

- Therapist–client relationship and concept of boundary violations

- Legal and ethical prohibitions against therapist–client sexual involvement

- Survey data: sexual feelings are normal; Acting out sexual feelings is abnormal, illegal and unethical; readings to contextualize sexual feelings in the therapist

- Proper management of eroticized transferences and counter transferences

- Discussion of Epstein & Simon's The Exploitation Index

- Gender issues and power imbalances in the clinical encounter, and in male–female relationships

- Client vulnerabilities

- Therapist vulnerabilities

- Readings on trauma that sexual boundary violations cause to clients

- State civil and criminal statutes on therapist–client sexual intimacy

Source: Adapted from Kay J, and Roman, B. Prevention of Sexual Misconduct at the Medical, Residency, and Practitioner Levels. In Bloom JD, Nadelson CC, Notman MT. (eds) Physician Sexual Misconduct, American Psychiatric Press Inc. Washington DC, 1999 pp. 153–177.

12.8 Experiential Learning: Trainee Epistemology

Supervisors wishing to promote the gradual expansion and increasing sophistication of trainee clinical thought first need to understand how beginning, intermediate, and advanced trainees think. Sophisticated clinical thought processes that come easily to supervisors are often the result of years of intellectual grappling with complex constructs and hundreds or thousands of hours of trial and error in employing clinical thinking in the consulting room. What can be automatic to the seasoned supervisor is not so for the trainee.

Sophisticated clinical thought is a form of complex reasoning that necessarily occurs in an environment of epistemic uncertainty. Inspired by Dewey's observation that reflective thinking is called for when problems are characterized by uncertainty, King and Kitchener [24] devised the seven-stage *Reflective Judgment Model*. The first three stages of the model demonstrate prereflective reasoning; then, growing in epistemic sophistication, come two quasireflective reasoning stages; the two most mature and sophisticated stages show reflective reasoning.

The model explains a thinker's assumptions about the process of knowing (his or her view of knowledge) and how it is acquired (the justification for his or her beliefs):

- In the *prereflective reasoning* stages, people believe that knowledge is gained through the word of an authority figure or through first-hand observation rather than the evaluation of evidence. People who hold these assumptions believe that what they know is absolutely correct and that they know it with complete certainty [24].

- In the *quasireflective reasoning* stages, people recognize that knowledge contains elements of uncertainty and have a basic notion that decisions and judgments are reached by evaluating evidence. However, conclusions are often more a function of the idiosyncrasies of the thinker (for example, choosing evidence that fits an established belief) rather than a more mature evaluation of the imperfect information [24].

- In the *reflective reasoning* stages, people accept that knowledge cannot be made with certainty, but are not immobilized by it; rather, they make judgments that are the "most reasonable" based on their evaluation of available data and about which they are "relatively certain". They believe they must actively construct their decisions and that knowledge must be evaluated in relationship to the context in which the knowledge is generated in order to determine its validity. They also readily admit their willingness to reevaluate the adequacy of their judgments as new data or new methodologies become available [24].

Owen, Tao and Rodolfa note the utility of the Reflective Judgment Model to the clinical situation, in particular to the trajectory of trainees as they move from less sophisticated to more sophisticated thinking and knowing regarding uncertain clinical material [25]. Beginning trainees may not yet have the tools to evaluate clinical data [25] and may thus need to rely fully on supervisors' beliefs and clinical thinking. Trainees in this pre-reflective stage of thinking will require more sensitive and attuned supervision that is tailored to assist them in learning to trust their own instincts (and authority) as they develop more tolerance for ambiguity and a greater reliance on their own capacity to have and contain expertise.

Many beginning, intermediate, and advanced trainees are in the quasireflective mode of thinking [25], and are prone to evaluating clinical material based on pre-existing theoretical positions and beliefs [24] and such personal factors as idealization and identification with the beliefs of favored professors and supervisors. Supervision with trainees in the quasi-reflective stage may involve encouraging the trainee to really listen to and to learn from his or her client and to stick closely to the clinical material. Encouraging quasireflectively thinking trainees to broaden their perspectives and entertain alternate clinical approaches may be useful in helping them reach more advanced stages of reasoning.

As trainees grow more comfortable with the inherent ambiguity of the clinical encounter and the uncertain data it yields, they may approach the reflective reasoning stage, in which they are less immobilized or overwhelmed by not knowing clinical data with certainty. Moreover, as trainees grow into reflective reasoners, they are better able to be clinically effective in a world where they must actively construct their decisions, in which knowing is inherently uncertain; and where knowledge is always subject to reevaluation when newer clinical material or more accurate working hypotheses present themselves.

Case 3

Mellisa was an attractive clinical psychology graduate student in her mid twenties. She had gotten a BA majoring in business and spent 2 years in the corporate sector where she had a nagging feeling of emptiness and dissatisfaction. On a whim she decided on a change in direction and jumped in to clinical psychology grad program. During her psychology practicum she frequently felt impatient, critical, and annoyed by the trivial concerns her student clients were discussing. One client, Cindy, had just been rejected by her boyfriend and was having trouble recovering. After 3 weeks where Mellissa had listened intently and given excellent advice, Mellissa felt sure that Cindy would walk in feeling chipper and chirpy and be appreciative of the good treatment. When Cindy was instead only more depressed, Mellissa felt angry and told her client that she needed to toughen up! Later that day, in supervision, Mellissa insisted that only people who have real issues belong in counseling; Cindy, with her selfish little love troubles was not one of them.

12.8.1 Understanding Today's Student

Kadison and Digeronimo [1] Grayson and Meilman [18] and pertinent chapters in this volume (e.g. Kay Chapter 1, Eichler and Schwartz Chapter 5) offer a thorough treatment exploring common stressors, common disorders, high risk groups, and the specific developmental phase shared by most college students. Seminar instructors will find it useful to introduce interns to today's student through the lens of forging an identity. College students are negotiating a life stage that may be challenging and confusing personally, professionally, and spiritually. The freedoms of Western culture and society can provide a backdrop against which students can explore identity, forge a comfortable self, and thrive or, if they are less sure of themselves, falter and find themselves in a state of painful confusion as they search for a meaningful and authentic self.

Many students lack the inner compass needed to negotiate this time successfully. Many are ill-prepared for the freedoms of college and lack in the critical life skills required to approach their academics with organization and purpose, tolerate disappointments, regulate affects, form new friendships, find their social place, and form secure romantic attachments. Lacking ability in any of these critical life skills can rapidly lead to anxiety, depression, and despair; surveys indicate that 43% of today's college students at times experience depression so severe they have difficulty functioning, and 9% seriously consider suicide [26].

For new trainees, it is useful to understand that no one has a single, unitary personality and that we all have distributed selves with areas of strength and weakness and differing aspects of identity. Among them are:

- The sphere of the *social self*, in which college can be an exhilarating time during which new confidence is gained, new friendships are forged, and social skills are honed. Alternatively, students may fail to develop a social self (often after lifelong difficulty with fitting in) and become increasingly withdrawn and socially isolated.

- The sphere of the *professional self*, in which students can gain professional competence and sophistication, choose a career direction with a sense of purpose, and begin the journey of becoming increasingly comfortable in their chosen professional direction.

However, less prepared students may wallow in a directionless state, suffering enormously from their painful confusion about who they are professionally.

- The sphere of the *academic self*. Here, students may experience the satisfaction of discovering that they can get the job done, participate in our meritocracy, and grow in the ability to solve problems effectively. Alternatively, they may struggle to get papers done on time, fail to delay gratifications, avoid regular and purposeful study, and live in a cycle of procrastination, guilt, and stress. The American College Health Association lists anxiety and depression among the top five impediments to academic performance [27].

- In the sphere of the *sexual self*, students may find a secure sexual orientation and an increasingly confident sexual identity, or may fail to find romance and/or develop as sexual beings, questioning their sexual orientation and using sex in maladaptive ways (e.g. promiscuity) as a form of affect regulation and coping.

- In the *cyber-self sphere*, technology is shaping identity, social interaction, language, habits, and how we operate in both space and time. Students may successfully negotiate this intriguing new world of chat rooms, instant messaging, cell phones, e-mail, and social networking sites with balance or they may have cyber-pursuits instead of real world interests and pleasures, and cyber-friendships instead of enjoying a growing capacity to get along with real people, Students may fall victim to temptations such as cybersex, internet gambling, and plagiarism, experiencing a numbing emptiness in the absence of the addictive high stimulation of ringing cell phones and the flashing computer screens.

12.9 Organization of Training

12.9.1 Principles of Experiential Learning

The principles of experiential education have much to offer trainers of mental health professionals. With philosophical roots dating back to the apprenticeship systems of medieval guilds, Sweitzer and King note that professional schools began including practical placements – experiential learning – as an integral component of their academic programs in the late nineteenth century, and cite an observation of educational philosopher John Dewey (1859–1952):

> An ounce of experience is better than a ton of theory, simply because it is only in experience that any theory has vital and verifiable significance [19].

Sweitzer and King [19] list several key principles for a successful internship program:

- Trainees need to be active participants in their learning

- Supervisors must guide, facilitate, and coach the trainee to learn from their clinical activities

- Training experiences need to be organized in order to facilitate a process of learning

- Active experimentation is a critical part of learning from experience

- Active reflection is the bridge that connects a trainee's work in the consulting room (concrete experience) to learning (abstract conceptualization).

As Baird has observed, an internship's focus is not on what you *know*, but what you *do*, an educational paradox he pithily sums up with the comment, "First, life gives the test, then the lesson [4]".

12.9.2 The Developmental Stages of Internship

Sweitzer and King [19] have identified a developmental stage model of the internship experience for trainees: anticipation, disillusionment, confrontation, competence, and culmination.

- The *anticipation stage* is characterized by excitement and anxiety (about competence, evaluation, supervisors, etc.); the rate of skills acquisition and learning in this stage is often relatively low.

- The *disillusionment stage* begins when disappointment in the training experience sets in. Disillusionment – with the organization, the clients, the supervisors, the "system", and so on – is most often directly related to the gap between what a trainee had expected of the internship and what he or she really experiences. Sweitzer and King refer to the disillusionment stage as a "crisis of growth" in which trainees can become stuck or blocked, with consequences ranging from a reduced capacity for learning and lingering disappointment to – in the worst cases – termination of the training.

- The *confrontation stage* occurs when the trainee acknowledges and confronts his or her disillusionment, reevaluating his or her expectations, goals, skills, and role in the agency. Just as failure to acknowledge and work through disappointments leads to stagnation, successful resolution leads to growing confidence and empowerment as a learner.

- The *competence stage* is usually characterized by a period of high morale and a newfound investment in learning, growth and skills acquisition as trainees begin to view themselves less as apprentices and more as emerging professionals.

- A trainee enters the *culmination stage* through a variety of feelings related to the ending of his or her training experience. They may range from a sense of pride in new skills to guilt over not having done enough for clients and sadness that the experience is ending. Sweitzer and King note that goodbyes are difficult – relationships reorganized to accommodate the demands of the training must now be reorganized again – and trainees in this stage may avoid dealing with their feelings or act them out through behaviors such as jokes, lateness, and absences [19].

Within each stage, according to the authors [19], trainee morale and learning will initially suffer, as trainees grapple with new difficulties, then pick up again as they are successfully resolved. Supervisors attuned to a trainee's ups and downs can maximize the learning experience as they journey through the training year.

Case 4

> After finishing in the peace corps, Abe worked for habitat for humanity and also temporarily looked after shelter animals awaiting adoption. Becoming a therapist and helping others was a no-brainer. It felt so natural to him. He enjoyed helping and found it deeply satisfying. He struggled though with clients who had more serious and intractable issues. As the session neared its end, Abe grew increasingly more frustrated. He felt he had to help; he hated a session ending without some real progress achieved, a well targeted intervention delivered, or the client feeling better. Several times, upon feeling no progress made after 45 minutes, he just extended the session for another 30. He hated these sessions and felt badly for the client. His supervisor suggested that he felt it was his responsibility to fix it, to provide some real relief. Abe partly agreed. On the other hand, he felt proud that his wish to help was a calling and a passionately held altruistic conviction. On a philosophical level, he wasn't sure he could embrace the supervisors caring but more dispassionate approach to psychotherapy.

12.9.3 Sequencing and Pacing of Training

The Association for State and Provincial Psychology Boards [3] argues that sequential training, gradually increasing in sophistication, is the proper model for practicum training. In a perfect world, it might be possible for trainees to be assigned cases that incrementally expand in complexity and match each trainee's developing consulting room capabilities. But in the real world of counseling centers, often overwhelmed by the huge volume of students needing care, it is likely that trainees will sometimes be assigned cases they are challenged to treat. Therefore, from the supervisory side, it is imperative that a thoughtful consideration of a trainee's competency level be made each time a new case is assigned [20]. On the other hand, speaking from the trainee's perspective, Baird urges trainees to immediately bring to their supervisor's attention any assignment that may be hazardous or otherwise beyond their competence [4].

Training directors will have more control in planning the pacing and sequencing of such didactic elements as group seminars and individual supervisions. In these settings, theories, constructs, and techniques can be introduced at an optimum pace for expanding trainees' overall development. Within this structure, however, care must be taken to match seminar and supervision content with trainee's capability: Introducing sophisticated concepts before the cohort is ready risks overwhelming them and/or unanticipated effects in the consulting room as trainees try out the new ideas; going too slowly risks infantilizing graduate students who need the tools of their trade in order to understand their clients as deeply as possible.

12.9.4 Demystifying Psychotherapy in the CAPS Setting

The theoretical constructs most useful in teaching trainees are those that almost automatically translate themselves into everyday experience – concepts intended for practical use in the consulting room can suffer from being overworked and being made unnecessarily complex. At one counseling center, for example, a trainee enamored with Lacanian constructs brought them into the consulting room and, while she struggled mightily to make them work, succeeded only in steadily mystifying and confusing her clients.

In a college setting, it is optimal to encourage trainees to speak English rather than jargon by helping them translate theoretical constructs into everyday language. For example, "defense mechanism" is simply a theoretically specific version of "a way of protecting yourself" or "a coping style"; "repression" can be translated as "not wanting to think about it", and so on. (A more thorough exposition of treatment approaches useful in the college counseling setting is available in Chapter 5.)

12.10 Teaching the Intake Interview in the College Setting

Intakes in the college setting have a number of important differences from the general intake interview.

12.10.1 The Student

Students who come to a counseling center are often interacting with a therapist for the first time and are likely to feel nervous, self-conscious, and embarrassed about the encounter. Students new to counseling are frequently also fearful of having to come to grips with potentially frightening emotions or worried about being perceived as weak. Not having any prior experience with counseling only exacerbates their anxiety. It is therefore useful for the intake interviewer to be warm, friendly, and supportive. Setting the student at ease begins to promote a working alliance and helps him or her feel comfortable and safe enough to report the difficulties that prompted the visit more efficiently.

12.10.2 The Trainee

If not the very first, an intake is frequently among the earliest clinical encounters for a counseling center trainee. New trainees are likely to be anxious to do well, self-conscious about how they are perceived, and worried about making a good impression on the client and later, the supervisor. Moreover, because most trainees are close in age and life circumstances to an interviewee, they are more likely to experience unbridled identification with their clients. These intense identifications lead to an ease of empathy that is beneficial, but can also lead to complications, such as assuming or overlooking important information about the client [28], or having difficulty confronting a student from a position of clinical authority.

12.10.3 Teaching the Initial Intake

It is imperative that sufficient time be spent on teaching the proper techniques for an initial intake, on alerting the trainees to their own counter-transference reactions and identifications [28], and on normalizing anxiety. Inexperienced trainees in particular need to rely on a well-taught and well-rehearsed method of interviewing that includes a formalized series of stages in which specific ground is covered.

Harry Stack Sullivan's classic *The Psychiatric Interview* (1954) [28] remains a remarkably relevant guide to the technique of psychotherapy. Nearly 60 years after its publication, the treatise is an outstanding and extensive reference that profitably anchors and organizes the teaching of intake interviews to counseling center trainees. Sullivan's work is full of amusing anecdotes and, more importantly, piercing insights and pragmatic prescriptions on conducting the initial interview. With its chapters on the interview's basic concepts, structuring the interview situation, general technical considerations, the early stages of an interview, the interview as a process, and the termination of an interview, counseling center supervisors will need to make only a few adjustments to customize the book to counseling center work.

Harry Stack Sullivan on Inexperienced Trainees

The experience of the trainee is synthesized into an aptitude to do nothing exterior to his awareness which will greatly handicap the development of the interview situation, or which will direct its development in an unnecessarily obscure way . . . many inexperienced interviewers, quite exterior to their awareness, communicate to the interviewee a distaste for certain types of data . . . until such interviewers realize they are rather unwittingly prohibiting, or forbidding, or shooing the interviewee away from a particular type of data, they continue not to encounter it. Thus, "learning how to act" (as an interviewer) is largely a matter of being aware of what one does, and aware of it in terms of how it affects the setting of the interview. As an interviewer does this, he stops doing those things which interfere with the fuller development of the interview [28].

Miller's work [29] on the first session is written specifically for counseling and psychotherapy trainees, and will provide a useful, albeit simplified, corollary to *The Psychiatric Interview* [28].

Noting the frequency with which counseling center intakes become crisis intervention, Hipple and Beamish [8] recommended that supervisors and trainees plan for this possibility in advance. Supervisors need to assess the competency level of the trainee and know his or her capacity to handle crisis situations [8]. Kleespsies advocates a mentoring relationship where trainees have multiple opportunities to observe supervisors conducting intakes [30]. The following pedagogical techniques may be useful in optimizing the CAPS training experience [15]:

- Viewing videotapes of master clinicians in the consulting room

- *In-vivo* observation of seasoned clinicians in the CAPS consulting room

- Detailed discussion of readings which include the actual "blow by blow" process notes of illustrative case write-ups.

12.10.4 Obtaining a Complete Initial Diagnostic Impression

An initial meeting with a new client is not complete without gathering sufficient information to gain an initial diagnostic impression and, consequently, it is critical to include elements of the mental status exam that are appropriate to the college setting. Asking a college student all the questions that are important in a hospital setting, however, is unnecessary and likely to be alarming. The questions related to schizophrenic and psychotic conditions should be asked only when indicated by data emerging from the interview. On the other hand, Schwartz [31] notes that a thorough evaluation of suicidality should always be included. Questions regarding a student's academic focus, satisfaction with the college experience, relationships with roommates, romances, and time spent on the internet, on the other hand, are important in a college setting. Questions about self-confidence, social skills, and self-consciousness will also make sense to the student while providing important data.

At a college counseling center, it is particularly important to teach trainees to contextualize and normalize students' presenting difficulties. Many college students are self-conscious and, still in the process of finding their identities, prone to wondering if they are "normal". The final stage of the interview should include a formulation and summary of the student's difficulties [28], a collaborative setting of goals that will focus and organize the treatment, and – where appropriate – a statement on the likelihood of progress toward the therapeutic goals that offers the student a realistic sense of hope.

12.11 Nurturing Competency, Addressing Deficiency

The Assessment of Competencies Benchmark Work Group Report [13], is an excellent and developmentally-based review of the attitudes, skills, knowledge, and competencies expected in beginning (i.e. ready for practicum) and more advanced (ready for internship) therapists-in-training.

Under this system, there are clear guidelines and expectations for the range of competencies to be attained by therapists-in-training, as well as the developmental levels expected pre- and post-practica, pre- and post-internship, and pre- and post-licensure. Setting guidelines on the range of competencies expected at each successive stage of training, in addition to preparing professional psychologists [16] and social workers [16], has the explicitly stated aim of protecting both the public and the profession. Increasing attention is now being focused on the legal, ethical, and pedagogical obligation of training centers to identify and, where possible, provide remediation for trainees who are struggling with incompetence and/or impairment.

Training sites are urged to have well-developed policies and procedures both for evaluating and nurturing competence and identifying and remediating gaps in competence [11,32]. Should issues of incompetence or impairment become irremediable, training sites also have an obligation to protect the public and the profession by reassigning or removing a trainee if necessary.[1] The Student Competence Task Force of the Council of Chairs of Training Councils (CCTC) developed a model policy; a section of the policy is below.

As such, within a developmental framework, and with due regard for the inherent power difference between students and faculty, students and trainees should know that their faculty, training staff, and supervisors will evaluate their competence in areas other than, and in addition to, coursework, seminars, scholarship, comprehensive examinations, or related program requirements. These evaluative areas include, but are not limited to, demonstration of sufficient: (a) interpersonal and professional competence (e.g., the ways in which student-trainees relate to clients, peers, faculty, allied professionals, the public, and individuals from diverse backgrounds or histories); (b) self-awareness, self-reflection, and self-evaluation (e.g., knowledge of the content and potential impact of one's own beliefs and values on clients, peers, faculty, allied professionals, the public, and individuals from diverse backgrounds or histories); (c) openness to processes of supervision (e.g., the ability and willingness to explore issues that either interfere with the appropriate provision of care or impede professional development or functioning); and (d) resolution of issues or problems that interfere with professional development or functioning in a satisfactory manner (e.g., by responding constructively to feedback from supervisors or program faculty; by the successful completion of remediation

---

[1] Roberts *et al.* have written a more thorough discussion of the shift to competency-based training [36].

plans; by participating in personal therapy in order to resolve issues or problems). http://www.apa.org/ed/graduate/cctcevaluation.pdf

12.11.1 Nurturing Competence: the Supervisory Relationship

It is important that trainees have the foundational competencies [16] of self-reflection, self-awareness, and self-evaluation prior to beginning supervision (Figure 12.3). Being

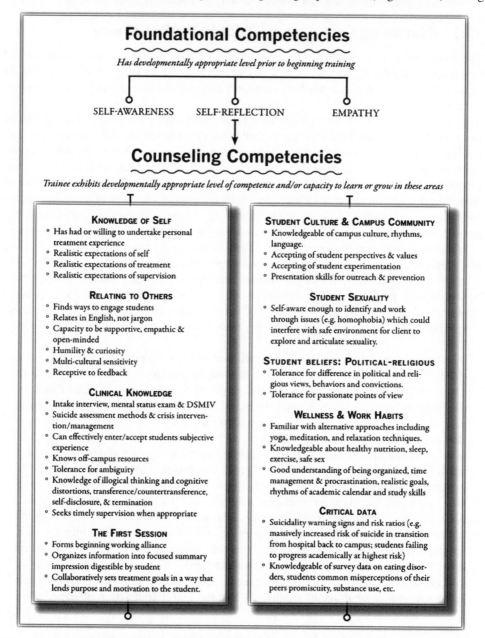

Figure 12.3 *Foundational and counseling competencies.*

receptive and open to supervisory feedback is one of Sweitzer and King's essential attitudes [19]. Numerous writers emphasize self-reflection as the key to growth as a clinician [4,16,19,25,33].

Supervisor and supervisee each have a role in constructing a stimulating and safe environment for learning and growth. Supervisees are expected to be curious and eager to explore new ideas, techniques and approaches, and open to constructive feedback. Supervisors are expected to nurture and hone the foundational competencies of self-awareness, self-reflection, and self-evaluation in the supervisee; to actively seek to construct a safe supervisory environment; and to supportively confront the supervisee when he or she may be lacking.

Shoshani-Rosenbaum cautions both supervisees and supervisors to avoid the hazards of trying to model the "ideal therapist" who is exceptional in every way and never deviates from textbook notions of therapeutic perfection [20]. Trainees who suffer from this common malady frequently hide any non-ideal aspects of their professional selves from supervisors and may ultimately develop and come to adopt a false professional self [20]. To combat this, it is important for supervisors to model the reality that even seasoned master clinicians often struggle to understand clients, often don't know exactly what to say, at times dislike difficult qualities in clients, and wrestle with their own feelings.

Harry Stack Sullivan noted the propensity of inexperienced clinicians to avoid clinical information or encounters that make them uncomfortable. Through becoming more self-aware, therapists-in-training can gradually learn to stop avoiding such issues in the consulting room [28]. In helping them to do this, however, supervisors need to avoid turning supervision into treatment [33]. It is challenging to find the balance between, on the one hand, constructively engaging and confronting the trainee, and, on the other hand, being mindful of the overarching supervisory task of facilitating a growing self-trust and clinical self-confidence.

This challenge can often be greater in a CAPS setting. Because of their usually limited budgets, CAPS frequently recruit newly licensed clinicians who may excel at supporting supervisees but struggle to confront their deficiencies, a problem that can be exacerbated by the relatively narrow differences in age among student-clients, therapists-in-training, and newly licensed supervisors. CAPS supervision therefore often occurs without the benefit of the life experience and wisdom a more seasoned supervisor might provide. Senior staff must help remedy this common issue informally through mentoring, and, formally via professional development and ongoing education in supervision [16], and professional staff meetings devoted to the study of supervision, training, and evaluation issues.

The Supervisory Encounter, written by Jacobs *et al.* [33], is a noteworthy text focusing on the modes of thinking and attitudes that need to be fostered in therapists-in-training regardless of the specific theoretical approach. The authors focus not on *what* approach is taught, but *how* it is taught. Among their core insights on supervision are:

- Though students' difficulties in learning and mastering are pointed out to them, a supervisor's potential difficulty in learning how to teach is not often discussed. More attention needs to be paid to helping supervisors learn to supervise.

- Supervisors fail to distinguish between training and treating the supervisee, and transplant such therapeutic concepts as defense and resistance into the educational realm. Supervisors often analyze a trainee's personality rather than the educational situation. Seeing the trainee's difficulty as stemming from his or her personality issues robs supervisors of the opportunity to see them as problems in teaching and learning.

- Feeling safe is central to the supervisory endeavor. The supervisor must titrate interventions in a way that is protective of the trainee's self-regard, while asking the trainee to expand his or her ways of knowing and feeling. The choice of supervisory intervention needs to be based on an assessment of the trainee's stage in learning, capacity to tolerate affect, and so on.

- In the initial phases of supervision, the supervisor tries to create an atmosphere in which a meaningful dialog can take place, but many supervisory hours inadvertently turn into interviews, with the supervisor playing the role of the interviewer. A major impediment to the creation of meaningful dialog is failure of the supervisor to appreciate the extent of anxiety and vulnerability felt by the trainee. Underestimating these feelings leads to difficulties in teaching and learning.

Jacobs *et al.* citing Flemming and Benedek (1966), point out that learning in supervision develops in three stages:

- The first stage, *learning by imitation*, is based primarily on identification with the supervisor. This echoes the pre-reflective stage in the reflective judgment model.

- In the second stage, *corrective learning*, different clinical techniques and approaches can be discussed based on the theoretical model of treatment the *supervisee* has chosen. This echoes the quasi-reflective mode of reflective judgment.

- The third stage, *creative learning*, is characterized by deeper understanding and integration of intrapersonal and interpersonal dynamics, resulting in more original clinical thinking and echoing the reflective stage in the reflective judgment model.

12.11.2 Nurturing Competence: Trainees Expectations of Treatment and of Themselves

Trainees often enter the field as well as the CAPS internship with unrealistic expectations of treatment, supervisors, and themselves. Trainees frequently expect that treatment can cure and cure quickly; that supervisors have all the answers; and that they can very quickly master the nuances of clinical practice which take many many years to learn. Such unrealistic expectations can lead to frustration and disappointment and impede the slow but steady increases in clinical confidence which effective training can instill. Consequently, it is imperative that supervisors pay attention to, confront and discuss their trainee's unrealistic expectations. Supervisors should pace their interventions with each trainee with the following matters of clinical growth in mind:

1. More realistic appreciation of the potentials, and the limits of treatment

2. More realistic expectation that learning to be a clinician is a life-long process where clinical growth and mastery is a slow and gradual rather than a rapid or dramatic process

3. Growing understanding and utilization of own strengths as a clinician

4. Growing appreciation of own limitations with corollary efforts to improve these areas

5. Gradually increasing epistemic sophistication in clinical thinking (e.g. tolerance for ambiguity) and decision-making

6. Growing capacity in foundational competencies of empathy, self-reflection, self-awareness

7. Increasing mastery and confidence in crisis intervention and management.

Though a more thorough exposition of issues in the supervision of counseling center trainees is beyond the scope of this chapter, supervisors working in college centers will benefit from matching their supervisory interventions to the trainee's developmental stage in the supervision [8,24,33]. Training directors and supervisors will also profit from a familiarity with the supervisory competencies now expected from supervisors [16]; from the teaching of inductive, associative, creative, and self-reflective modes of thought that are so essential to psychotherapists [33]; from training in the supervision of crises in the college counseling environment [8]; from a mastery of suicide assessment competencies [34]; from an awareness of the sexual attraction trainees commonly feel toward their student-clients [22]; and from supervision in the era of evidence-based practice [25].

12.12 Recognizing and Addressing Deficiencies

National surveys of academic programs and training sites [10,11] have consistently found significant rates of trainee impairment among graduate students in clinical, counseling, and school psychology and, in their review of the literature on trainee impairment, Huprich and Rudd [9] conclude that it is a serious concern in the mental health profession.

Academic programs and training sites have a responsibility to identify and then work to remediate impairments and deficiencies in trainees. Significant attention has now been devoted to the creation of benchmarks and best practices; both academic programs and training sites have a responsibility to:

- Identify deficiencies in trainee competence

- Identify psychological impairments interfering with and/or preventing competent professional practice among trainees

- Implement fair and consistent evaluation procedures that include a detailed explanation of the expectations and time frames for remediating gaps in competency as therapists, and for the remediation of psychological impairment

- In accordance with their duty to protect the public and the profession, implement sanctions up to and including involuntary leave of absence or termination on trainees incapable or unwilling to adequately ameliorate impairment and/or meet minimal standards of developmentally appropriate competence.

12.13 Social Work and Psychology Therapists-in-Training

Social work and psychology therapists-in-training arrive at college counseling centers partially socialized [16] with the core philosophies of their respective disciplines. There is much in common, but some difference between the two philosophies. Both share a commitment to human welfare and dignity, to ethical standards and to respecting difference and diversity; both disciplines view self-reflection and commitment to life-long learning as core values; both are moving toward competency-based training; both emphasize evidence-based practice; both emphasize supervision and consultation; and both emphasize evaluation of trainees. In social work, there is more of a tradition of social advocacy and action. In psychology there is the scientist-practitioner model and more of an emphasis on scholarly research.

Social worker therapists-in-training may enter college counseling settings more prepared to understand, negotiate, and think about organization and system dynamics [16]; they may also be more inclined to focus on individual strengths. Psychologist therapists-in-training may arrive more prepared to think about individual dynamics and psychopathology and are usually prepared to conduct psychological testing. Social work accreditation standards call for 900 hours of fieldwork typically acquired over a two-year MSW program [35]. Psychologists-in-training usually go on to complete a doctorate and may enter the counseling setting at a more advanced level of clinical training.

Both the similarities and the differences in how social work and psychologist therapists-in-training are acculturated and educated are likely to show up in all phases of the CAPS training experience, including the didactic elements of the seminar and case conference, approaches to the counseling center as an organization, and experiences in supervision and in the consulting room with student-clients.

12.14 Conclusion

Training programs in university CAPS have many advantages, including aiding the recruitment of talented clinicians, and providing for a larger pool of clinicians to provide evaluation and treatment to many more students than would otherwise be possible. Running a training program requires careful attention to best practices in CAPS training, and demands thoughtful consideration of how to balance the dual roles of providing competent care to students in need, and providing diverse training experiences to clinicians-in-training.

Trainees move through predictable stages in their internship and practicum experiences. The excitement of the anticipation stage precedes the disappointment stage; next is the confrontation stage, wherein trainees confront the often unrealistic expectations and/or maladaptive attitudes that lead to disappointment. Successful resolution of disappointments leads to more efficient learning and to the competence stage, wherein the trainee begins to function more like a junior professional than a hesitant trainee.

Trainees move through predictable stages of clinical thought. Beginning with relatively rudimentary clinical thinking, trainees move through a trajectory towards epistemically more nuanced and sophisticated ways of thinking about ambiguous clinical material. Beginning trainees typically struggle with the inherent uncertainty of the material and often rely on the judgments of their supervisors in clinical decision-making. Trainees with a little more experience develop more tolerance for epistemic uncertainty, but often rely on pre-existing theories or positions for their clinical thinking. Advanced trainees learn to be comfortable with uncertainty, and to think creatively and reflectively as they understand that clinical thinking and decisions are probabilistically constructed (not absolutely known).

The internship seminar and case conference are important means for teaching CAPS trainees. Setting ground rules for the seminar and periodically reviewing these expectations will maximize learning as it ameliorates the tendencies of trainees to use seminar time to compete with other trainees, show off their wonderful ideas, and impress the instructor. The sexual attraction and sexual feelings that CAPS trainees feel towards their student-clients is a crucial topic - to date largely neglected in academic programs and training sites. The appropriate professional management of sexual feelings, as well as their contextualization within available theory, can be profitably taught in the CAPS seminar.

Supervision competencies are a relatively neglected area in the helping fields. This has placed supervisors at a disadvantage as they point out the learning needs of their supervisees while nobody points out the developmental needs of the supervisors. Supervisees often move through predictable stages in the supervisee relationship, and supervisors' familiarity with these stages will optimize learning. Supervisors commonly make two unfortunate supervisory interventions. First, supervisors are prone to analyzing the trainee's personality instead of analyzing the educational situation; this moves the supervisory relationship into a treatment and personality-focused direction instead of keeping it properly rooted in an educationally-focused approach. Second, supervisors are prone to falling into an interviewing style of supervision in which they ask questions and supervisees produce answers. Keeping the supervision as a true dialog and exchange of ideas is educationally far superior.

A culture shift is under way in training. Training is moving into an era of competency-based training wherein attention is focused on broad *foundational* competencies, such as empathy and capacity for reflection, as well as the more specific *functional* competencies necessary in the CAPS setting. These functional competencies include understanding the CAPS mission, competencies for evaluating and treating students, crisis management and suicide-management competencies, cultural sensitivity competencies, and outreach and prevention competencies.

Finally, both academic programs and training sites have a duty to provide competent training but also a duty to protect the profession and the public. As such, rigorous evaluation procedures including clear protocols for addressing incompetence and deficiency are essential aspects of best practice in today's CAPS training programs.

Appendix A: Sample Syllabus for Counseling Center Trainees

Fall: Basic concepts/treatment approaches in college mental health

Topic 1	Developmental perspectives: psychotherapy with college students. *Reading*: Grayson, P. (2005) Overview. In *College Mental Health Practice*. (eds P. Grayson, and P. Meilman,), Routledge, New York, pp. 1–20 Eichler, R. (2005) Developmental perspectives. In *College Mental Health Practice*. (eds P. Grayson, and P. Meilman,), Routledge, New York, pp. 21–41
Topic 2	Basic principles in the college counseling therapeutic encounter. *Reading*: Sullivan, H.S. (1954) *The Psychiatric Interview*. WW Norton, New York
Topic 3	Brief dynamic and relational treatment Safran, J.D. and Muran, J.M. (2000). The therapeutic alliance reconsidered, In: *Negotiating the therapeutic alliance: a relational treatment guide*. Guilford Press, New York, pp. 1–29

Topic 4   Solution focused psychotherapy

Topic 5   Prescription medication and stimulant use in college students
                 Reading:
                 Schwartz, V. (2006). Medications. In *College Mental Health Practice*.
                 (eds P. Grayson, and P. Meilman,), Routledge, New York

Topic 6   CBT for depression

Topic 7   CBT for anxiety

Topic 8   Eating disorder treatment
                 Reading:
                 Bruch H. *Eating Disorders*. (1973) Obesity, Anorexia Nervosa, and the Person within.
                 Basic Books.

Topic 9   Substance abuse treatment with a college population
                 Readings:
                 Washton, A.M. (1996) Clinical assessment of psychoactive substance use.
                 In *Psychotherapy and Substance Abuse: A Practioners Handbook*
                 (ed. Washton, A.M.) The Guilford Press, New York.
                 Prochaska, J.O., DiClemente, C.C. and Norcross, J.C. (1992). In search of
                 how people change. *American Psychologist*, **47**, 1102–1112

Topic 10   Multicultural psychotherapy

Topic 11   Working with LGBT students

Topic 12   Transference and counter transference in short-term treatment

Spring: Advanced concepts in college counseling

Topic 13   Mindfulness relaxation training

Topic 14   DBT with college students

Topic 15   Short-term expressive psychodynamic psychotherapy

Topic 16   Working with reluctant students

Topic 17   Suicide assessment with students
                 Reading:
                 Silverman, M. (2006). *Suicide and Suicidal Behaviors* In College Mental Health Practice.
                 Routledge New York, pp. 303–323.
                 Rudd, M.D. *Core Competencies In Suicide Assessment.*

Topic 18   Towards a career in college mental health: administrative, clinical, and training
                 competencies for the college counseling professional

Topic 19   Towards a career in college mental health: competencies in the Va. Tech era.
                 Dangerousness assessments; re-entry evaluations; college counseling in
                 the mass media era.

Topic 20   Sexual attraction to clients
                 Readings:
                 Pope K.S., Keith-Spiegel P., Tabachnick B.G. (2006) Sexual attraction to clients:
                 The human therapist and the (sometimes) inhuman training system. *Training and
                 Education in Professional Psychology*, **11**(2), 96–111.
                 Epstein R.S., Simon R.I. (1990) The Exploitation Index: An early warning
                 indicator of boundary violations in psychotherapy. *Bulletin of the Menninger
                 Clinic*, **90**;54(4), 450.

References

1. Kadison, R. and DiGeronimo, T.F. (2004) *College of the Overwhelmed*, Jossey-Bass. San Francisco.

2. Boyd, V., Hattauer, E., Brandel, I.W. *et al.* (2003) Accreditation standards for university and college counseling centers. *Journal of Counseling & Development*, **81**(2), 168–177.

3. Association of State and Provincial Psychology Boards (2009) Guidelines on practicum experience for licensure.

4. Baird, B.N. (1998) *The Internship, Practicum, and Field Placement Handbook*, Prentice Hall. Upper Suddle River, NJ.

5. Rockland-Miller, H.S. and Eells, G.T. (2006) The implementation of mental health clinical triage systems in university health services. *Journal of College Student Psychotherapy*, **20**(4), 39–51.

6. Falvey, J., Caldwell, C. and Cohen, C. (2002) *Documentation in supervision: The focused risk management supervision system*, Brooks/Cole: Pacific Groves, CA.

7. Freeman, B. and McHenry, S. (1996) Clinical supervision of counselors-in-training: A nationwide survey of ideal delivery, goals, and theoretical influences. *Counselor Education and Supervision*, **36**(2), 144–157.

8. Hipple, J. and Beamish, P.M. (2007) Supervision of counselor trainees with clients in crisis. *Journal of Professional Counseling: Practice, Theory, & Research*, **35**(2), 1–16.

9. Huprich, S.K. and Rudd, M.D. (2004) A National survey of trainee impairment in clinical, counseling, and school psychology doctoral programs and internships. *Journal of Clinical Psychology*, **60**(1), 43–52.

10. Procidano, M.E., Busch-Rossnagel, N.A., Reznikoff, M. and Geisinger, K.F. (1995) Responding to graduate students' professional deficiencies: A national survey. *Journal of Clinical Psychology*, **51**(3), 426–433.

11. Lumadue, C.A. and Duffey, T.H. (1999) The role of graduate programs as gatekeepers: A model for evaluating student counselor competence. *Counselor Education and Supervision*, **39**(2), 101–109.

12. Kay, Jerald. (2009) *Interview Rating Form*, Wright State University.

13. American Psychological Association Board of Educational Affairs (2007) *Assessment of Competencies Benchmark Workgroup Report*, APA (American Psychological Association) Washington, DC.

14. Hunter, G.A., Delgado-Romero, E.A. and Stewart, A.E. (2009) What's on your training program's web site? Observations and recommendations for effective recruitment. *Training and Education in Professional Psychology*, **3**(1), 53–61.

15. Kay, J.,Training in College Mental Health. Personal Communication via Email from Kay, received by Davar 2009 May 11.

16. Birkenmaier, J. and Berg-Weger, M. (2006) *The Practicum Companion for Social Work*, Allyn and Bacon.

17. Kaslow, N.J., Borden, K.A., Collins, F.L. Jr *et al.* (2004) Competencies Conference: Future Directions in Education and Credentialing in Professional Psychology. *Journal of Clinical Psychology*, **60**(7), 699–712.

18. Grayson, P.A. and Meilman, P.W. (2006) *College Mental Health Practice*, CRC Press, Boca Raton, FL.

19. Sweitzer, H.F. and King, M.A. (2008) *The Successful Internship*, Brooks/Cole Cengage Learning. Belmont, CA.

20. Shoshani Rosenbaum, Michael (2009) *Dare To Be Human: A Contemporary Psychoanalytic Journey*, Routledge, New York.

21. Kahn, Michael (2003) The Seminar [Internet]. The Seminar. Available from: http://www.sonoma.edu/users/m/mccaffry/libs320A_Immigrant/seminar.kahn.html.

22. Pope, K.S., Keith-Spiegel, P. and Tabachnick, B.G. (2006) Sexual attraction to clients: The human therapist and the (sometimes) inhuman training system. *Training and Education in Professional Psychology*, **S**(2), 96–111.

23. Epstein, R.S. and Simon, R.I. (1990) The Exploitation Index: An early warning indicator of boundary violations in psychotherapy. *Bulletin of the Menninger Clinic*, **54**(4), 450.

24. King, P.M. and Kitchener, K.S. (2004) Reflective judgment: theory and research on the development of epistemic assumptions through adulthood. *Educational Psychologist*, **39**(1), 5–18.

25. Owen, J., Tao, K. and Rodolfa, E. (2005) Supervising counseling center trainees in the era of evidence based practices. *Journal of College Student Psychotherapy*, **20**(1), 67–77.

26. American College Health Association (2009) The American college health association national college health assessment (ACHA–NCHA) Spring 2008 reference group data report. *Journal of American College Health*, **57**(5), 477–488.

27. American College Health Association (2006) American college health association national college health assessment (ACHA-NCHA) Spring 2005 reference group data report (Abridged). *Journal of American College Health*, **55**(1), 5–16.

28. Sullivan, H.S., Perry, H.S. and Gawel, M.L. (1970) *The Psychiatric Interview*, W. W. Norton & Company, New York.

29. Miller, Riva (2006) The first session with a new client: five stages, in *The Trainee Handbook: A Guide for Counseling and Psychotherapy Trainees*, Sage, London.

30. Kleespies, P.M. (2000) *Emergencies in Mental Health Practice*, Guilford Press, New York.

31. Schwartz, V. (2009) Mental Status Exam in the College Counseling Center. Personal Communication via Email from Schwartz, received by Davar 2009 May 11.

32. Student Competence Task Force of the Council of Chairs of Training Councils (2004) The Comprehensive Evaluation of Student-Trainee Competence in Professional Psychology Programs [Internet]. Available from: http://www.apa.org/ed/graduate/cctc.html.

33. Jacobs, D., David, P. and Meyer, D.J. (1997) *The Supervisory Encounter*, Yale University Press.

34. Rudd, M.D., Cukrowicz, K.C. and Bryan, C.J. (2008) Core competencies in suicide risk assessment and management: Implications for supervision. *Training and Education in Professional Psychology*, **2**(4), 219–228.

35. Council on Social Work Education (2008) Educational Policy and Accreditation Standards.

36. Roberts, M.C., Christiansen, M.D., Borden, K.A. and Lopez, S.J. (2005) Fostering a culture shift: assessment of competence in the education and careers of professional psychologists. *Professional Psychology: Research & Practice*, **36**(4), 355–361.

13 Special Populations

Beverly J. Fauman[1] and Marta J. Hopkinson[2]

[1]University of Michigan School of Medicine, Department of Psychiatry, Ann Arbor, MI, USA

[2]University of Maryland, University Health Center, College Park, MD, USA

13.1 Introduction

There are a number of unique student populations in American colleges and universities that pose distinct challenges for college mental health services. This chapter/presentation will try to identify those challenges and suggest ways they have been approached and can be improved. These students share some characteristics that warrant special attention, because they can increase the student's stresses and impede the student's ability to recognize and seek help for mental health issues.

What are some of the unique features common to these populations? First of all, they have an identity which makes them stand out from the general campus population. By manner, accent, age, appearance and dress, they are recognizable as "different".

What are some of the problems they encounter? The predominant common issue is the lack, or perceived lack, of a cohort. Language, lifestyle, age, and lack of a support system may add to the stress of the college experience. They may have experienced discrimination; they may feel or actually be older than their classmates. Their school experiences prior to entering college or graduate school may vary significantly from the public primary and secondary schools most students in the US have attended. They may have traveled or lived in other countries, often to a greater degree than the average college student.

13.2 Athletes

The link between the high rates of exercise that athletes participate in and the reduction in rates of depression and hopelessness is well documented [1]. However, the collegiate sports atmosphere is quite insular and does produce some unique stressors [2]. The freshman college athlete enters the NCAA having been the star of his or her high school team, only to find themselves at the bottom of the status hierarchy in an atmosphere that is much more business-like and less emotionally supportive than their high school experience. This sudden change can be shocking and demoralizing to the athlete, and many in this situation have said they find their sport "no fun anymore". This level of disappointment can lead to depression, anxiety, or substance use [3] (typically alcohol abuse which is easier to hide from detection by random urine drug screens). In turn, this demoralization can lead

Mental Health Care in the College Community   Edited by Jerald Kay and Victor Schwartz
© 2010 John Wiley & Sons, Ltd.

to declines in athletic performance, which exacerbates the negative feedback received from coaches and can result in a negative spiral out of collegiate sports altogether.

Athletic practice schedules are often grueling and highly structured, leaving little time for leisure or even homework. Additionally, the physical demands of the sport often put pressure on the athlete to maintain a certain weight, which can lead to eating disorders or other stress-related illnesses. The student athlete's social structure is often limited to other athletes, and if someone leaves the sport for some reason he or she can feel abandoned and isolated. Conflicts with coaches can upset an athlete's entire social support system and result in divisive team dynamics, especially in smaller teams.

Aside from social and work stressors, athletes are also vulnerable to becoming seriously injured, sometimes several times, during their college career. Joint and muscular injuries can progress to chronic pain disorders or can end an athlete's career in sports, and closed head injuries can lead to mood disorders, irritability, and decreased academic functioning [4].

Athletes may avoid seeking help when symptoms of emotional distress appear. Often the athlete is accustomed to being independent and wants to appear "together", therefore avoiding dealing with emotional distress. Additionally, stigma against mental illness remains strong among many coaches and fellow athletes, causing fear of reprisal or negative judgment if help is sought. Sometimes coaches or athletic trainers will want to know intimate details of mental health treatment, causing tension between the mental health professional who wants to honor the athlete's confidentiality and the authorities who want to know if their athlete is fit to participate. Usually this tension can be resolved to the benefit of the athlete and the team while the athlete's personal information is protected, but it requires careful communication between the mental health professional and the athlete to ensure that only the required information is shared. Regular liaison activity between the mental health staff and the athletic staff and students is helpful in order to keep the lines of communication open and to provide educational opportunities that help to reduce stigma, inform staff and students about the confidentiality issues, and encourage more help-seeking.

One of the mental disorders that athletes are vulnerable to is an eating disorder, which is typically characterized by resistance to treatment and lack of insight, especially before treatment is sought or mandated [5]. When an athlete is reluctant to seek or accept treatment, intervention can be extremely difficult. Engaging coaching staff to encourage or mandate treatment can be helpful, but again the relationship must be carefully negotiated to avoid splitting and triangulation while building a therapeutic relationship with the athlete. While the threat of losing scholarship support or being removed from the team can be motivating for accepting treatment, the need for coercion is not conducive to building therapeutic rapport. The position that the therapist finds him or herself in can also engender negative countertransference that must be carefully monitored. Peer consultation and support is crucial in these instances.

Another aspect of mental health treatment of athletes that should be mentioned here is use of medications. Athletes are often concerned about possible interference with their athletic performance by psychotropic medications, and careful attention to these concerns is warranted. Additionally, NCAA drug testing rules must be followed, and documentation of prescribed medications is needed. New rules regarding the prescription of stimulants for attention deficit disorder took effect in September 2009. These rules require significant documentation of the diagnostic procedures, and athletes who do not have this documentation will be considered out of compliance if stimulants are found during drug testing [6].

In sum, since there are many issues unique to athletes, it is helpful for a college mental health or counseling service to have one or two "specialists" who are familiar with these issues to work with athletes seeking help.

13.3 International Students

International students comprise a significant portion of the student body, especially in major research-oriented universities. "The number of international students at colleges and universities in the United States increased by 7% to a record high of 623 805 in the 2007–2008 academic year, according to the *Open Doors* report published annually by the Institute of International Education (IIE) with support from the US Department of State's Bureau of Educational and Cultural Affairs. This 2007–2008 growth builds on a 3% increase reported for 2006–2007, and the total number now exceeds by 6% the previous all-time high of 586 323 reported in 2002/03" [7]. More than 62% of the international student population is Asian, with India and China being the top two countries of origin of these students. At the University of Michigan approximately 10% of the enrollment is foreign, predominantly Asian, and primarily graduate students. Although we describe them all as "international", they are a very heterogeneous group. At the University of Michigan 115 countries are represented most years, and at many of the top 20 U.S. universities students are from more than 150 countries.

The changing political and economic climate in recent years around the world affects international students in substantial ways. The treatment of students from Arab countries after the attacks of 11September 2001 and the global economic problems beginning in 2008 impact this group in terms of their ability and willingness to access the educational opportunities of the United States.

Some of the issues facing international students include distance from home, with trips home during school vacations or just to "recharge" extremely costly and sometimes impossible. Some graduate students are unable to return home for visits for many years. After the events of 11 September 2001, some of these students found they could not return to their home countries without jeopardizing their return to school. Dorm closings over holidays put them at a disadvantage; semester or summer breaks require some accommodation for their belongings, as they cannot simply pile their books, bedding and clothes into a car and drive home. As one international student told me, "I felt like a homeless person" at the end of the term.

Language skills are often a hindrance to social interaction, even when an international student is very competent in the classroom. One student from another country explained how frustrating it was when she used words inaccurately, because she appears to be very fluent in English. Others assume she is fluent, and then become annoyed with her when she fails to understand a figure of speech, or mispronounces a long word. This difference between "educational fluency" and "social fluency" in English interferes with a student's willingness to speak to a professor, even to answer questions in the classroom, and additionally when speaking to a therapist.

Unlike most American students, international students generally have no opportunity to visit the school they come here to attend prior to actual enrollment. Visas may limit their ability to travel home periodically, and the changing political climate in some countries may preclude travel in general. International students report that educational visas often provide very limited opportunity to arrive at school with time to acclimate before the start of the school year, resulting in a foreshortened "orientation", as well as limited time to find a peer group.

International students have varying degrees of sophistication regarding higher education, ranging from students whose parents may also have attended school in the United States, and/or are professionals or educators themselves, to students who grew up in rural regions of third world countries, and may be the first in their family to seek a higher education, especially abroad. While a range as broad as this certainly occurs among United States citizens, the familiarity of the English language and closeness to home makes that accommodation somewhat easier. International students have experienced a wide range of educational settings prior to coming to the United States; often very large classrooms, significant competition for educational opportunities, with an emphasis on rote learning and supporting the peer group, rather than on individual effort. On the other hand, in countries such as the United Kingdom and Canada, preparation for college commonly exceeds that in the United States public school system. These variables can lead to large gaps in the preparation level of students, contributing to higher stress and frustration levels, as well as variability in competititiveness with their American peers.

Sophistication regarding psychiatric illness and treatment also varies widely. The acknowledgment or recognition of the symptoms of a mental illness may be difficult for a student from a country where depression is considered a moral weakness, and academic struggles to be a sign of laziness. Students who do poorly academically or have to take a medical leave of absence may not be able to stay in this country to remediate or get treatment. Furthermore, they may fear that a psychiatric diagnosis compromises the possibility of returning to this country (or a particular school). Information about a prior mental illness may not be revealed prior to admission, and in addition, in some countries and some cultures a psychiatric illness is so shameful that treatment either in their country of origin or in the United States is avoided. For example, many Asian students have commented in sessions that "mental illness is not dealt with" in their country of origin. Comments such as these have also been made by Middle Eastern students. Additionally, many international students may be reluctant to accept Western medication treatment for mental disorders, and beginning the alliance by recommending alternative therapies like acupuncture or meditation can be a helpful first step.

A student from a fairly homogeneous country with a strong belief system, especially with regard to religious beliefs, can be overwhelmed by the range of races, religions and lifestyles they encounter in the U.S. Homosexuality, alcohol abuse, even dating, and especially interracial dating may be frightening or abhorrent to the naïve international student. An international student who became aware of homosexual preference avoided returning home for several years, anticipating that he will meet with strong disapproval from his family. At the same time, he anticipates pressure to marry once studies are completed.

Other international students may feel relief from the openness and tolerance of American lifestyle.

Many schools provide an International Center to help these students adapt to the cultural and academic demands of the school, but these cannot address every issue that may confront these students. The problem of greatest concern for college mental health centers is the strategy for facilitating help-seeking behaviors for students in distress. Orientation needs to be structured to address this issue at the beginning of the term, but also periodically during the year. At orientation, international students are deluged with the tasks of registering for classes, finding their way around campus, and identifying a peer group academically, religiously, culturally or interest-wise. They may not hear or want to hear about potential psychological problems or how to access help at the beginning of their experience in the United States. The University of California, San Francisco, promotes a series of "social get-togethers" throughout the year for international students, and recognizing the fact that these students are generally very conscientious about following rules, makes them mandatory. Another strategy to promote help-seeking is to form alliances between counseling services and international student advisors and clergy. Programs organized and attended by each of these groups can help destigmatize help-seeking as well.

13.4 Returning Students

Older (i.e. students matriculating after the traditional undergraduate college age group of 18–22) and returning students are non-traditional in a number of ways. Many factors can cause someone to delay their college education after high school. Some students start a family early and choose to stay home with their children until they are older. Some individuals join the workforce first, either because they didn't want to go to college right away, or because financial or family concerns delayed their entry into higher education. Still other students start college, and for various reasons choose to or are forced to leave academia only to return at a later date. This group includes those who start college with poorly defined career goals or poor study habits who are academically dismissed for poor performance. Another reason for taking an extended leave from college is illness, either of self or a family member – or perhaps death of a loved one. Upon returning to college, the student is older than his or her peers, immediately causing a separation in experience from peers.

Additionally, the reason for leaving college may continue to be a stressor for the returning student. Poor performance or personal illness may cause fear of failure a second time, and if an illness recurs or relapses this can lead to another withdrawal from school. Sometimes the reason for failure the first time was undiagnosed attention deficit disorder, and the returning student may still be undiagnosed. Often this student can present for mental health services with initial complaints of anxiety or depressed mood which turn out to be secondary to executive functioning difficulties.

Whatever the reason for returning or starting school later, most of these students will have a few things in common: their older age and more life experience may alienate them from their younger and more naïve peers. The older student may feel that the younger students are not taking college seriously or that they are immature and "party" too much. Conversely, the older student may either be more academically successful because they are more experienced and serious about school, or they may struggle more academically than their younger peers because of being "out of practice" with studying or due to interference by their illness or outside obligations such as family or full-time work.

All these factors can lead the returning student to need counseling and mental health support as they find their niche in the undergraduate college life. Additionally, they may need academic or learning services support in order to compete with the younger students.

Although undergraduates, these students often have more in common socially with graduate students because of their age, life experience, higher likelihood of being partnered and/or a parent, and general outlook on life. These students are often referred to the graduate student therapy groups because of their commonalities.

Students returning to school after an illness may require extra support, especially if the illness is a mental illness. Students with self-identified mental illness tracked by the

University of Maryland College of Behavioral and Social Sciences are less likely to complete college, more likely to take at least one leave of absence, more likely to need several exceptions to policies on dropping courses, and likely to have lower grade point averages. The average time to complete a degree for these individuals was 12.6 semesters. Many of these students would not have attended college before the advent of the newer psychotropic medications, but many require extensive mental health treatment and support in order to be successful.

Returning students with physical illnesses (such as multiple sclerosis, lung disorders, diabetes, severe physical injuries, etc.) may also suffer relapses and need more time off, medical and emotional care and support, and/or reduced course loads in order to complete their degree. While these students can tax the college support systems designed for healthy students, they are a crucial part of a diverse student body and offer a wealth of information and experience to enrich the college experience for everyone. Universities must adjust to this changing climate in order to comply with civil rights laws and to improve retention of these important students, while remaining competitive in the college ranking system.

13.5 Students with Chronic Illnesses

There are several chronic illnesses that present specific difficulties for college mental health services. Physical disabilities began to be addressed a number of years ago, driven ultimately by the Americans with Disabilities Act (ADA), which was signed into law in 1990. Accommodations for wheelchair bound and hearing or sight-impaired students have been in place for a number of years. While these arrangements do respond to the physical limitations of a student, they may not protect the psyche of a student who can so clearly be recognized as "different". Many students with long-term physical limitations have learned to make others comfortable with them; this is often a result of good parenting. However, when the disability is more recent and/or temporary, the student may not have developed the coping skills to maneuver campus, interpersonal relationships, or classroom demands effectively. Furthermore, a student with a recently acquired disability has often not processed the meaning of this limitation; they can become discouraged and depressed over the limitations imposed by needing to eat special foods, at specific times; having limited access to a bathroom or even the privacy they may desire. Because of the ADA, campuses are required to provide accommodations for students who have a defined disability. However, offices charged with this responsibility are increasingly taxed with developing creative ways to address the disabilities of students who in prior years would never have made it into college. Many institutions are preparing for the enrollment of students who carry the diagnosis of Asperger's syndrome and have developed specific programs to enhance socialization and intercept potential difficulties in dorms and class-rooms for these students. Finding other individuals with this same problem seems to be very helpful for many of these students [8].

Chronic mental illness is particularly problematic. College mental health service directors report a significant increase in students who have a history of serious psychiatric problems, including prior psychiatric hospitalizations and suicide attempts [9]. College seems to be somewhat protective, in that college students are about half as likely as their age-matched peers to commit suicide; however, the headline suicides of college students are very distressing to classmates and dorm-mates. The administrative issues around identifying, treating, allowing medical leave and deciding when a seriously mentally ill student who has left school to obtain treatment and may return to campus are very complex. And of course the age of onset for some of these disorders corresponds to the age at which students arrive on campus. Sometimes it is hard to tell how much of a student's distress is simply a result of making the transition to college. It is widely felt among college mental health clinicians that the development of the newer antidepressants and the efforts of the mental health profession to de-stigmatize mental illness have resulted in increased numbers of students attending college who formerly would not have been able to do so. Certainly "adult" attention deficit disorder or attention deficit hyperactivity disorder did not appear to the degree we see it now. College health services are conflicted about how to diagnose and whether to prescribe medications for these students, recognizing the amount of diversion of stimulant medications for recreation or for exams. In 2008, nearly 7% of US college students reported using stimulants non-medically(not for prescribed use, or not prescribed to them) [10].

Eating disorders and associated body image issues afflict a large number of college students, predominantly female. Surveys suggest the incidence is as high as 1 in 5 among female students, and almost 1 in 10 among male students. 50% of women and 35% of men report dieting to lose weight [11]. There are a number of factors that contribute to this; competition with other students for attractiveness, being away from home and making their own decisions about meals, including when and what to eat; ready availability of exercise equipment, and the usual stresses of college. The need to have some mastery in their lives, when grades, coursework, or relationships seem so unpredictable is a more powerful driving force than food and weight. College health services increasingly are enhancing programs to treat this chronic (and potentially fatal) disease, with provision of groups, nutritionists, and educational programs in the dorms. Often it is helpful for a group of interested clinicians, including a social worker, a dietician, and a primary care physician to meet regularly to discuss mutual patients and to develop additional strategies to identify and treat eating disordered patients. Organizations have been created on campuses consisting of interested students, health educators and clinicians who are highly visible during orientation, and have developed a series of programs to educate students and faculty on the recognition of eating disorders. One necessary component of identification is education of housekeeping staff in the dormitories and classroom buildings; interestingly, a custodian recently helped identify a woman who was seriously bulimic, because she had noted repeated evidence of this behavior in a bathroom she cleaned regularly, and suspected a particular student. Anorexia can be particularly pernicious. When body weight falls too low, a patient's thinking becomes clouded, affecting not only their academics but even the ability to acknowledge his or her problem and to make use of treatment. Residential or partial hospital programs may be necessary, requiring the student to take a medical leave from campus. At least one private university went so far as to demand proof of treatment and weight gain in a severely anorectic patient before allowing the student to return to classes. However, this approach can be difficult to generalize, since many universities do not have specific policies to accommodate this approach. Administrators must be careful not to violate students' civil rights by discriminating against them because of mental illness. Sometimes a student may be pushed into treatment by invoking student conduct rules such as the ability to remove a student from campus for "Engaging in disorderly or disruptive conduct on University premises or at University-sponsored activities which interferes with the activities of others" [12]. Usually, however, colleges deal with students who refuse treatment by involving the parents when life-threatening situations are present. When a mental illness is of sufficient severity that there is a threat to the life of the student, parents of dependent students can be contacted. However, if the severity of the illness is not immediately life-threatening, administrators and clinicians must monitor the student regularly and continue to attempt to engage him or her in treatment.

Late adolescence is a period of enormous change in self-awareness. Exposure to new situations and ideas may enable a formerly quiet and self-conscious student to blossom, and to master coursework and other stresses that the home environment would not have allowed or facilitated. Students' own and their families' experiences with mental health may color their willingness to access college mental health services, and their ability to make use of such services. Chronic medical or psychiatric illness may impede progress in school, but on the other hand these illnesses may improve with treatment and maturity, or may be of less significance than the field the student is studying, the student's academic abilities, or extracurricular skills and activities. At all times, it is important to find out how the student views their disability, and what accommodations they feel they need, rather than making assumptions a priori about the student's limitations.

While students with chronic medical illness such as Crohn's disease, diabetes, cystic fibrosis or cardiac problems generally arrive on campus with good health insurance in place, it is less common for families to understand or recognize the need for coverage for psychiatric illness. In states without mental health parity laws, insurance plans may not provide very good coverage for illnesses such as bipolar disorder, eating disorders, major depressive disorder or generalized anxiety disorder. Even with this coverage, if a student is forced to leave school because of severe depression or incapacitating eating disorder, or needs residential treatment for an eating disorder or substance abuse problem, they may lose their insurance coverage if it is defined as coverage under a parent's policy only while a full-time student. Campus resources such as student health and campus counseling centers are also no longer available to a student who has had to withdraw from school. Some schools have attempted to address this by special arrangement to provide a student with campus resources such as student health or campus counseling services, for six months to a year while they are taking medical leave.

13.6 Graduate Students

Depending on the field they are in, students enter graduate school with certain expectations, such as how they will be mentored, how long their course of study will be, and what their colleagues will be like. In the sciences, there may be competition for the lab in which they'll eventually work. In the arts, there may be an expectation of collaboration with classmates or faculty. Because graduate students have completed college, many universities do not direct as much effort towards apprising them of mental health resources; there is the assumption that they will require fewer social and emotional resources than undergraduates. In fact, graduate students may be more or less motivated, prepared, respectful of faculty, and looking for a community of like-minded colleagues, depending on their previous experience. Significantly, graduate students complete their studies at a very individualized rate; they may complete their requirements in the middle of an academic year, actually leave campus and begin new positions prior to fully completing their degree, or decide to take a "terminal master's" when it appears to them or to their advisors that they are not likely to complete requirements/expectations for a doctorate. Because it may take several years to complete a thesis in the humanities, it is not uncommon for a graduate student to find their major advisor leaving for another position or taking a sabbatical before the student has finished; sometimes this necessitates a change in their thesis, or at least collaboration with an advisor who now lives elsewhere (and has other priorities). Even in medical school, which generally is thought to be a four-year curriculum, a significant portion will not finish in the same cohort they began with, taking time for master's degrees in public health or a basic science, or medical or academic leave. At the same time, they have concerns about finding partners, getting a job, financing their studies and possibly meeting obligations of family of origin. All of these factors tend to isolate the graduate student at one point or many times in their educational experience.

Towards completion of their degree, graduate students may find departmental expectations have become less well-defined. Graduate students in the sciences may have difficulty meeting the demands of the department when a paper is not accepted or needs to be revised, research results are not forthcoming, or an advisor simply seems to find it hard to "let go" of a promising colleague and sets out additional requirements for graduation. If they had difficulty with separation from home very early in life, even though they appear to have mastered that, separation issues may reemerge. The challenges of financial support and health care coverage loom large; as well as the realization that they will soon have to pay back loans.

Common entry points for graduate students to seek help from College Mental Health services are:

1. within the first year, when they may experience disappointment with the program, their mentors, or their classmates, and have not yet established a community of friends;

2. after they have qualified, or finished their coursework and find difficulty defining the focus of their doctoral work; or are discouraged from pursuing their specific interest;

3. after their fourth year, when they become increasingly isolated as they pursue the specific topic they have chosen; coursework and preliminaries are behind them, and classmates have begun to "peel off", as they graduate or otherwise discontinue graduate school.

At the University of Michigan, there are over 2000 international students in our graduate school, the sixth largest number of international students among research universities in the United States. The majority of them are from Asian countries, where traditionally, recognizing, talking about psychiatric illness and seeking psychiatric services is discouraged. Most of our international students are in engineering programs; even among United States citizens, engineering students tend not to feel comfortable talking about emotions.

Of major concern to college mental health services is that the highest risk of suicide among our patients is in upper-class and graduate students; this is compounded by the fact that suicide is highest among Asian students. A study completed at UC Berkeley in 2000 and repeated in 2004 outlines some of the significant issues graduate students face (see Box 13.1) [13,14].

An excellent publication is available for further reading on this topic. "Helping Students Adapt to Graduate School: Making the Grade", put out by the College Student Committee of the Group for the Advancement of Psychiatry (GAP) [15].

Box 13.1   Berkeley Graduate Student Mental Health Survey April 2004

- 45.3% of grad students had experienced an emotional or stress-related problem that significantly affected their well-being or performance

- 52% considered using university counseling services; less than 33% actually did

- nearly 25% of grad students were unaware of campus mental health services; nearly 40% of international grad students unaware

- 9.9% seriously considered suicide

- estimated suicide completion rate of 2.3–7.2 per 10 000, compared with 1.48 in general population, and 0.75 per 10 000 for undergraduates.

13.7 Transfer Students

Transfer students represent a widely divergent group, with a few general issues defining them. Students who have transferred from a community college to a four year school do so because that was their plan all along, to save money and/or to start college at a slower pace; or they may not have even considered the possibility of going to a four-year college initially. Time management may be a new skill they have to master if they attended community college on a part-time basis.

Community college may have allowed them to live at home. However, this can present a problem when they transfer, because they are dealing with the issue of leaving home at a time when their classmates have already addressed this in the past, so they don't have the support of a group of peers going through the same thing. They may have transferred from another four-year college for personal reasons, for economic ones, or because they have changed their minds about a major and determined that the second school suited their purposes better. These students may be frustrated by the fact that not all of their credits transfer, the coursework at the second school is harder, and that registering for the classes they want is complicated by the fact that many of these classes are already closed. They also will not have the advantage of the "grapevine" regarding which professors or classes are attractive, and which ones are to be avoided. If they also transferred because of unpleasant or even traumatic experiences at the first school, they must process that even while they are learning their way around the new school.

Transfer students often choose to live off-campus. Unfortunately, this further isolates them because they miss the socialization that occurs in the dorms; if they do live on campus, they are often placed in the least desirable dorms, the preferred ones having already been selected by entering or returning students. Even finding their way around campus presents a stress, especially since they are in upper level courses so are more likely to need to get to several buildings, as opposed to freshmen, who may have most of their classes in the same building.

Once again, transfer students have a difficult time finding a cohort. It may be hard to find interest groups as a junior; many organizations are already crystallized by then. If they started school at a community college, they may not be prepared for the rigors or the competition of a four-year college, and find therefore that they don't have the time to devote to a club or interest group. There is good evidence that joining groups helps in retention and grades [16].

It is helpful to orient and include transfer students into the campus community as quickly as possible. At the University of Michigan, orientation for transfer students is offered during the summer, many weeks before the start of the academic year. It consists of a 2-day visit to the campus, with tours and question-and-answer sessions. Additional strategies for enabling the transition to go smoothly include research opportunities on campus for community college students prior to their enrollment, even going so far as to court promising and talented community college students on their own campus. Certain components of the usual orientation that occur when they arrive on campus are repeated later on in the semester, once they have settled in. This is done because the administration recognizes that incoming transfer students often feel they "know everything they need to know about college", but only later discover what they didn't know. At that point they are more receptive to hearing about helpful resources on campus, including of course college mental health services, but also mentoring programs, special groups such as OATS (the Organization for Adult and Transfer Students), study groups, and receptions soon after the beginning of fall and winter terms for transfer students to meet other transfer students.

Solutions for transfer students that the University of Michigan is still working to address include possible floor or wing specific areas in the dormitories that would be offered to incoming transfer students, and, for the large number of transfer students that are commuting to campus, student resources such as a lounge, lockers, kitchen, and special parking privileges.

13.8 Lesbian, Gay, Bisexual, Transgendered and Questioning Students

Lesbian, gay, bisexual, transgendered and questioning (LGBTQ) students are often called the "invisible" minority, because one often cannot tell by looking at a person what her or his sexual or gender orientation is. In converse to what many racial and ethnic minorities face, like being assumed to be "black" or "Hispanic" or "Middle-eastern" because of their physical characteristics, LGBTQ individuals are often assumed to be one of the dominant group, that is, heterosexuals. While it can be said that there are benefits to blending in with the dominant social group, it is also true that currently it is not socially acceptable to be openly racist [17]. On the other hand, the LGBTQ community continues to face overt discrimination as evidenced by the passage of state laws and constitutional amendments during every national election cycle since 2004 that strip them of either the right to marry, adopt or foster children, or even enter into other legal contracts. For example, 28 states have adopted constitutional amendments since 2004 banning same-sex marriage, Alaska adopted the amendment in 1998, and another 11 states have state laws restricting marriage to between one man and one woman; 18 of those 40 states have further legislation that limits or bans other legal relationships such as domestic partnerships and civil unions. Only 10 states and the District of Columbia provide state-wide for same-sex adoption of children, while five states openly ban same-sex or second-parent adoption, and another five state courts have declared that same-sex or second-parent adoption is not allowed by state law [18]. There has even been resistance to adding this population to hate crimes laws, despite the brutal murder in 1998 of University of Wyoming student Matthew Shepard. President Barack Obama signed into law the Matthew Shepard Act on October 28, 2009 [19].

On a more positive note, however, several states are also passing state laws and handing down court decisions declaring discriminatory laws such as marriage bans to be unconstitutional. These states now include Massachusetts, Connecticut, Iowa, Maine, and Vermont.

Several states and the District of Columbia (California, Oregon, New Hampshire, and New Jersey) now allow for domestic partnership or civil unions. Several other states either offer some same-sex couple legal rights or are currently in the process of considering legislation.

The legal and civil rights battles going on nationwide can be seen as a metaphor for what many young LGBTQ college students are going through. While social and legal acceptance of sexual minorities has come a long way since the Stonewall riots of 1969, considerable prejudice against the LGBTQ community still exists. Religious conservatives take the view that homosexuality is a "choice" that is morally "wrong", while the American Psychiatric Association removed it from the listing of mental disorders in 1973, and the World Health Organization voted to remove it from the International Classification of Diseases (ICD) in 1990. Both the American Psychiatric Association and the American Psychological Association, along with former Surgeon General David Satcher, hold the position that sexual orientation cannot be changed. This landscape of conflicting views, messages, and laws contribute to the difficulty that many LGBTQ youth face in coming to terms with their sexuality. Often these individuals are conflicted within themselves about how to proceed with their lives, and many fear rejection or outright abandonment by their family and other loved ones if they reveal their sexual or gender orientation. Youth from a religious family may also fear judgment by clergy or even God. All of these pressures contribute to the high suicide rate of LGBTQ youth. These youth have up to four times the risk of attempting suicide compared to their heterosexual counterparts, and those from unaccepting or very judgmental families have up to eight times the suicide attempt rate [20]. Some estimates state that up to 30% of youth completing suicide are LGBT [21]. Aside from the suicide risk, LGBT youth are also at risk for substance abuse, depression, and anxiety disorders. Welcoming counseling and mental health resources on campus are crucial in order to offer a safe place in which to explore and process their new experiences.

Many times college is the first opportunity a closeted youth has to explore his or her sexuality in an environment away from parental and family pressures. This can be liberating, but also frightening and stressful, especially for youth who have significant internalized homophobia. Although college students today are relatively accepting of LGBTQ lifestyles, depending on the region of the country and nature of the particular campus community, significant overt disdain and negative pressure can exist. LGBTQ youth can feel very isolated, not knowing whom to trust. LGBTQ youth also may not seek counseling or mental health assistance, either due to their own fears, stigma against seeking mental health treatment, or fear of negative judgment by the mental health professional due to a past history of negative behavior on the part of some mental health professionals. It is especially important for college mental health services to do aggressive outreach to the LGBTQ community to encourage help-seeking behavior and as part of the service's suicide prevention strategy. Open support groups are an essential part of the treatment spectrum, as is easy access to sensitive and competent counseling and psychiatric services. Often these services are provided by clinicians who are either LGBT themselves or have a particular interest in the service. However, many colleges and universities also have LGBTQ equity offices that offer training to interested parties. All mental health clnicians should avail themselves of these trainings whenever possible in order to minimize their own internalized homophobia or negative countertransference toward LGBTQ individuals. The Gay and Lesbian Medical Organization (GLMA) has developed a handbook to assist medical professionals in developing a sensitive treatment environment (Box 13.2). The publication is available online at: http://www.glma.org/_data/n_0001/resources/live/Welcoming%20Environment.pdf [22].

Box 13.2   Creating a Welcoming Environment for LGBTQ Clients

- Display rainbow flags or other LGBTQ-friendly symbols

- Hang posters depicting multiracial and same-sex couples

- Post or disseminate prominently a non-discrimination policy

- Display brochures on pertinent health concerns such as HIV/AIDS, hormone therapy, and so on

- Acknowledge dates of observance such as world AIDS day, gay pride, and so on

- Display LGBT-specific media

- Educate all staff on sensitivity to LGBT concerns and make it clear that discrimination will not be tolerated.

13.9 Veterans

Veterans are a unique group of students (Box 13.3), and for them the ground is changing even as they try to gain their footing. The combination of a prolonged war, a faltering economy, and enhanced educational opportunity has led to greater numbers of veterans entering college. This group of students is recognizably distinct; they have been in the service. Because they have spent time after high school in the armed forces, they are older, and often more focused or goal-directed in their pursuit of higher education. They may have elected to join the service in order to be able to attend college ultimately and are often the first ones in their family to attend college. The majority of veterans are from lower to middle-income families, sometimes finding it hard to accept and to be accepted by their more carefree and privileged classmates. Their political orientation tends to be conservative and very patriotic; they may clash with views of classmates and professors who tend towards being more liberal.

Box 13.3   Veterans

Two hundred and fifty thousand GIs are attending college under the new, more generous GI Bill – the largest number since the return from Vietnam [23].

Veterans may have been victims of, or witness to very traumatic experiences, beyond what most of us can imagine. This may lead some of them to abuse drugs and alcohol, but it also may give them a healthier perspective on the college experience. One veteran told his advisor, "My roommate is upset he didn't get into the fraternity he wanted to; I'm just glad I didn't get shot at today!" They are generally unwilling to discuss their service experiences, particularly with people who have not had similar experiences. Thus, ghosts of PTSD remain hidden, causing greater or lesser degrees of stress and a desire to isolate. There is certainly mounting evidence for serious psychiatric problems in returning veterans, including PTSD and an increased suicide rate. Closed head injury may impact their ability to make the most of the college opportunity [24].

Another trauma that women veterans may experience during their tour of duty is sexual assault, often by men in their own unit [25]. CBS News reported in March 2009 that women in the military are twice as likely as their non-military counterparts to be raped during their service. Very few of these crimes are prosecuted, even when they are reported to military authorities. It is important for campus mental health clinicians and services to be prepared for this issue with returning veterans, and to actively educate veterans about services available on campus, as well as services made available off-campus for veterans.

College is a huge transition for many veterans. In the military all needs are met, including food, shelter, and salary; all decisions come from commanders, there is a shared sense of purpose and built-in camaraderie, especially in deployment, where each soldier knows how necessary it is to watch his buddy's back. In college, many decisions are difficult, partly due to the veteran's background but significantly because the choices the veteran is now making are individual.

Those veterans who decide to attend college find numerous challenges in this transition; the length of time since they were last in school, their age, the experiences they had in service, the loss of their peer group, and the need to assume responsibility for themselves, often with a wife and children as well. They report feeling conflicted about whether to reveal that they are veterans. They may get questions from classmates such as "Did you kill anyone?" If they did, this certainly sets them apart, but more significantly they may not want to reveal this to anyone or have not yet even fully processed it themselves. Some veterans report that the generally more liberal faculty may openly or subtly be critical that they were in the military.

Their generally lower to working-class background commonly means they are less comfortable seeking mental health services, although they have access to veteran's hospital treatment programs. Here again, however, they do not fit in with veterans who are severely impaired, and/ or much older, who remain relatively less educated. On several campuses across the United States, student veteran's organizations have been formed in the last few years.

13.10 Victims of Sexual Assault

College is the riskiest time for sexual assault. One in four women will be sexually assaulted while in college, a staggering statistic. This rate is at least 3 times higher than that of the age-matched general population [26]. Most of these assaults will be perpetrated by a male acquaintance, and alcohol is involved more than half of the time [27]. The severity of these incidents varies from coerced or unwanted fondling or intercourse by a friend to brutal gang rapes by several casually known men which can include beatings and use of foreign objects in the assaults. The overwhelming majority of these crimes will not be reported to police, and most are not even reported to advocacy centers. Still, those that are reported either to police or to advocacy centers must also be reported to the campus community since the rape and murder in her residence hall room of Jeanne Clery in 1986 prompted the Crime Awareness and Campus Security Act of 1990 (also known as the Clery Act). Campuses are required to report violent crimes committed on or near campus to the campus community in an effort to warn students of violent crimes. For more information on the Clery Act and its reporting, see the web site http://www.securityoncampus.org.

Even with this mechanism in place, many pressures contribute to women remaining silent about their experiences. These include shame and guilt, especially for women who were intoxicated at the time of their assaults; they often feel and are told by others that they "shouldn't have been drinking", or "should have known better than to trust that guy". Women are often given the message that if they drink, wear attractive or sexy clothing, or go out at night that they are "asking for it". Additionally, law enforcement personnel who face the realities of the difficulty of prosecution of these cases may aggressively question a victim such that she is re-traumatized by that experience. Until January 2009, law enforcement personnel were allowed to refuse to authorize collection of evidence and a forensic exam if they felt that the case was too weak to prosecute; hence, if the evidence wasn't collected, the victim had no recourse to pursue legal action even if she chose to. However, the Violence Against Women and Department of Justice Reauthorization Act of 2005 ("VAWA 2005"), 42 USC. § 3796gg-4(d), provides that states may not:

> require a victim of sexual assault to participate in the criminal justice system or cooperate with law enforcement in order to be provided with a forensic medical exam, reimbursed for charges incurred on account of such an exam, or both (the "VAWA 2005 forensic examination requirement").

This portion of the law took effect 1 January 2009. This means that a victim of sexual assault may now ask for evidence to be collected without the authorization of law enforcement, or even without revealing her or his name or other identifying information. It is hoped that more women will choose to get evidence collected after a sexual assault, and that more women will choose to report to police. However, especially on college campuses there are other pressures in play to discourage women from reporting sexual assault. Many sexual assaults happen in the Greek community on college campuses. This is a very secretive and insular group, and as such there is extraordinary pressure not to get a "brother" or a fraternity in trouble. A sorority member or pledge who is assaulted will often face pressure not just from the fraternity involved, but from her own sorority sisters. Often the relationship between the two houses takes priority over the individual traumas. Young women raped in these circumstances have been quoted as hearing their "sisters" say "he's really hot; you should be honored" when discussing a sexual assault by a "brother". Aside from this pressure, sometimes women are just not believed when they discuss a sexual assault, or are overtly shunned or even dismissed from the sorority for accusing a fraternity member of assault. More heinous crimes such as gang rape also happen at some fraternity parties [28]. These crimes are virtually never reported to police due to the amplified shame of this sort of trauma. At The University of Maryland, roughly five to seven gang rapes are reported to campus advocacy staff yearly, but none are reported to police. Some of these assaults result in serious physical injury, and virtually all are life-changing traumas. Many victims leave school after such an assault, and most are unable to complete their semester.

Regardless of the "severity" of the assault, most victims of sexual assault are not ready to process their emotional response to it for several weeks or months afterward. Sometimes victims will seek medication to deal with the anxiety, panic, and nightmare symptoms in the immediate aftermath. Prescription of small quantities of mild hypnotic medication can be very helpful for these symptoms. Other mental health services are always offered to victims in the aftermath of an assault, but most do not take advantage of these services until about 3–4 months after the assault. This phenomenon has been described as the acute phase of the "rape trauma syndrome" [29,30]. Victims are often numbed to the emotional aspects of their trauma, or may have patchy or incomplete memories of the events. Defenses some women use at this time include denial and minimization as they attempt to cope with the aftermath of the trauma. It is often during the following phase, labeled the "outward adjustment phase" that women experience an unbearable increase in their symptoms. Although many women will not avail themselves of treatment immediately after the attack, it is crucial to educate women about the resources available as soon as possible so that when they are ready they can enter treatment immediately. At that time, it is helpful to have individual psychotherapy as well as support groups to assist the healing process. Post-trauma symptoms can persist for several months to a year after a sexual assault, and can persist in the long term in some cases.

13.11 Conclusion

What are the obligations of college mental health services towards these special populations? It is important to recognize that each of the groups described above has some reluctance to access services, either out of fear that they will not be understood, or ignorance of the services that can be provided. Information offered at orientation needs to be repeated during the year; printed material or general e-mails to the student body can remind and reinforce the availability of help. Mental health services, possibly with the help and support of administration, should make every effort to facilitate the formation of affiliative groups. As noted above, there is good evidence that joining groups helps in retention and grades. Directors of college mental health services should make it a point to be available to these groups, possibly meeting with them during each academic year. Within their frame of reference, some of the problems students have in college need to be "normalized", and acceptable, as is the appropriateness of seeking help for them. Members of these groups should be consulted regarding their needs and concerns. Materials designed for the specific cohorts described in this chapter should be available at orientation and subsequently in several locations around campus, and reviewed regularly for relevance to each group. Mental health clinicians need to be flexible and to provide some services in a variety of settings. When a graduate student died unexpectedly, several members of the counseling service went to that department the next day and met with a group of students who had known her, to provide an opportunity to process their feelings. An interactive performance about eating disorders was followed by a question and answer session with the actress; a therapist from the counseling service and a psychiatrist from the student health service were also present. Mental health services must be prepared to do outreach such as educational programs at orientation and throughout the year, be willing to come into the dorms or visit groups of students with particular issues or concerns, and be readily available to consult with faculty and administration. College mental health leaders need to have their "finger on the pulse" of campus, by maintaining an open dialog with faculty, student leaders, and administration.

In the face of rising numbers of students with persistent mental illnesses on campus, colleges and universities must continue to evolve and find creative ways to provide comprehensive treatment and support to the campus community. Aggressive outreach efforts must be undertaken to educate students about services available and about the warning signs for depression, suicidality, and other signs of distress. Peer education and health promotion programs geared toward suicide prevention, stress management, and recognition of the signs of depression and anxiety are vital components of a good outreach program. Usually theses programs are given by students themselves under the guidance of clinicians, and often students are more willing to make the first contact with another student when they are in distress. A well-trained cadre of student "ambassadors" for mental wellness is an excellent method of reaching large numbers of students.

Finally, outreach and training efforts should be directed at multiple groups of faculty and staff, including advisors, teaching assistants, dining and housekeeping services, resident life, police and student affairs professionals. A comprehensive approach to college mental health must be the responsibility of the entire campus in order to "connect the dots" and ensure troubled students are identified and offered state of the art assistance (Box 13.4).

Box 13.4 Elements of a Comprehensive Approach to College Mental Health

- Multidisciplinary treatment teams
  - Psychotherapists
  - Psychiatrists
  - Trainees
  - Close liaison with primary care, health center.

- Services and materials targeted at special populations:
  - Athletes
  - Racial and ethnic minorities
  - Transfer students
  - Returning students
  - International students
  - Graduate students
  - Students with chronic health or psychiatric illnesses
  - LGBTQ students
  - Veterans
  - Sexual assault victims.

- Liaisons with multiple departments, providing
  - Nimble crisis intervention
  - Regular liaison and consultation
  - Staff education
  - Interaction with student media.

- Health promotion and peer education programs:
  - Suicide prevention gatekeeper training
  - Stress management
  - Sleep hygiene
  - Depression and anxiety recognition and referral.

References

1. Taliaferro, L.A., Rienzo, B.A., Pigg, R.M. Jr *et al.* (2009) Associations between physical activity and reduced rates of hopelessness, depression, and suicidal behavior among college students. *Journal of American College Health*, **57**(4), 427–436.
2. Thompson, R.A. and Trattner Sherman, R. (2007) *Managing Student-Athletes' Mental Health Issues*, NCAA Handbook.

3. Miller, B.E., Miller, M.N., Verhegge, R. *et al.* (2002) Alcohol misuse among college athletes: self-medication for psychiatric symptoms? *Journal of Drug Education*, **32**(1), 41–52.

4. Chen, J.-K., Johnston, K.M., Petrides, M. and Ptito, A. (2008) Neural substrates of symptoms of depression following concussion in male athletes with persisting postconcussion symptoms. *Archives of General Psychiatry*, **65**(1), 81–89.

5. Greenleaf, C., Petrie, T.A., Carter, J. and Reel, J., (2009) Female collegiate athletes: prevalence of eating disorders and disordered eating behaviors. *Journal of American College Health*, **57**(5). 489–496.

6. NCAA Banned Drugs and Medical Exceptions Policy Guidelines Regarding Medical Reporting for Student-Athletes with Attention Deficit Hyperactivity Disorder (ADHD) Taking Prescribed Stimulants, The National Collegiate Athletic Association, January 30, 2009.

7. Press Briefing – November 17, 2008 – 9:30 a.m. National Press Club – Washington DC by the Institute of International Education (IIE).

8. Weidle, B., Bolme, B. and Hoeyland, A.L. (2006) Are peer support groups for adolescents with Asperger's syndrome helpful? *Clinical Child Psychology and Psychiatry*, **11**(1), 45–62.

9. Gallagher, R.P. *National Survey of College Counseling Center Directors 2008*, International Association of Counseling Services, Washington, DC.

10. Substance Abuse and Mental Health Services Administration, Office of Applied Studies (April 7, 2009) The NSDUH Report: Nonmedical Use of Adderall among Full-Time College Students. Rockville, MD.

11. American College Health Association-National College Health Assessment (ACHA-NCHA) (2009) *II: Reference Group Data Report Fall 2008*, American College Health Association, Baltimore.

12. University of Maryland Code of Conduct, Approved by the Board of Regents January 25, 1980; amended effective September 4, 1990; December 18, 2001; April 22, 2004; November 18, 2005, April 5, 2006.

13. Berkeley Graduate Student Mental Health Survey, Report by the Berkeley Graduate and Professional Schools Mental Health Task Force http://www.ocf.berkeley.edu/~gmhealth Released: 9 December 2004.

14. Kuo, W.H., Gallo, J.J. and Tien, A.Y. (2001) Incidence of suicide ideation and attempts in adults: the 13-year follow-up of a community sample in Baltimore, Maryland. *Psychological Medicine*, **31**(7), 1181–1191; Silverman, M.M., Meyer, PM, Sloane, F. et al. (1997) The Big Ten Student Suicide Study: a 10-year study of suicides on midwestern university campuses. *Suicide and Life-Threatening Behavior*, **27**(3), 285–303.

15. The Committee on the College Student Group for the Advancement of Psychiatry (GAP) (2000) *Helping Students Adapt to Graduate School: Making the Grade*, Haworth, New York.

16. Laanan, F.S., TI: Transfer student adjustment New Directions for Community Colleges Volume 2001 Issue 114, Pages 5–13 Special Issue: Transfer Students: Trends and Issues Published Online: 4 Apr 2002.

17. Eduardo, Bonilla-Silva (May 2003) *Racism without Racists: Color-Blind Racism and the Persistence of Racial Inequality in the United States*, Rowman & Littlefield Publishers, Inc. Lanham MD.

18. Chris, Edelson (Dec 2008) Equality From State to State: A Review of state legislation in 2008 affecting the lesbian, gay, bisexual, and transgender community, and a look ahead to 2009, Human Rights Campaign Foundation, Washington, DC.

19. Lynsen, Joshua (13 June 2008) "Obama renews commitment to gay issues". *Washington Blade* (Window Media LLC Productions). http://www.washblade.com/2008/6-13/news/national/12766.cfm.

20. McDaniel, J.S., Purcell, D.W. and D'Augelli, A.R. (2001) The relationship between sexual orientation and risk for suicide: Research findings and future directions for research and prevention. *Suicide and Life-Threatening Behavior*, **31**(1), (Suppl.), 84–105.

21. Russell, S.T. and Joyner, K. (2001) Adolescent sexual orientation and suicide risk: Evidence from a national study. *American Journal of Public Health*, **91**, 1276–1281.

22. Gay and Lesbian Medical Association (GLMA) (2006) *Guidelines for care of LGBT patients*. San Francisco, CA 94102.

23. The Associated Press College-bound vets getting help: Many find colleges, universities are only beginning to figure out how to help; July 22, (2008.).

24. Schacter, D.L. and Crovitz, H.F. (1977) Memory function after closed head injury: a review of the quantitative research. *Cortex*, **13**(2), 150–176, Veterans Administration Hospital, Durham, North Carolina 27705, USA.

25. http://www.cbsnews.com/stories/2009/03/17/eveningnews: Sexual Assault Permeates US Armed Forces – CBS Evening News.

26. Fisher, Bonnie S., Sloan, John J., Cullen, Francis T. and Lu, Chunmeng (1998) Crime in the ivory tower: the level and sources of student victimization. *Criminology*, **36**(3), 671–710.

27. Fisher, B., Cullen, F. and Turner, M. (2000) *The Sexual Victimization of College Women*, US Department of Justice, National Institute of Justice and Bureau of Justice Statistics, Washington, DC.

28. Sanday, P.R. (1990) *Fraternity Gang Rape: Sex, Brotherhood, and Privilege on Campus*, With New Introduction and Afterword 2007, 2nd edn, New York University Press, New York.

29. *Rape, Abuse & Incest National Network* (http://www.rainn.org) Rape Trauma Syndrome.

30. Chivers-Wilson, K.A. (2006) Sexual assault and posttraumatic stress disorder: A review of the biological, psychological and sociological factors and treatments. *McGill Journal of Medicine*, **9**(2), 111–118.

14 Using A Public Health Approach to Address Student Mental Health

Laurie Davidson[1] and Joanna H. Locke[2]

[1]*Suicide Prevention Resource Center, Education Development Center, Inc., Newton, MA, USA*
[2]*The Jed Foundation, New York, NY, USA*

Health care is vital to all of us some of the time, but public health is vital to all of us all of the time. (C. Everett Koop)

14.1 Introduction

Other chapters in this book examine best practices for providing mental health services to students with a range of psychological problems. While most 4-year and some 2-year colleges and universities provide low- or no-cost mental health treatment services to their students, and/or facilitate access to off-campus services, student survey data shows that many students who need help are not asking for it directly. For example, the majority of students who report being depressed are not in treatment [1,2], and most students who die by suicide are not clients of the counseling center [3]. These data show that, while increasing help-seeking and providing effective treatment are critical, campuses must not rely solely on the counseling center to address student suicide prevention and mental health promotion.

Many colleges are going beyond simply providing treatment services by expanding efforts to *prevent mental health problems from arising* and to *promote the mental health of all students*. In other words, they are adopting a public health approach to address the social and environmental risk factors that influence student mental health [4].

For example, there may be opportunities to address the risk of suicide and mental health problems *before* intensive and costly treatment services are required. In one study, students

Parts of this chapter were adapted from The Jed Foundation/Education Development Center Inc.'s *CampusMHAP (Mental Health Action Planning)* webinar series and accompanying written guide.

with current financial problems were more likely to be depressed or suicidal [5]. An early, non-clinical intervention to help these students deal with financial issues more effectively may be sufficient. (Note: The term "intervention" refers to an activity, policy, practice, or service that is designed to result in some change in people or in the environment. In public health, the term is sometimes used interchangeably with "program", which may be used to describe an integrated set of multiple interventions.)

Another study found that certain groups of students who experience a lower quality of social support are six times more likely to experience depressive symptoms [6]. This might suggest an effort to intervene with specific student populations rather than waiting until students have developed problems requiring clinical care.

A comprehensive, multi-component effort to reduce these and other risk factors may actually produce a decline in the number of students requiring intensive clinical services over time. Rather than focus on the small number of students who need counseling, a public health approach to campus mental health aims to create conditions to support the mental wellness of all students.

14.2 A Public Health Approach to Campus Mental Health

The recent Institute of Medicine (IOM) report *Preventing Mental, Emotional, and Behavioral Disorders Among Young People: Progress and Possibilities* [7] provides an extensive rationale for a public health approach, suggesting that "behavioral health could learn from public health in endorsing a population health perspective" [2009, p. 21].

In contrast to a treatment-focused perspective, the core focus of public health is on preventing health problems and promoting health in the overall population. Public health practitioners rely on data about health problems, including their frequency and impact, to plan interventions. Perhaps the most important assumption in public health is that risk and protective factors for health problems occur not only within individuals but also at the interpersonal, institutional, community, and public policy levels [8,9]. Known as a *social ecological model*, this approach asserts that health- and safety-related behaviors are shaped not only by the individual but also by that individual's environment.

The social ecological model acknowledges that context – the social, physical, economic, and legal environment – is as important a determinant of an individual's behavior as internal knowledge, attitudes, and behavioral intentions. The model is used as a framework for examining and planning prevention programs to address a wide range of health and safety problems throughout the world.

On college and university campuses, the public health approach, including the social ecological model, is at the foundation of successful alcohol prevention [10] and violence prevention [11]. Mental health promotion and suicide prevention efforts should include activities across the continuum of the social ecological model and address the complex interplay among all of the levels.

Table 14.1 lists general factors that contribute to mental health problems at each level.

The IOM report outlines the spectrum of mental health interventions that should be included in a public health approach: mental health promotion, prevention of mental illness, treatment, and maintenance [2009]. Definitions of "prevention" and "promotion" in the context of mental health are similar to those offered in the World Health Organization's (WHO) reports on each topic [12,13].

Table 14.1	General factors contributing to mental health problems

Individual factors: Attitudes and beliefs about mental illness, help-seeking, and treatment efficacy; biological factors and family history; skills in problem-solving, relationships, and conflict resolution. Strategies addressing this level of influence are designed to affect an individual's behavior.

Interpersonal processes: Group norms regarding suicidal or help-seeking behavior; responses to individuals in distress; discrimination toward those with mental health problems. Strategies addressing this level of influence promote social support through interaction with others.

Institutional/organizational factors: Policies and procedures; existence of and availability of methods for self-harm or suicide; access to quality mental health services; high levels of alcohol consumption. Strategies addressing this level of influence are designed to change institutional conditions and environments that influence individual behavior.

Community factors: Access to quality mental health services (e.g. outpatient, inpatient, emergency hospitalization.) Strategies addressing this level of influence are designed to change conditions and environments that affect the institution; group/family/peer behavior; and individual behavior.

Public policy and societal influences: Existence of federal, state, and local laws and regulations related to restriction of lethal means, health insurance, and confidentiality; cultural contributors such as media images that portray those with mental health problems in a derogatory way or glamorize suicidal behavior [7]. Strategies at this level are designed to have wide-reaching impact through actions affecting communities, organizations, and entire populations.

McLeroy, K.R., Bibeau, D., Steckler, A. and Glanz, K. (1998) An ecological perspective on health promotion programs. *Health Education & Behavior*, **15**(4), 351–377.

Mental health promotion focuses on well-being as an end in itself rather than on preventing illness. However, there is evidence that mental health promotion is key to reducing mental health disorders as well as related problems [7].

Preventing mental disorders entails efforts to reduce the risk conditions for a mental illness; the incidence, prevalence, and recurrence of mental disorders; and the length of time that an individual experiences symptoms. Prevention also includes activities to prevent or delay recurrences of mental disorders and decrease the impact of illness on the affected person, family, and society [14]. A comprehensive prevention approach would include *universal, selective, and indicated* interventions. Universal interventions address the population at large; selective interventions target groups or individuals with an elevated risk; and indicated interventions target individuals with early symptoms or behaviors that are precursors for disorder but are not yet diagnosable [14]. In other words, a comprehensive prevention approach would include "a balance between approaches aimed at those at imminent risk, those at elevated risk, and those who currently appear risk free but for whom specific interventions have been demonstrated to reduce future risk" ([7], p. 64).

While treatment can prevent the exacerbation of symptoms, the emergence of new or comorbid symptoms, and relapse, the IOM report suggests that a key feature of public health prevention is that it can take place at any or all levels of the social ecological model. This type of prevention also focuses on preventing new disorders and targets a specific population for an intervention [7].

Table 14.2 summarizes the goals of promotion, prevention, treatment, and maintenance and provides examples of campus programs in each category.

14.2.1 Risk and Protective Factors for College Students

A public health approach aims to improve the health and safety of all students by identifying the risk and protective factors associated with mental health problems and suicidal behavior. Risk factors include traits, events, conditions, and situations that increase the likelihood that

Table 14.2	Types of public health interventions	
Intervention type	**Goal**	**Campus examples**
Promotion	"[T]o enhance individuals" ability to achieve developmentally appropriate tasks (competence) and a positive sense of self-esteem, mastery, well-being, and social inclusion and to strengthen their ability to cope with adversity' ([7], p. 66).	Opportunities to develop skills in relationships, conflict resolution, problem solving; courses about the first-year college experience; creation of a physical and social environment conducive to social connection
Prevention -Universal	To prevent disorders from developing by targeting entire population in an effort to reduce risk factors and build protective factors for all students. Focus should also be placed on preventing distress/subclinical disorders and harmful behaviors (e.g. heavy episodic drinking) [7].	Strategies to change the environment that supports high risk alcohol consumption [15,16]; restricting access to potentially lethal means of suicide
-Selective	To prevent disorders from developing in a person or group at higher risk of developing mental health disorders [7].	"Postvention" program for friends of a student who has recently died.
-Indicated	To prevent disorders from developing in individuals showing early signs or symptoms or to prevent exacerbation of existing problems [7].	Screening and referral systems; "feel better fast" psycho-educational groups
Treatment	To reduce the length of time an individual has a disorder, reduce disorder severity, and prevent recurrence [14].	Evidence-based use of psychotherapy and/ or medication
Maintenance	To decrease disorder-related disability [14].	Support groups for students living with depression

an individual will develop a specific illness or behavior. Protective factors make the occurrence of the problem or behavior less likely. Risk and protective factors can be psychological, biological, social, environmental, or cultural.

Like many chronic diseases, mental health problems tend not to have a single cause, with many different factors contributing to increased risk and no single factor being either necessary or sufficient to cause a disorder [7]. Multiple risk and protective factors for mental health problems or suicide have been identified in research studies (see Table 14.3). However, the identification of a risk factor in a particular population or group does not mean that all members of the group will experience the disorder or become suicidal. Similarly, identifying a protective factor does not ensure that the population will be protected from these problems.

It is worth emphasizing one risk factor in particular: More than 90% of people across the lifespan who die by suicide meet the criteria for a psychiatric diagnosis with the majority having more than one condition, most often mood disorders and alcohol abuse [17]. Despite the key role that mental illness plays, prevention programs still need to be comprehensive, as suicide is generally the outcome of multiple risk factors.

Interventions to change these risk factors and increase protective factors are described later in this chapter. Given the range of interventions suggested – targeting the social and physical environment, campus systems, academics, and family and peer relationships – it becomes clear that addressing student mental health problems and suicidal behavior needs to be the responsibility of the entire campus community, not just the counseling center staff. Launching a campus-wide effort requires that some key infrastructure be put in place to build and sustain an effective mental health promotion and suicide prevention effort.

Table 14.3	Risk and protective factors relevant to college students	
	Risk factors	**Protective factors**
Suicide	• Biopsychosocial	• Strong connections to family and other supports
		• Access to effective clinical interventions
	• Previous suicide attempt	• Restricted access to lethal means
	• Untreated or under-treated mental illness	• Skills in problem-solving, conflict resolution
	• Chronic physical illness	
	• Alcohol or other drug use and abuse	• Frustration tolerance, ability to regulate emotions
		• Positive beliefs about future, ability to cope, and life in general
	• Hopelessness	• Cultural/religious beliefs discouraging suicide
	• Impulsivity or aggressiveness	
	Sociocultural and environmental	
	• Barriers to effective clinical care	
	• Isolation, lack of social support	
	• Unsupported financial/social loss	
	• Stigma associated with seeking care	
	• Access to lethal means	
	• Exposure to media normalizing/ glamorizing suicide	
	Demographic	
	• Completions: male; white race; Native American youth	
	• Attempts: female; Hispanic female youth; lesbian, gay and bisexual youth	
Mental health disorders	*Individual and family-related determinants*	*Individual and family-related determinants*
	• Academic failure	• Ability to cope with stress
	• Emotional immaturity	• Adaptability
	• Excessive substance use	• Autonomy
	• Loneliness	• Exercise
	• Family conflict	• Feelings of mastery and control
	• Personal loss	• Problem-solving skills
	• Poor work skills and habits	• Self-esteem
	• Social incompetence	• Social conflict management skills
	• Stressful life events	• Stress management
		• Social support of family and friends
	Social and environmental determinants	*Social and environmental determinants*
	• Access to drugs and alcohol	• Positive interpersonal interactions
	• Isolation and alienation	• Social participation
	• Peer rejection	• Social support and community networks
	• Work stress	

US Department of Health and Human Services (2001) National Strategy for Suicide Prevention: Goals and Objectives for Action, US Department of Health and Human Services, Substance Abuse and, Mental Health Services Administration, Rockville, MD.

National Research Council and Institute of Medicine (2009) Preventing Mental, Emotional, and Behavioral Disorders Among Young People: Progress and Possibilities, in *Committee on Prevention of Mental Disorders and Substance Abuse among Children Youth and Young Adults: Research Advances and Promising Interventions. Board on Children, Youth and Families, Division of Behavioral and Social Sciences and Education* (eds M.E. O'Connell, Thomas Boat and K.E. Warner), The National Academies Press, Washington, DC.

14.3 Building Momentum and Infrastructure

A public health approach requires support from senior administrators and a broad base of key stakeholders (e.g. staff in decision-making roles, faculty who can be change agents). Promoting the mental health of all students is everyone's concern because of the relationship between mental health problems and academic success. In one study, approximately 44% of undergraduates reported that mental health issues had affected their academic performance during the past four weeks [5]. Mental health problems, specific symptoms, and possible risk factors for or consequences of both have an impact on performance as well. Stress, sleep difficulties, anxiety, depression, concern for a troubled friend or family member, and relationship difficulties are among the top factors affecting students' individual academic performance [1]. For example, 16% of students indicated that anxiety/depression/seasonal affective disorder affected their academic performance during the past 12 months [1].

There are a few essential capacities that campuses must have in place before adding new efforts to increase the identification of students at risk and/or increase help-seeking behavior. Some will take more effort to put in place than others, but all of the following are essential to ensure that demand does not outpace capacity.

- A crisis protocol is in place and key players (e.g. resident assistants) are trained in its use [18].

- Local, state, and national 24-hour hotlines are widely publicized on campus, including the National Suicide Prevention Lifeline number 1-800-273-TALK.

- Sufficient mental health services are available on- and off-campus to handle an increase in the number of students who ask for help.

- Counseling and health services clinicians are trained to assess and manage suicide and other urgent risk.

Every campus should have a dedicated office or staff person to coordinate programs, policies, and services that address suicide prevention and mental health promotion. The ability of a program coordinator to exercise leadership depends a great deal on whether there is active support from the president and other senior administrators for a campus-wide effort [10].

A key step in building momentum is to establish a mental health task force to lead a strategic planning process and oversee ongoing program efforts. Such efforts are more likely to succeed when there is broad participation and a shared commitment to meet common goals.

Many senior administrators have created the impetus for mental health promotion and suicide prevention themselves by asking health promotion and counseling staff to expand their efforts or by establishing a task force to study campus problems. In other cases, staff members have assembled data and anecdotal information and presented it to the senior student affairs administrator or the president along with a recommendation to create a task force [19]. On one campus, a student who was passionate about mental health got an appointment to meet with the president and enlisted his support for increased attention to the issues [19].

If a campus is not ready to start a task force, an individual can simply invite conversations with faculty, staff, and students to hear their concerns. Campus or national data showing the prevalence of mental health problems and suicidal behavior can also help convince senior administrators that a formal task force should be formed.

When there is widespread buy-in for a public health approach with many partners participating in an integrated set of activities and policies rather than isolated ones, it is much more likely that programs will continue to attract financial and staff support from senior administrators. And, if the activities and policies show results, key stakeholders are more likely to want to be involved. Using a strategic planning process will ensure that planners are prioritizing problems and choosing and designing programs that are likely to have the greatest impact.

14.4 Thinking and Planning Strategically

Interventions to promote emotional health and prevent mental health problems should be chosen in the context of a strategic thinking and planning process such as the one presented in Figure 14.1. Campuses should follow the steps described below when developing and implementing a public health approach.

14.4.1 Describe the Problem and Its Context

Without a clear definition of campus-specific problems, colleges run the risk of implementing interventions prematurely and could fail to achieve desired changes (e.g. fewer depressed and anxious students, less suicidal behavior) as a result.

A thorough problem assessment gives campus leaders objective data about the problems students experience, risk and protective factors linked to these problems, and estimates of prevalence. An examination of existing data, such as campus-specific National College Heath Assessment (NCHA) data from ACHA, is a good starting point. If campus-specific data is not available, data from the most recent national NCHA administration and the National Research

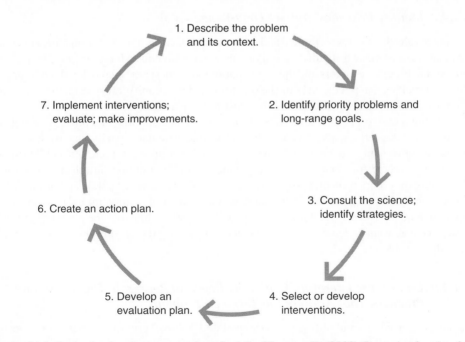

Figure 14.1 *Strategic planning process. Langford, L., Wootten, K. (2009) Strategic planning for suicide prevention. Presentation delivered at American Association for Suicide Prevention Annual Conference, San Francisco, CA, 16 April 2009.*

Consortium of Counseling Centers in Higher Education's 70-campus study on suicidal crises [20] can be informative.

Information from focus groups and one-to-one interviews with faculty, staff, and students can supplement survey data and yield a deeper understanding of student mental health needs on campus. For example, NCHA data shows that students are not seeking help for depression, but it does not provide insight into the reasons for this finding. Focus groups conducted with students can reveal some of the barriers and facilitators to help seeking and either confirm or challenge planners' assumptions.

A problem assessment can also help campuses identify which programs are already in place, how effective they are, and what gaps may exist. Campuses that are very decentralized in decision-making may find that many offices and departments are implementing program elements related to student mental health, so planners should be sure to investigate beyond counseling, health services, and health promotion. The Suicide Prevention Resource Center's (SPRC) *Inventory of Programs, Policies and Services* can assist planners with this part of the assessment. The *Inventory* and other strategic planning tools are available as part of the *CampusMHAP (Mental Health Action Planning)* webinar series archived on TJF's web site.

An assessment of the campus climate and other contextual issues provides information to round out an overall problem description. This should include an honest assessment of the individual and institutional factors that are likely to facilitate or resist change. A readiness assessment does not need to take a great deal of time, but it can help to identify community support for and obstacles to accepting mental health promotion and suicide prevention as issues that need attention [21].

14.4.2 Identify Priorities and Set Long-Range Goals

Resources are almost always limited and every campus has multiple and competing concerns, so planners must make difficult decisions about which problems to focus on first. Having data on risk and protective factors and those populations at highest potential risk will help support decision-making, but planners should be sure to consider risk and protective factors across the entire social ecological model rather than just individual factors.

Creating good problem definitions from the outset supports the process of setting appropriate long-term goals. A goal statement should articulate specific, measurable goals whose achievement can be readily observed and measured. A focus on conditions or behaviors targeted for change will help planners avoid a common pitfall in goal-setting: describing the completion of a program as a goal, such as "conduct gatekeeper training". A more useful goal statement would be "increase the number of faculty trained to identify and refer students in distress". Achieving many goals may take time, but the planning group or task force may want to demonstrate early successes by prioritizing some quick fixes to easily remedied problems.

14.4.3 Consult the Literature to Identify Relevant Research, Theory, and Best Practices That Address the Targeted Problem

Identifying problems and setting goals (Steps 1 and 2 above) provide the basis for choosing programs that will make desired changes. It is important to choose evidence-based practices whenever possible to ensure that you are investing time and other resources on programs that are likely to achieve those changes. Section 14.5 below will discuss specific interventions.

Although practitioners at other campuses can be a valuable source of ideas for programs, planners should keep in mind that programs and policies from other campuses need to be critically examined. Before adopting a program that may be popular, well-known, or seem promising, campus leaders should determine whether it has strong empirical or theoretical support and addresses the specific problems of students on their campus.

The research on mental health promotion and prevention for adolescents and young adults, in both the college and non-college populations, is limited. The online Best Practices Registry (BPR), a collaboration of SPRC and the American Foundation for Suicide Prevention (AFSP) is one helpful tool. The BPR provides information about three categories of practices: (1) those that have been reviewed for the quality of the scientific evidence to support their use; (2) consensus statements that summarize the best knowledge in the field in the form of guidelines or protocols; and (3) programs and materials that have been reviewed by experts and determined to adhere to current program development standards and recommendations.

An evidence-based program may not exist for certain identified needs, target populations, and/or campus cultural contexts. In this case, campus planners can get assistance in several areas. A fundamental principle in developing any new program is to base the program content and process on health behavior change theory, which attempts to explain and predict health behaviors. Planners should look at what has worked in other areas of campus health promotion, such as the prevention of high-risk alcohol use or violence prevention. Best practices in these two areas of campus health and safety highlight the environment as an influence on individual behavior, and approaches developed in those fields can inform mental health promotion and suicide prevention efforts. Programs tested in community settings can also be adapted to the campus environment.

14.4.4 Select or Develop Programs

Regardless of the source of program ideas, planners should choose programs based on the likelihood that the activities, policies, messaging campaigns, or other interventions will achieve the defined goals and objectives.

As with any area of campus health and safety, many campus teams find it useful to create a "logic model", a diagram illustrating how each planned activity will contribute to their long-term goals (e.g. reduce mental health problems, suicidal behavior, and suicide) [11]. By using a logic model, campuses can articulate how and why each activity will result in specific outcomes, increasing the likelihood that these outcomes are achieved. There are several logic model formats planners can use as a guide, including the one shown in Figure 14.2.

The term *inputs* refers to the investment of resources in the program (e.g. staff time, volunteers, and funds). *Activities* are the actual programs to be implemented, such as a training, screening program, or awareness campaign. *Outputs* refers to the number of activities or the level of activity achieved. If the activity is a communications campaign, for example, then outputs might be the number of public service announcements (PSAs) aired, the number of brochures distributed, and the number of students exposed to the message [22].

Short-, intermediate-, and long-term outcomes are the attitudes, knowledge, skills, and behaviors that are expected to change as a result of inputs, activities, and outputs.

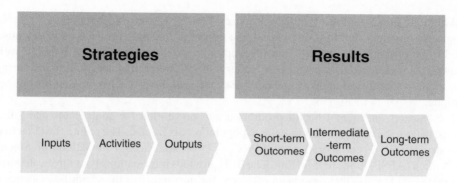

Figure 14.2 *Logic model format. W.K. Kellogg Foundation (2004) Using Logic Models to Bring Together Planning, Evaluation, and Action: Logic Model Development Guide, W.K. Kellogg Foundation, Battle Creek, Michigan; University of Wisconsin-Extension (2009) Enhancing Program Performance with Logic Models. Online self-study module accessed 19 June 2009 at http://www.uwex.edu/ces/lmcourse/.*

There should be a *logical* connection between program activities and desired results [11].

14.4.5 Develop an Evaluation Plan

To be most effective and useful, the evaluation should be planned as the program is being developed [11], with the logic model as a foundation. Including a professional evaluator – perhaps a faculty member in public health, health education, psychology, or social work – on a project team helps to ensure that outcome-based thinking is an integral part of the project's design and implementation [23].

There are myriad reasons to evaluate campus programs, including to:

- Add to the body of knowledge about which interventions work.
- Show that programs are achieving their intended outcomes, thereby demonstrating that campus resources are being used wisely.
- Determine whether a program was implemented as intended and provide information to revise and improve its quality.
- Communicate successes to key stakeholders and senior administrators.
- Attract long-term financial support for programs.

14.4.6 Create an Action Plan

Given the expectation that no single program will reduce risk and provide protection for mental health problems and suicide, campus planners will need to integrate a somewhat complex set of interventions to make an impact. To stay on track, campuses may want to create a detailed work plan that lists specific tasks, who is responsible for each, and a timeline for completing those tasks.

14.4.7 Implement Programs, Evaluate, and Make Improvements

Following all of the previous steps should make it possible to implement high quality programs and allows planners to answer the basic questions that senior administrators and other stakeholders are likely to ask [24]:

- What activities were implemented?
- What were the strengths and weaknesses of the implementation?
- Was the program implemented as planned?
- Was the program implemented with quality?
- Was it effective?
- Should we continue the program?
- What can be modified to make the program more effective?
- What evidence proves that funders should continue to spend their money on this program?

Using a strategic planning process to adopt a public health approach helps to ensure that campus efforts will be effective in addressing student mental health problems. When selecting interventions, as described in 14.4.3, colleges should include a continuum of programs that address multiple levels of the social ecological model. Having a combination of activities, policies, and interventions working together is more likely than any single intervention to produce results and sustain mental health promotion, prevent and treat mental health problems, maintain mental wellness, and prevent suicide over time.

14.5 Strategies for Promoting Mental Health and Preventing Suicide Among College Students

To guide colleges in developing a campus-wide, public health approach, TJF and SPRC have formulated a *Comprehensive Approach to Suicide Prevention and Mental Health Promotion* that comprises seven strategic areas for intervention (see Figure 14.3). Each strategic area is discussed in detail below.

This comprehensive approach is drawn primarily from the overall strategic direction of the United States Air Force (USAF) Suicide Prevention Program, a population-based strategy to reduce risk factors and enhance protective factors for suicide. The program components included: commitment of Air Force leadership to suicide prevention and communication about this commitment throughout the ranks; efforts to strengthen social support and promote the development of adaptive coping skills; training non-health professionals in identifying and referring at-risk individuals; and changing policies and norms to encourage effective help-seeking [25].

By implementing eleven initiatives and policy changes, the program reduced the rate of suicide among USAF personnel by 33% during the first 5 years of the program [26]. The program also reduced homicides by 51% and accidental deaths by 18% [26]. In short, "[as] a "model of cultural change', the Air Force prevention program potentially serves as the first demonstration of the relevance of Rose's Theorem for preventing suicide: improving overall

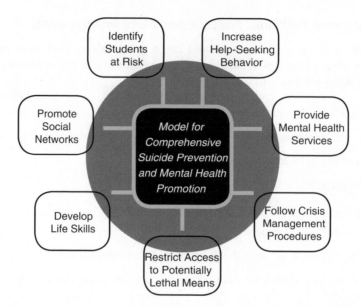

Figure 14.3 *Comprehensive approach to suicide prevention and mental health promotion. Silverman, M.M., Locke, J., Davidson, L. (2007) Using a campus task force to develop a comprehensive, strategic approach to mental health promotion and suicide prevention. Presentation delivered at National Association of Student Personnel Administrators Mental Health Conference, Houston, TX January 12, 2007.*

community mental health can reduce the events of suicide more effectively than extensive efforts to identify the imminently suicidal individual' [27].

In addition to drawing on lessons from the USAF program, the TJF/SPRC approach is also based on decreasing risk factors and increasing protective factors for mental health and suicide among adolescents, college students, and the general population; an understanding of the student mental health problems that campuses face; and existing best practices.

While some examples of programs that fall under each strategic area have been provided below, campuses are encouraged to implement programs that are appropriate to their campus-specific problems. Campus planners are cautioned to ensure that adequate institutional capacity exists and that linkages to community services are in place before they create programs that will significantly increase the number of students seeking services (see p. 243 for a bulleted list of critical capacities).

14.5.1 Promote Social Networks That Reinforce a Sense of Community on Campus and Strengthen Social Relationships Among Students, Faculty, and Staff

In both the general and college student population, research has consistently shown that loneliness and isolation are risk factors for suicide, suicidal behavior, and mental health problems, while supportive social relationships serve as a protective factor against these outcomes [4,6,7]. In adolescents, feeling connected to their school is also protective against suicidal thoughts and behaviors [28]. The CDC considers "connectedness" to be so critical that its 5-year strategic direction for preventing suicidal behavior is focused on "building and strengthening social bonds within and among persons, families and communities" [p. 1].

According to one study, experiencing a higher quality of social support is more protective than having a large number of social contacts [6]. For example, students who perceived a higher quality of social support were less likely to be depressed, anxious, or suicidal, independent of how frequently they interacted with their social contacts [6]. Notably, certain subgroups of students reported lower quality of social supports including men, Asian/Asian-American students, those who classified themselves as being in "multiple" racial/ethnic categories, international students, and those with financial problems [6].

Efforts to facilitate social connection should go beyond simply encouraging individual students to "get involved". For example, many campuses have developed smaller "living and learning communities", where students have the opportunity to live with other students who share their interests and have increased interactions with faculty outside the classroom. Other schools have dedicated space in their student unions or equivalent for specific groups (e.g. international students) to meet and socialize together.

14.5.2 Help Students Develop Skills to Face Life Challenges in College and Beyond

Table 14.4 lists some of the key life skills that students should be developing or refining during their time in college. Whether or not students have these skills can either confer protection against or increase the risk for suicide and mental health problems (see Table 14.3). In the college population specifically, relationship difficulties and financial problems have been identified as risk factors for both depression and suicidal behavior [5,20]. Even so, one survey found that 40% of seniors say that their college or university does not place much importance on helping them cope with non-academic life [29].

Since the college experience serves to develop more than just the intellect and professional skills, colleges are increasingly making efforts to foster the development of necessary life skills in all students. For example, programs for first-year students, sometimes in the form of a semester-long course, are now offered by hundreds of campuses. Many campuses also offer health education workshops around developing a variety of life skills.

Table 14.4	Examples of critical life skills

Interpersonal communication/human relations
- Establishing and maintaining relationships

Physical fitness/health maintenance

Problem solving/decision making
- Assessing and analyzing information
- Identifying and solving problems
- Setting goals
- Managing time
- Resolving conflicts

Identity development/purpose in life
- Developing awareness of personal and emotional identity
- Maintaining one's self esteem
- Clarifying values
- Developing meaning of life

Picklesimer, B.K., Miller, T.K. (1998) Life-skills development inventory-college form: An assessment measure. *Journal of College Student Development*, 39(1), 100–110.

In addition, campuses should consider how day-to-day experience itself offers students opportunities to develop their ability to cope with and respond to an array of challenges. Students frequently encounter situations where they can learn adaptive ways to negotiate conflict, solve problems, or handle financial responsibilities. The expectations for how students will behave academically or personally, and the consequences for not meeting these expectations, may have an even more profound effect on developing students' life skills than formal workshops and courses.

An increased focus on life skills development may also ease the burden on counseling centers. Providing students early assistance with life problems may prevent them from becoming acutely distressed and experiencing depression or anxiety at the level that would require mental health treatment. This type of assistance can be provided by non-clinical staff such as health educators, student affairs staff, or financial services staff.

14.5.3 Identify Students Who May Be at Risk for Suicide, Have Untreated Mental Health Problems, or Exhibit Early Signs of Mental Health Problems

Research on the college student population has shown that many students who need help do not, for a variety of reasons, seek it out on their own. For example, according to one study, 36% of students who screened positive for major depressive disorder had not received medication or therapy during the past year [2]. Therefore, the responsibility for identifying students at risk cannot fall only on the shoulders of campus mental health professionals. On a daily basis, more students come in contact with student personnel staff, residence hall staff, academic deans and advisors, faculty, campus clergy, coaches and cafeteria workers than with counseling center staff. Every member of the campus community can help to identify and refer a student in distress to the people best able to help that student.

Campuses are using a variety of methods to identify and reach out to at-risk students including:

- Asking questions about mental health on medical history forms completed by incoming first year students to identify high-risk or potentially high-risk students and encourage help-seeking.

- Participating in screening activities such as Screening for Mental Health's College Response program (http://www.mentalhealthscreening.org/college/), which includes National Depression Screening Day.

- Screening students for symptoms of depression or other mental health problems when students seek primary care services [30,31].

- Creating an interface between the disciplinary process and mental health services in order to identify students who may need treatment and promote help-seeking.

Gatekeeper training (GKT) is perhaps the most common campus program designed to identify and refer students in distress. The term is used to describe a range of activities from a one-hour presentation on the warning signs for suicide to an 8-hour skills-based workshop where attendees participate in role plays.

Syracuse University's *Campus Connect* gatekeeper training, created specifically for college campuses, is a 3-hour experientially-based crisis intervention and suicide prevention training program for resident assistants (RAs) [32]. After the training, RAs reported an increase in their ability to connect to students in crisis, comfort in asking students about suicidal thoughts, and ability to help distressed students to find available resources [32]. The program evaluation also found that the RAs demonstrated significant improvement in their suicide intervention skills [32]. Of course, campus staff must state clearly the expectation that student gatekeepers are not meant to provide counseling and other assistance that health and mental health professionals are trained to do offer. The aim is for students to help their peers access those services.

It is important to be realistic about the desired outcomes from a GKT program before designing one. For example, a recent study assessed the impact of providing a GKT program to staff at middle and high schools in Georgia [33]. After one year, trained staff members were no more likely than non-trained staff members to ask students about suicide or refer them for help, even though trained staff members had demonstrated significantly improved gatekeeper knowledge, preparedness, and efficacy over non-trained staff members [33]. In fact, the program was found to benefit only those staff that were asking students about their distress or thoughts of suicide prior to the training [33]. Short-term goals related to gains in knowledge and confidence are appropriate, but the end result of GKT should be increased referrals, help-seeking, and utilization of appropriate services [34].

Another method of identifying students at risk is the use of a case management team, also known as a student-at-risk response team or a behavioral intervention team. A case management team "promotes information-sharing and coordinated action to address students who may be in distress or at risk for harming themselves or others" [35]. Key members generally include representatives from student affairs, health services, counseling center, residence life, disabilities services, campus security, and campus legal counsel [36].

A case management team differs from a planning task force, which creates and implements a campus-wide plan for addressing the mental health and wellness of all students [35]. A case management team also differs from a threat assessment team, which assesses threats of violence toward others and includes members with appropriate expertise in this area [35]. The three types of groups may have overlapping membership and, on small campuses, be less formal [35]. Nevertheless, it is important for each group to have a clear mandate that differentiates its purpose and methods [35].

14.5.4 Increase the Number of Students Who Seek Help for Emotional Distress

The process of help-seeking is complex with many possible factors influencing whether or not someone takes steps to get help. For example, one model breaks down seeking treatment into four related steps: acknowledging that one feels badly enough to need treatment and that the problem is a medical or mental health one; deciding to get help and from whom; getting treatment; and deciding to continue treatment [37]. When designing programs to increase student help-seeking, campuses should seek to understand the barriers and facilitators to students taking each of the four steps listed above. Eisenberg and colleagues [2] found that predictors of college students not receiving care include not perceiving a need, being unaware of available mental health services or insurance coverage, skepticism about the effectiveness of treatment, low socioeconomic (SES) status growing up, and identifying as Asian or Pacific Islander.

The research data as to whether stigma prevents college students from seeking help is limited and the findings are inconsistent [38]. For example, one survey found that while 50%

of college students would encourage a friend to seek help for emotional issues, only 22% would seek help themselves [39]. Almost 60% of students in another study thought that people would see someone in a less favorable light if they knew that the person had been in treatment for psychological problems [38]. This same study found that perceived public stigma, "the extent to which an individual perceives the public to stereotype and discriminate against a stigmatized group", ([38] p. 392) is higher among men, older students, Asian or Pacific Islanders, international students, students with current mental health problems, those without family and friends who have used mental health services, students with low SES backgrounds, and students who do not think treatment is effective [38]. However, among students with probable depression or anxiety disorders, perceived stigma was not associated with whether or not the students sought treatment [38].

Multiple studies have shown that students go first to friends, family, or a significant other when they are struggling, rather than seeking professional help [1,20,37]. Understanding the reasons for this *on a particular campus* will help program planners better address their students' barriers to help seeking. Many schools have instituted peer counseling or peer education programs to take advantage of students' willingness to talk to their peers. Active Minds, a national peer-to-peer organization dedicated to raising awareness about mental health among college students and encouraging students to get help, has chapters on approximately 200 campuses (www.activeminds.org).

Campuses are engaging in a variety of activities designed to increase the likelihood that a student who needs supportive services or counseling will seek out and secure assistance. The Interactive Screening Program developed by the American Foundation for Suicide Prevention targets students who may be reluctant to seek traditional psychological services but who may respond to offers of anonymous assessment and counseling via the internet (www.afsp.org). ULifeline, TJF's online resource, provides an anonymous screening tool and information about campus resources (www.ulifeline.org).

Many campuses are also using communication campaigns that include brochures, posters, and a variety of web-based content to increase help-seeking. Prior to creating a campaign, campuses should embark upon a strategic planning process, using campus-specific data if possible, to focus the campaign goals and identify specific target audiences. The National Cancer Institute's *Making Health Communication Programs Work*, also known as the "pink book", is one of the best resources available to guide health communication planning and evaluation (http://www.cancer.gov/pinkbook).

Several national campaigns, targeting the general public or college students specifically, promote student help-seeking behaviors and attempt to reduce the stigma associated with mental health issues. One example is TJF's Half of Us campaign, which features public service announcements, personal stories from students and high-profile artists, and information about different mental health problems (http://www.halfofus.com/). Other examples include SAMHSA's Campaign for Mental Health Recovery, which aims to decrease negative attitudes surrounding mental illness by encouraging young people to support friends with mental health problems (http://www.whatadifference.samhsa.gov/).

14.5.5 Restrict Access to Potentially Lethal Means of Self-Harm and Suicide

An individual's intention is only one factor in whether he or she attempts suicide. The availability and acceptability of various methods of self-harm and the attempter's knowledge about how lethal different methods may be also play a role in the decision.

In the general population, guns are the most lethal means of suicide, resulting in a fatality rate of more than 90% compared to a 3% fatality rate for suicide attempts by drug overdose [40]. One reason the rate of suicide among college students is only half the rate of same-age peers who are not in college [41] may be that firearms are not allowed on the vast majority of campuses. For college students who die by suicide, firearms and overdose are the most commonly used methods [41]. In a study that asked students who had thought about attempting suicide what method they considered using, 51% of students named overdosing but only 15% named firearms [20].

Researchers have investigated the possible effect of alcohol availability on suicide. Between 1970 and 1990, the suicide rate of 18–20-year-old youths living in states with an age-18 minimum legal drinking age was 8% higher than the suicide rate among 18–20-year-olds in states where the drinking age was 21 [42]. Researchers estimate that lowering the drinking age from 21 to 18 in all states could increase the number of suicides in the 18–20-year-old population by approximately 125 each year [42]. Alcohol abuse may facilitate suicidal behavior by promoting depression and hopelessness, impairing problem solving, and facilitating aggression [43]. In studies of deaths by suicide, alcohol use was a proximate risk factor – found to be present in more than 50% of deaths [44].

Limiting students' access to sites, weapons, and agents that may facilitate their ability to harm themselves or others are all methods of means restriction. Specific efforts may include restricting access and/or erecting fences on roofs of buildings, replacing windows or restricting the size of window openings, restricting or denying access to chemicals like cyanide that are often found in laboratories, prohibiting guns on campus, and reducing consumption of alcohol and other drugs (e.g. enforcing underage drinking policies).

The specific setting of the campus can influence the type of means restriction needed, so each campus should do an "environmental scan" for potential access to lethal means. One campus is working with facilities management, the campus safety committee, and student groups to review institutional and national data about the most common means used in suicide attempts and studying other colleges" firearms policies. The campus is also conducting an inventory of toxic chemicals, including reviewing policies for their storage, and surveying buildings to identify where students have access to high places. Since hanging was a method that students had been most likely to use in prior suicide attempts, the campus group researched break-away clothes rods for residence hall closets.

Colleges and universities wishing to conduct an environmental scan can find guidance on the web site of the *Means Matter Campaign*, a national effort to reduce access to lethal means. The "Taking Action" section of the web site includes recommendations for colleges and universities provided by the Suicide Prevention Resource Center (http://www.hsph. harvard.edu/means-matter/recommendations/colleges/index.html).

14.5.6 Develop Policies and Procedures That Promote the Safety of all Students on Campus and Guide the Response to Campus Crises

When a student is acutely distressed or suicidal, it is important that clear protocols are in place for addressing the crisis. It is also critical that all of the administrators and staff who have a role in addressing the needs and safety of the student and the campus community understand what actions they are expected to take.

TJF's *Framework for Developing Institutional Protocols for the Acutely Distressed or Suicidal College Student* [18] provides a blueprint for campus officials to use in developing or revising crisis procedures in three key areas: safety, emergency contact notification, and leave of absence and re-entry. With the proliferation of "threat assessment" and other emergency preparedness procedures, administrators should ensure that all protocols are appropriately linked but that efforts to address suicidal behavior and other mental health problems do not suggest that mentally ill students are a threat to the campus community.

Crisis procedures should also include a comprehensive "postvention" program designed to help students deal with their grief and confusion, and prevent suicide contagion, following the death of a student by suicide. Postvention involves coordinated, rapid outreach to help specific students and the entire community, which may involve "community support meetings" to facilitate the grieving and recovery process [45].

Campus-wide dissemination of state or local 24-hour hotlines, plus the National Suicide Prevention Lifeline (800-273-TALK), is also a critical part of every campus crisis management effort. In addition, colleges should ensure that all faculty and staff understand the laws and professional guidelines that can affect decision-making around students at risk. One resource is TJF's *Student Mental Health and the Law: A Resource for Institutions of Higher Education* [35]. This report provides guidance in the following areas: privacy and confidentiality, disability law, delivering mental health services, and liability for student suicide and violence. The document also contains related good practice recommendations. (Chapter 7 provides discussion of legal issues in college mental health.)

14.5.7 *Increase Student Access to Effective Mental Health and Other Support Services*

Although the counseling center is central to providing treatment to students with mental health problems:

> [students] from cultures that do not understand or acknowledge mental illness, or that discourage revelations of personal problems, are not likely to seek services, so colleges need to develop creative approaches to respond to those students in ways that they will find helpful and nonthreatening [46].

These students may seek help at health services or from a tribal elder, cultural healer, clergy, academic advisor, or staff member in international services or student culture centers.

Many campuses are collaborating with both on- and off-campus religious leaders to ensure that students receive appropriate and helpful services and clergy members know how to assess suicide risk. Engaging in activities that fall under all six strategic areas discussed above is critical to ensuring that these students do not fall through the cracks.

Other students may be experiencing "life" problems that, if left unresolved, could put them at risk for a mental health disorder or suicide. For example, in one study, 59% of students who had seriously considered attempting suicide during the past year reported romantic relationship problems as having a large impact on thinking about the attempt [20]. Efforts should be made to help those students who have experienced a recent loss, such as an important relationship, as a potential way to prevent the development of depression or suicidality. Similar logic can be applied to helping students experiencing other stressors, such as academic difficulties.

As stated earlier, the counseling and/or health center plays a critical role in providing treatment to students who need it. Although many campuses express the need to hire additional counseling staff, "simply adding more therapists isn't always the best way to improve access to high-quality services" [46]. Approaches campuses can employ to meet service demand while using existing staff and resources more efficiently while strengthening service delivery include:

- Instituting brief, same-day appointments by phone or in person for quick assessment and referral to either campus or community providers based on established criteria [47].

- Offering four-session psycho-educational groups – sometimes called "Feel Better Fast" – for students who may not need more intensive therapy [John Hoeppel, personal communication].

- Ensuring that mental health clinicians are adequately trained to:

  – Accurately diagnose students and provide appropriate treatment or referral

  – Use goal-oriented, time-limited treatment modalities

  – Assess and manage suicide risk

  – Follow laws and professional guidelines that govern student privacy and confidentiality.

- Partnering with wellness/health promotion staff who can assume outreach duties.

- Complementing campus resources with longer-term treatment services available in the community.

Treatment services should be viewed within the context of the continuum of campus-wide efforts toward promotion, prevention, treatment, and postvention. Counseling centers should consider a stepped care model frequently employed to address many behavioral health issues including the reduction of college student alcohol use [48,49]. The premise of stepped care is to provide the most effective yet least resource-intensive intervention first [50]. For some students, a "minimal intervention" will be enough, while others will need to "step up" to increasingly more intensive levels of care. For example, a mailed intervention providing students with personalized feedback and information about their symptoms for depression was inexpensive to implement yet reduced depressive symptoms and feelings of hopelessness [51]. Of course, criteria must be carefully crafted to facilitate decision making about which students need more intensive care [49].

14.6 Conclusion

Untreated mental illness on the nation's campuses is problematic. An increasing number of institutions of higher learning are correctly taking the position that treatment alone is not the answer and asserting that the burden of solving student mental health problems should not be solely on the shoulders of the college mental health service or counseling center.

An approach that focuses solely on getting more students into treatment, no matter how effective the services, relies on the flawed assumption that counseling centers will be provided the resources to support an expanding number of students seeking care. Student mental illness is a public health problem, and promoting the mental wellness of students is the responsibility of everyone on campus.

Changing how administrators respond to student mental health problems requires a paradigm shift much like the one that campuses have experienced regarding alcohol and other drug prevention during the last 20 years. We must go beyond simply providing education and treatment services by adding efforts to prevent mental health problems from arising and promote the mental health of all students.

References

1. American College Health Association (2008) *National College Health Assessment: Reference Group Executive Summary Spring 2008*, American College Health Association, Baltimore, MD.
2. Eisenberg, D., Golberstein, E., Gollust, S. and Hefner, J. (2007) Help-seeking and access to mental health services in a university student population. *Medical Care*, **45**(7), 594–601.
3. Gallagher, R.P. (2006) *National Survey for Counseling Center Directors*, International Association of Counseling Services, Arlington, VA.
4. Suicide Prevention Resource Center (2004) *Promoting Mental Health and Preventing Suicide in College and University Settings*, Education Development Center, Inc., Newton, MA.
5. Eisenberg, D., Golberstein, E., Gollust, S. and Hefner, J. (2007) Prevalence and correlates of depression, anxiety and suicidality among university students. *American Journal of Orthopsychiatry*, **77**(4), 534–542.
6. Hefner, J. and Eisenberg, D. (2009) Social support and mental health in a university student population. *American Journal of Orthopsychiatry*, (in press).
7. National Research Council and Institute of Medicine (2009) Preventing Mental, Emotional, and Behavioral Disorders Among Young People: Progress and Possibilities, in *Committee on Prevention of Mental Disorders and Substance Abuse among Children Youth and Young Adults: Research Advances and Promising Interventions. Board on Children, Youth and Families, Division of Behavioral and Social Sciences and Education* (eds M.E. O'Connell, Thomas Boat and K.E. Warner), The National Academies Press, Washington, DC.
8. DeJong, W. and Langford, L. (2002) A typology for campus-based alcohol prevention: Moving toward environmental management strategies. *Journal of Studies on Alcohol*, (Supp 14), 140–147.
9. McLeroy, K.R., Bibeau, D., Steckler, A. and Glanz, K. (1998) An ecological perspective on health promotion programs. *Health Education & Behavior*, **15**(4), 351–377.
10. Higher Education Center for Alcohol and Other Drug Abuse and Violence Prevention (2007) *Experiences in Effective Prevention: The US Department of Education's Alcohol and Other Drug Prevention Models on College Campuses Grants*, US Department of Education, Office of Safe & Drug Free Schools, Washington, DC.
11. Langford, L. (2006) *Preventing Violence and Promoting Safety in Higher Education Settings: Overview of a Comprehensive Approach*, US Department of Education, Higher Education Center for Alcohol, and Other Drug Prevention, Washington, DC.
12. World Health Organization (2004) *Promoting Mental Health: Concepts, Emerging Evidence, Practice: Summary Report*, World Health Organization, Geneva.
13. World Health Organization (2004) *Prevention of Mental Disorders: Effective Interventions and Policy Options: Summary Report*, World Health Organization, Geneva.
14. Institute of Medicine (1994) Reducing Risks for Mental Disorders: Frontiers for Preventive Intervention Research, in *Committee on Prevention of Mental Disorders, Division of Biobehavioral Sciences and Mental Disorders* (eds P.J. Mrazek and R.J. Haggerty), National Academy Press, Washington, DC.

15. DeJong, W., Vince-Whitman, C., Colthurst, T. *et al.* (1998) *Environmental Management: A Comprehensive Strategy for Reducing Alcohol and Other Drug Use on College Campuses*, US Department of Education, Higher Education Center for Alcohol, and Other Drug Prevention, Washington, DC.

16. The Higher Education Center for Alcohol and Other Drug Abuse and Violence (2002) *Prevention Updates: Environmental Management: An Approach to Alcohol and Other Drug Prevention*, US Department of Education, Washington, DC.

17. Goldsmith, S.K., Pellmar, T.C., Kleinman, A.M. and Bunney, W.E. (2002) *Reducing Suicide: A National Imperative*, National Academy Press, Washington, DC.

18. The Jed Foundation (2006) *Framework for Developing Institutional Protocols for the Acutely Distressed or Suicidal College Student*, The Jed Foundation, New York, NY.

19. The Jed Foundation (2006) Unpublished study.

20. Drum, D.J., Brownson, C., Denmark, A.B. and Smith, S.E. (2009) New data on the nature of suicidal crises in college students: Shifting the paradigm. *Professional Psychology*, **40**(3), 213–222.

21. Edwards, R.W., Jumper-Thurman, P., Plested, B.A. *et al.* (2008) Community readiness: Research to practice. *Journal of Community Psychology*, **28**(3), 291–307.

22. Horn, L. and Downs, M. (2009) Is Stigma Preventing College Students from Seeking Help? Presentation delivered at National Association of Student Personnel Administrators Mental Health Conference, Boston, MA, January 23, 2009.

23. Langford, L. and DeJong, W. (2001) *How to Select a Program Evaluator*, U.S. Department of Education, Higher Education Center for Alcohol, and Other Drug Prevention, Washington, DC.

24. Chinman, M., Imm, P. and Wandersman, A. (2004) *Getting to Outcomes™ 2004: Promoting Accountability Through Methods and Tools for Planning, Implementation, and Evaluation*, RAND Corporation, Santa Monica, CA.

25. National Registry of Evidence-based Programs and Practices (2006) United States Air Force Suicide Prevention Program, reviewed July 2006. US Department of Health and Human Services, Substance Abuse and Mental Health Services Administration, Washington, DC. Accessed June 19, 2009 at http://www.nrepp.samhsa.gov/programfulldetails.asp?PROGRAM_ID=68.

26. Knox, K.L., Litts, D.A., Talcott, G.W. *et al.* (2003) Risk of suicide and related adverse outcomes after exposure to a suicide prevention programme in the US Air Force: cohort study. *British Medical Journal*, **327**, 1376.

27. Knox, K.L., Conwell, Y. and Caine, E.D. (2004) If suicide is a public health problem, what are we doing to prevent it? *American Journal of Public Health*, **94**(1), 37–45.

28. Centers for Disease Control and Prevention, National Center for Injury Prevention and Control (2008) Promoting Individual, Family, and Community Connectedness to Prevent Suicidal Behavior. Retrieved 20 June 2009 from http://www.cdc.gov/ViolencePrevention/pdf/Suicide_Strategic_Direction_Full_Version-a.pdf.

29. The National Survey of Student Engagement (NSSE) Annual Report 2007: Experiences That Matter: Enhancing Student Learning and Success. Retrieved 20 June 2009 from http://nsse.iub.edu/NSSE_2007_Annual_Report/docs/withhold/NSSE_2007_Annual_Report.pdf.

30. Chung, H. and Klein, M. (2007) Improving identification and treatment of depression in college health. *Student Health Spectrum*, June, 13–19.

31. Klein, M.C. and Chung, H. (2008) The CBS-D Project: Transforming depression care on college campuses – Part II. *Student Health Spectrum*, Spring, 3–8.

32. Syracuse University Counseling Center, Research Findings. Retrieved 19 June 2009 at http://counselingcenter.syr.edu/index.php/campus-connect/research-findings/.

33. Wyman, P., Brown, D.H., Inman, J. *et al.* (2008) Randomized trial of a gatekeeper program for suicide prevention: 1-year impact on secondary school staff. *Journal of Consulting and Clinical Psychology*, **76**(1), 104–115.

34. Wallach, C. and Steward, D. (2009) Training Gatekeepers to Identify At-Risk Students: Research, Utility, and Implementation. Presentation delivered at National Association of Student Personnel Administrators Mental Health Conference, Boston, MA, January 24, 2009.

35. The Jed Foundation (2008) *Student Mental Health and the Law: A Resource for Institutions of Higher Education*, The Jed Foundation, New York, NY.

36. Davidson, L. and Ayash, C. (2008) Case Management Teams: Early Intervention for At-Risk Students. Presentation at 7th Annual Massachusetts Suicide Prevention Conference. Sturbridge, MA, 13 May 2008.

37. Sussman, L.K., Robins, L.N. and Earls, F. (1987) Treatment-seeking for depression by black and white Americans. *Social Science & Medicine*, **24**(3), 187–196.

38. Golberstein, E., Eisenberg, D. and Gollust, S. (2008) Perceived stigma and mental health care seeking. *Psychiatric Services*, **59**, 392–399.

39. The Jed Foundation & mtvU (2006) College Mental Health Study: Stress, Depression, Stigma & Students. Executive Summary. Retrieved on 20 June 2009 from http://www.halfofus.com/_media/_pr/mtvuCollegeMentalHealthStudy2006.pdf.

40. Miller, M., Azrael, D. and Hemenway, D. (2004) The epidemiology of case fatality rates for suicide in the Northeast. *Annals of Emergency Medicine*, **43**(6), 723–730.

41. Silverman, M.M. *et al.* (1997) The big ten student suicide study: A 10-year study of suicides on Midwestern university campuses. *Suicide and Life-Threatening Behavior*, **27**(3), 285–303.

42. Brickmayer, J. and Hemenway, D. (1999) Minimum age drinking laws and youth suicide, 1970–1990. *American Journal of Public Health*, **89**, 1365–1368.

43. Hufford, M.R. (2001) Alcohol and suicidal behavior. *Clinical Psychology Review*, **21**(5), 797–811.

44. Hall, R.C.W., Platt, D.E. and Hall, R.C.W. (1999) Suicide risk assessment: A review of risk factors for suicide in 100 patients who made severe suicide attempts. *Psychosomatics*, **40**, 18–27.

45. Meilman, P.W. and Hall, T.M. (2006) Aftermath of tragic events: The development and use of community support meetings on a university campus. *Journal of American College Health*, **54**(6), 382–384.

46. Silverman, MM. (2008) Campus security begins with caring. Chronicle of Higher Education, 18 April 2008, Commentary.

47. Rockland-Miller, H.S. and Eells, G.T. (2006) The implementation of mental health clinical triage systems in university health services. *Journal of College Student Psychotherapy*, **20**(4), 39–51.

48. Marlatt, G.A., Baer, J.S., Kivlahan, D.R. *et al.* (1998) Screening and brief intervention for high-risk college student drinkers: Results from a two-year follow-up assessment. *Journal of Consulting and Clinical Psychology*, **66**(4), 604–615.

49. Borsari, B. and O'Leary Tevyaw, T. (2004) Stepped care: a promising treatment strategy for mandated students. *NASPA Journal*, **42**(3), 381–397.

50. Sobell, M. and Sobell, L. (2000) Stepped care as a heuristic approach to the treatment of alcohol problems. *Journal of Consulting and Clinical Psychology*, **68**, 573–579.

51. Geisner, I.M., Neighbors, C. and Larimer, M.E. (2006) A randomized clinical trial of a brief, mailed intervention for symptoms of depression. *Journal of Consulting and Clinical Psychology*, **74**(2), 393–399.

15 Magnitude and Prevention of College Alcohol and Drug Misuse: US College Students Aged 18–24

Ralph W. Hingson and Aaron M. White

Division of Epidemiology and Prevention Research, National Institute on Alcohol Abuse and Alcoholism, Bethesda, MD, USA

15.1 Introduction

National surveys have focused attention on the heavy drinking patterns of many college students. In 1993, 1997, 1999, and 2001, the Harvard School of Public Health College Alcohol Survey (CAS) monitored among college students heavy or binge drinking, defined as having five or more drinks in a single drinking session for males or four or more for females [1–3]. From 1999 to 2002, the proportion of college students ages 18–24 who drank five or more drinks on an occasion in the previous 30 days increased from 41.7% to 43.2%. This represents a 4% increase per population from 3,615,550 to 3,842,208 college students [4]. The proportion of college students ages 18–24 who in the past year reported driving under the influence of alcohol also increased significantly from 26.5% to 31.4%, reflecting an 18% increase from 2,297,550 to 2,792,716 college students [4]. It has been estimated that in 2001 1700 college students died from alcohol-related unintentional injury deaths, over 1400 from alcohol-related traffic deaths. Further, more than 690,000 college students between ages 18 and 24 are assaulted by another student who had been drinking, and 97,000 were victims of alcohol-related sexual assaults or date rapes [4].

The purpose of this review is to examine (1) the magnitude of morbidity and mortality associated with college drinking and drug use among 18–24-year-old students, (2) trends in those indices from 1998 to 2005, and (3) interventions established through scientific research to reduce alcohol and drug use among college students.

15.2 Methods: Calculating Changes in Alcohol-Related Mortality

This review compares the number of alcohol-related traffic and other unintentional injury deaths in 1998, 2001, and 2005 among 18–24-year-olds in the United States who are full- or part-time college students attending either 2- or 4-year colleges. Information was integrated from multiple data sets. First, the Centers for Disease Control and Prevention (CDC) annually records the numbers and ages of unintentional injury deaths [5], but they do not record whether these deaths are alcohol-related. Second, a meta-analysis of 331 medical examiner studies [6] from 1975 to 1995 revealed that 84% of unintentional non-traffic injury fatalities were tested for blood alcohol concentrations (BACs). Of those tested, 38% had positive BACs and 31% had BACs of 0.10% or higher, exceeding legal limits for intoxication nationwide [6]. This analysis provides the best available estimates for alcohol involvement in injury deaths (other than motor vehicle crash deaths), but it does not provide information on annual changes in the proportions of those deaths that are alcohol-related.

Third, the National Highway Traffic Safety Administration's (NHTSA) Fatality Analysis Reporting System (FARS) records all motor vehicle crash deaths in the United States [7,8] and the proportion that are alcohol-related, defined as involving a driver or pedestrian with a positive BAC. The ages of decedents are recorded, as are their BACs. Because BACs are not drawn on all motor vehicle crash deaths, an imputational formula projects the likelihood of alcohol involvement in those crashes for which test results are not available.

Fourth, the Department of Education's National Center for Education Statistics [9–12] reports the number of undergraduate college students in the United States. In 1998, of the 26,155,000 18–24-year-olds living in the United States [13], 7,809,387 (30%) were enrolled as full- or part-time students in either 2- or 4-year colleges – 24% in 4-year colleges and the balance in 2-year colleges. In 2001, of the 28,058,000 18–24-year-olds living in the United States, 8,580,318 (31%) were enrolled as either full or part-time college students. In 2005, of the 29,155,000 18–24 year olds, 9,628,069 (33%) were enrolled as full- or part-time students in two or four year colleges. Of the students enrolled as undergraduates in 1998, 2001, and 2005, 62%, 63%, and 64%, respectively, were ages 18–24.

Fifth, the National Household Survey of Drug Abuse in 1999, 2002, and 2005 surveyed 18–24-year-olds regardless of whether they were college students [14–16]. In each survey, college students were more likely than same-age non-college respondents to report drinking five or more drinks on at least one occasion in the past month and driving under the influence in the past year. On the basis of those survey results, we projected that the proportions of traffic and other unintentional injury decedents testing positive for alcohol would be as high among college 18–24-year-olds as same-age non-college persons. Because college students comprised 30% of the 18–24-year-old population in 1998, 31% in 2001, and 33% in 2005, we estimated that in 1998 18–24-year-old college students accounted for 30%, in 2001 31%, and in 2005 33% of traffic and other unintentional injury deaths experienced by the 18–24-year-old US population. Calculation of other alcohol-related risks and methods for analyzing survey results are described in detail elsewhere [17].

15.3 Study Results

15.3.1 Heavy Episodic Drinking and Driving Under the Influence of Alcohol

As can be seen in Table 15.1, from 1999 to 2005, based on the SAMSHA national surveys [14–16], the proportion of 18–24-year-old college students who drank five or more drinks on an occasion in the previous 30 days increased from 41.7% to 45.2%, a significant 8% proportional increase. Increases were statistically significant from 1999 to 2002 and 2005 ($p < 0.05$), as well as from 2002 to 2005. The number of college students ages 18–24 who

Table 15.1	Past month heavy episodic drinking in past year and driving under the influence of alcohol among US 18–24-year-olds in college and not in college, 1999–2005

	1999		2002		2005		Percent change (1999–2005)
	Percent	Number	Percent	Number	Percent	Number	
Drank 5+ drinks on an occasion in the past 300 days							
College students	41.7	3 256 514	43.2	3 706 697	45.2	4 351 887	↑8%
Non-college persons	36.5	6 696 147	39.8	7 732 639	40.2	7 884 398	↑10%
Drove under the influence of alcohol in the past year							
College students	26.7	2 609 487	32.7	2 805 763	29.2	2 811 396	↑12%
Non-college persons	19.8	3 252 431	24.4	4 752 554	22.8	4 471 748	↑15%

consumed at least five drinks on an occasion increased from 3,256,514 in 1999 to 4,351,887 in 2005.

During the same years, the proportion of 18–24-year-olds not in college who consumed five or more drinks on an occasion in the previous 30 days increased from 36.5% to 40.2%, a significant proportional 10% increase.

A greater percentage of 18–24-year-old college compared with non-college respondents drank five or more drinks on an occasion [14–16]. However, because the number of 18–24-year-olds not in college greatly exceeded those in college, the number who consumed five or more drinks on an occasion also greatly exceeded the numbers of college students who did so. The number of non-college heavy episodic drinkers ages 18–24 was 6,696,147 in 1999 and 7,884,398 in 2005.

From 1999 to 2005, the proportion of college students ages 18–24 who drove under the influence of alcohol increased significantly from 26.1% to 29.2%. A similar pattern was observed among non-college 18–24-year-olds; the proportion who drove under the influence of alcohol increased from 19.8% in 1999 to 22.8% in 2005.

Of note, the increases from 1999 to 2005 in binge drinking and driving under the influence of alcohol occurred among respondents ages 21–24, not those 18–20. In each year examined, a greater percentage of 21–24-year-olds than 18–20-year-olds engaged in these behaviors. Among both 21–24 and 18–20-year-olds, college students were more likely than same-age respondents not enrolled in college to report these behaviors [17].

15.3.2 Alcohol-Related Traffic Deaths

From 1998 to 2005, the rate of alcohol-related traffic deaths per 100 000 college students declined 3% from 14.5 to 14.1, a non-significant decline [17]. In Figure 15.1, among persons ages 18–24, 3783 (51%) of 7452 traffic deaths in 1998, 4219 (51%) of 8253 traffic deaths in 2001, and 4114 (49%) of 8510 traffic deaths in 2005 were alcohol-related [17]. On the basis of the deliberately conservative assumption that college students (30% of the US population of 18–24-year-olds in 1998, 31% in 2001, and 33% in 2005) experienced alcohol-related fatalities at the same rate as the entire 18–24-year-old population, we estimate that, of the alcohol-related traffic deaths in that population, 1134 (30%) in 1998, 1308 (31%) in 2001, and 1357 (33%) in 2005 would have been college students. This assumption is conservative because a higher percentage of 18–24-year-old college students than those not in college reported driving under the influence of alcohol in the past year.

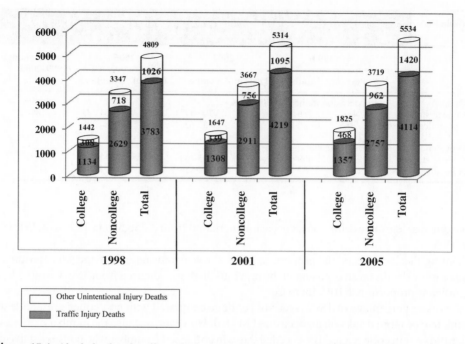

Figure 15.1 *Alcohol-related traffic and other unintentional injury deaths, 18–24-year-olds in college vs. not in college, 1998, 2001, 2005.*

Of note, among persons 18–20, there were 1528 alcohol-related traffic deaths in 1998, 1799 in 2001, and 1533 in 2005, reflecting a 6% decline per 100,000 population from 1998 to 2005. Among persons 21–24, the numbers were, respectively, 2195, 2420, and 2581, reflecting a 1% increase per 100,000 population from 1998 to 2005.

15.3.3 Alcohol-Related Unintentional Non-Traffic Deaths

From 1998 to 2001 to 2005, the rate of unintentional alcohol-related non-traffic injury deaths among 18–24-year-old college students increased from 3.9 to 4.0 to 4.9 per 100 000 college students, a significant 25.6% increase. According to the CDC [13], the numbers of unintentional non-traffic injury deaths among 18–24-year-olds were 2513 in 1998, 2849 in 2001, and 3993 in 2005 [17].[1] There were 1026 alcohol-related non-traffic injury deaths among 18–24-year-olds in 1998, 1095 in 2001, and 1420 in 2005. We estimate 308 college students aged 18–24 died from alcohol-related unintentional non-traffic injuries in 1998, 339 in 2001, and 468 in 2005. It should be noted that, relative to other unintentional injury deaths, poisoning deaths increased much more sharply among 18–24 year olds between 1998 and 2005, from 779 to 2290, nearly tripling during that

---

[1] Among persons 18–20, there were 1058 non-traffic injury deaths in 1998, 1104 in 2001, and 1427 in 2005, a 27% increase per 100,000 population. Among persons 21–24, the respective numbers were 1445, 1745, and 2566, a 51% increase per 100,000 population. The increases were because of increases in poisoning deaths. Excluding poisonings, non-traffic injury deaths declined 15% per 100,000 18–20-year-olds from 1998 to 2005 and 9% among 21–24-year-olds.

period. Unintentional injury deaths other than poisonings actually declined slightly about 2%.

15.3.4 Total Alcohol-Related Unintentional Injury Deaths

Among 18–24-year-old college students, deaths from all alcohol-related unintentional injuries, including traffic and other unintentional injuries, increased from 1442 in 1998 to 1647 in 2001 to 1825 in 2005, corresponding to increases in rates of death from 18.5 to 19.2 to 19.0, a 3% increase per 100,000 college population that approached but did not reach statistical significance, RR = 1.03 (95% CI 0.96, 1.1) [17]. Among all 18–24-year-olds, alcohol-related unintentional injury deaths increased from 4809 in 1998 to 5314 in 2001 to 5534 in 2005. Each of those years they exceeded the total number of deaths experienced by US soldiers in the entire second Iraq War (as of date of publication).

15.3.5 Other Alcohol-Related Health Problems

From 1999 to 2001 to 2005, the numbers of full-time, four-year students ages 18–24 increased from 5,496,000 to 5,709,000 to 6,200,000 [9–12]. Because there were no changes from 1999 to 2001 in the proportions of college student respondents in the CAS ages 18–24 who reported being hurt or injured because of drinking (10.5%), hurt or assaulted by another drinking college student (12%), or sexually assaulted or date raped by another drinking college student (2%), the projected numbers of students who experienced these alcohol-related problems increased at the same rate as the population. We estimated that 599,000 were injured because of drinking, 696,000 were assaulted or hit by a drinking college student, and 97,000 experienced a sexual assault or date rape perpetrated by another drinking college student in 2001 [4].

The 2005 follow-up study of the CAS at colleges with the highest percentages of heavy episodic drinkers revealed that the proportions of students who drank five or more drinks on an occasion in the past 2 weeks did not significantly change from the 2001 survey, nor did the proportions who had been hurt or injured because of drinking, who had been assaulted by another drinking college student, or who had been a victim of a sexual assault or date rape perpetrated by another drinking college student. Thus, estimates of the numbers of students who were injured because of drinking, assaulted, or sexually assaulted or date raped by another drinking college student in 2001 remain the best available, and the numbers experiencing these events in 2005 are probably similar [17].

Drug use among us college students

The National Survey on Drug Use and Health (NSDUH) [14–16] collects data on drug use among college students and others ages 18–25. Past 30-day use of any illicit drug or prescription drugs used illicitly tended to be slightly higher among persons ages 18–20 than those 21–25 (20% vs. 14%). By 2002 and 2005, those differences narrowed to 21.1% and 19.8% and 21.1% and 18.8%, respectively (differences between persons in college and not in college in those age groups were small).

Marijuana was by far the most commonly used illicit drug. It was consumed by 18% of college students 18–20 in 1999, 2002, and 2005. Among college students 21–25, use rose slightly from 14% in 1999 to 17% in 2002 to 16% in 2005. Use of drugs other than marijuana was reported by 7% of 18–20-year-old college students in 1999, 9% in 2002, and 8% in

2005. Corresponding percentages for college students 21–25 for these years were 5%, 8%, and 8%.

Data from the NSDUH [18] suggest that recreational use of prescription stimulants, such as Adderall, is a growing problem among college students. Analyses of combined data from 2006 and 2007 revealed that full-time college students were twice as likely to use Adderall recreationally in the past year than their non-college peers. The majority of college students, 90%, who used Adderall recreationally in the past year were also binge drinkers. Students who used Adderall recreationally were more likely than their peers to use other drugs. Specifically, they were:

- 3 times more likely to use marijuana (79.9% vs 27.2%)

- 8 times more likely to use cocaine (28.9% vs. 3.6%)

- 8 times more likely to use tranquilizers recreationally (24.5% vs. 3%)

- 5 times more likely to use pain relievers recreationally (44.9% vs. 8.7%).

Given the addictive potential of prescription stimulants and the relationships that exist between recreational use of stimulants, heavy drinking and use of other drugs, this is an issue that should be monitored closely.

According to the CDC [13], poisonings claimed the lives of 3170 18–25-year-olds in 2004, with 94.7% (3002) attributed to drug overdoses. Because the percentages of those who use illicit drugs are similar among 18–24-year-olds in college and not in college, college students probably account for approximately one-third of the poisoning deaths in that age group.

Clearly, while an important problem among college students, much smaller proportions of college students use illicit drugs than engage in heavy episodic drinking. Further, the percentages who use drugs did not increase in the college population over age 21 relative to 18–20-year-olds. In contrast, heavy episodic drinking occurs in a higher percentage of persons 21–24 relative to 18–20-year-olds, and the percentages of 21–24-year-olds engaging in this behavior increased from 1999 to 2005.

15.4 Discussion: Estimates of the Magnitude of College Drinking Problems

From 1998 to 2005, the nationwide number of alcohol-related deaths among 18–24-year-olds rose at a rate that significantly exceeded that age group's proportional population increase. Whereas the population increased 12% from 26,155,000 to 29,241,000, alcohol-related unintentional injury deaths rose 15% from 4808 to 5534. Thus, alcohol-related deaths per population of 18–24-year-olds rose 5% from 1998 to 2005.

From 1998 to 2005, among college students ages 18–24, the population increased 23% from 7,809,382 to 9,628,069, whereas unintentional alcohol-related injury deaths increased 24% from 1442 to 1825. Thus, similar to the overall 18–24-year-old group, alcohol-related unintentional injury deaths among college students, per population, rose 3%, an increase that approached statistical significance. In 2001, nearly 600,000 college students were injured because of drinking, and 696,000 were assaulted by another drinking college student [19].

Although the numbers are disturbingly high, we believe our estimates of alcohol-related college deaths are conservative. First, we focused only on unintentional injury deaths, not homicides and suicides, many of which are also alcohol related. Second, the proportion of 18–24-year-olds who engage in heavy episodic drinking and driving under the influence of alcohol is higher among persons that age who are enrolled in college. Consequently, our projection that college and non-college 18–24-year-olds experience traffic alcohol-related injury deaths at the same rate per population in each group was intentionally conservative.

Third, the meta-analysis of coroner studies [6] did not provide age-specific estimates of alcohol involvement in non-traffic unintentional injury deaths. We estimated the proportion of non-traffic unintentional injury deaths was the same among 18–24-year-old college students as among adults all ages, even though persons 18–24 are known to drink more than other adults. A higher proportion of traffic fatalities are alcohol related in the 18–24-year-old population (51%) than among all age groups (38%). It is therefore possible, if not likely, that our estimates of the number of unintentional alcohol-related non-traffic injury deaths among 18–24-year-olds are also conservative.

Fourth, if respondents underreport illegal behaviors like driving under the influence of alcohol, our estimate of the numbers of students who engage in those behaviors may be low. Fifth, response rates for the NHSDA and CAS were low. Thus, students may under- or over-represent problems associated with alcohol. In 1999 a short form of the CAS was sent to non-responding students, and there was no significant difference in rates of previous year alcohol use for those answering the short survey compared with the full questionnaire. Of note, the estimates of heavy episodic drinking reported by college students in the NHSDA and the CAS are very similar to those obtained by other major national surveys that include college students, for example, the Monitoring the Future Survey [20,21].

Sixth, this analysis focused only on college students ages 18–24, who comprise less than two-thirds of all undergraduate college students.

15.5 Implications

The magnitude of problems posed by excessive drinking among college students should stimulate both improved measurement of these problems and efforts to reduce them. We believe every unnatural death in the United States should be tested for alcohol. The average cost of such testing would be approximately $50 per deceased person [22] or an annual cost of $8.6 million for 171 637 unintentional deaths, homicides, and legal intervention and suicide deaths of all ages recorded in 2005 [13]. Congress, in its 2006 STOP Act legislation [23] and the Surgeon General's 2007 *Call to Action to Prevent and Reduce Underage Drinking* [24], recommended all injury deaths under age 21 be tested for alcohol. The annual costs for this testing would be less than $1 million. In comparison, the National Academy of Sciences [25] reports $71.1 million are spent annually to reduce underage drinking. Even though this review used cautious assumptions to estimate the numbers of alcohol-related deaths among college students and other 18–24-year-olds, direct systematic alcohol test results would be preferable. Also, mortality data sets (e.g. the Department of Transportation's FARS and CDC's Vital Statistics Mortality File) should include occupation and student status categories so that the absolute number of annual college student deaths can be tabulated.

Progress has been made over the past two decades to reduce alcohol-related crash deaths. This process has occurred in part because a sufficiently high and consistent level of fatally injured drivers in crashes are tested for alcohol that statistical models based on crash factors, vehicle factors, and person factors have been developed and used to estimate the annual numbers of alcohol-involved fatal crashes in all states [26]. The data on the numbers of alcohol-related fatal crashes annually in each state has proven invaluable to researchers seeking to study the effects of state-level legislative interventions to reduce alcohol-related traffic deaths.

Unfortunately, without comprehensive testing for alcohol and determination of college student status of all persons who die from unnatural deaths, we lack the most dependable yardstick by which to measure the magnitude of alcohol-related injury death among college students, and whether this figure is changing over time.

15.6 Interventions to Reduce College Drinking

The increase in the past 7 years in alcohol-related traffic and other unintentional injury deaths among 18–24-year-olds both in college and not in college underscores the need for colleges and their surrounding communities to expand and strengthen interventions demonstrated to reduce excessive drinking among college students and their same-age non-college counterparts.

Of note, heavy-drinking college students not only place their own health at risk, but also they jeopardize the well-being of others. As many as 46% of the 4553 people killed in 2005 in crashes involving 18–24-year-old drinking drivers are persons other than the drinking driver, and the total deceased has increased 33% from 3425 to 4553 between 1998 and 2001. Further, surveys both in 1999 and again in 2001 indicate annually over 600,000 college students nationwide were hit or assaulted by a drinking college student, and in 2001, 97,000 students were the victim of a date rape or assault perpetrated by a drinking college student [19]. Colleges and surrounding communities have an obligation to protect people from potential harm contributed by excess college drinking.

The recent report on college drinking [27] and its background reports [28], updated in 2007 [19], and the National Academy of Sciences' *Report on Underage Drinking* [25] identified numerous individually oriented counseling approaches, environmental interventions, and comprehensive community interventions that can reduce drinking and related problems among college students and the college age population. These documents summarize scientifically valid approaches for effective prevention, and some believe they establish a new legal standard by which the adequacy of any college or university's efforts can be judged [29].

15.6.1 Individually-Oriented Interventions

Information/knowledge change interventions
Larimer and Cronce's 2007 review [30] of individually-oriented interventions covered studies published between 1999 and 2006. Like their earlier report [31], this update also found no support for the effectiveness of information/knowledge approaches alone [32–34]. Seven additional studies include an information/knowledge condition as a comparison group against which to evaluate other interventions (LaChance, 2004, unpublished doctoral dissertation, University of Colorado; [35–40]). None found effects on drinking or

consequences from the information condition. Three of those studies also included values clarification in the comparison group [38,41,42], and one found behavioral changes attributable to values, clarification, and information interventions in combination.

Normative re-education interventions

Research suggests that college students often overestimate the amount of alcohol consumed by fellow students. Misperceptions of normative drinking behavior lead some students to consume more alcohol in an effort to reflect what they perceive to be normal group behavior. A growing body of literature has explored whether informing students of the true norms for alcohol consumption on their campus leads some students to curtail their drinking. This general approach is known as *normative re-education* or *social norms marketing*.

Eight studies in the updated review by Larimer and Cronce [30] examined normative re-education interventions [41–50]. The authors concluded that, taken together, findings indicate normative re-education interventions are efficacious in modifying both behavioral and attitudinal normative perceptions, but evidence was mixed regarding the impact of an in-person normative re-education component on drinking behavior or consequences. Personalized normative feedback resulted in drinking reductions in four studies [45–47,50].

Turner and colleagues [51] examined the effectiveness of social norms feedback for reducing alcohol consumption on college campuses. During a 6-year period, data were collected from roughly 2500 students from a single campus who completed a web-based survey after exposure to a social norms initiative. Students who recalled being exposed to the social norms initiative were less likely to suffer negative alcohol-related consequences and were less likely to exceed a BAC level of 0.08 than those who did not recall being exposed to the initiative. However, without a comparison group, one cannot discern whether only more cautious students recalled the social norms messages.

DeJong and colleagues [52] provided compelling evidence of the effectiveness of social norms marketing campaigns in their report on a randomized trial involving 18 colleges. They examined alcohol-related behaviors on all 18 campuses before and three years after the assignment of schools to either control or intervention conditions. The presence of a social norms marketing campaign was associated with lower levels of alcohol consumption.

In a more recent report, DeJong and colleagues [53] called the effectiveness of campus-wide social norms marketing interventions into question. The researchers designated 14 college campuses as control sites or intervention sites. As in the previous study, they examined alcohol-related behaviors on all campuses before and three years after the assignment of schools to either the control or intervention conditions. No significant reductions in alcohol consumption or the discrepancy between perceived and actual campus norms for drinking were observed, suggesting that social norms marketing campaigns are not always effective at reducing consumption on college campuses.

In two separate studies, Labrie and colleagues [54,55] demonstrated that providing immediate normative feedback to specific campus groups, rather than the campus as a whole, can aid in reducing high risk drinking. In the first study, Labrie *et al.* [54] assigned 20 campus organizations to either intervention or assessment only conditions. Those in the intervention group were asked to provide responses to alcohol-related questions via wireless keypads. These data were used to provide immediate feedback to the group regarding discrepancies between perceived and actual levels of consumption on campus. Reduced levels of consumption and corrected misperceptions were observed at both 1- and 2-month follow-ups for those in the intervention condition. Similarly, Labrie *et al.* [55] observed reductions in consumption in college athletes following the use of the same procedure.

The social norms marketing campaign utilized at Michigan State University (MSU) since 2001 serves as an example of the impact such approaches can have on alcohol consumption and alcohol-related outcomes (for more details, see http://socialnorms.msu.edn). Consistent with traditional social norms marketing approaches, MSU developed print materials, including posters, highlighting normative behaviors related to alcohol consumption (e.g. "56% [of MSU students] consume 0–4 drinks when partying and/or socializing") and the use of protective strategies (e.g. "92% of those who choose to drink, eat food before or while consuming alcohol"). Between 2000 and 2006, the average number of drinks consumed per occasion by MSU undergraduates decreased from 5.42 to 4.97. The frequency of alcohol-related harms such as sexual assaults decreased and the percentage of drinkers utilizing protective factors to minimize the risk of harm increased.

Expectancy challenge interventions

Research suggests that having positive expectations regarding the effects of alcohol can lead to higher levels of alcohol consumption and that challenging these expectations can lead to lower levels of consumption. This general approach is referred to as "expectancy challenge". Seven articles in the review by Larimer and Cronce [30] examined expectancy challenge interventions (Hunt, 2004, unpublished doctoral dissertation, University of Southern Florida) [36,56–61]. Larimer and Cronce [30] concluded that, taken as a whole, expectancy challenge interventions are associated with reductions in drinking for men but only one study [60] demonstrated effects in women.

In a subsequent study, Lau-Barraco and Dunn [62] observed reductions in consumption for both men and women following a single session in-person expectancy challenge. Moderate to heavy drinking college students were assigned either to the expectancy challenge condition or one of two control conditions. In a laboratory bar setting, those in the expectancy challenge group were given either real alcoholic beverages or placebo drinks and were then asked to identify which subjects in the group were drinking real alcohol and which subject were given placebos. A discussion regarding alcohol expectancies followed. One-month following the experiment, subjects in the expectancy challenge group, both males and females, exhibited decreases in consumption relative to baseline. No such changes were seen in either control group. The findings suggest that even single session, relatively brief applications of expectancy challenge can compel students to reduce their consumption.

Brief motivational interventions

Brief motivational interventions (BMI) had received strong support in the initial review by Larimer and Cronce [31]. This approach was found to be effective in reducing drinking problems in all eight studies that examined that approach in their initial review. Fourteen studies examined this approach in their follow-up review [30]. Of those, 10 reported significant reductions on outcome measures, prompting the conclusion that research continues to strongly support BMI with personalized feedback delivered individually in groups or as stand-alone feedback with no in-person contact (Gregory, 2001, unpublished doctoral dissertation, Florida Atlantic University; LaChance, 2004, unpublished doctoral dissertation, University of Colorado) [63–69].

Schaus, in an experimental study of college students attending a student health service clinic, found that students screened for heavy episodic drinking who received a two session brief motivational counseling intervention had significant reductions in typical BAC, peak BAC, and several other drinking outcome measures at 3- and 6-month follow-up. This is important because most college students at that university went to the student health service at least annually. Routine screening in that setting could have population-wide effects [70].

Among BMIs recently identified by Larimer and Cronce [30], eight new studies of mailed, written, or computerized motivational feedback were identified [35,39,64,68,71–75]. All but McNally et al. [64] reported reductions in drinking.

Of note, seven studies of mandated populations were reviewed. Mandated populations consist of students instructed to undergo BMIs due to violating alcohol policies. Five of the seven studies examining brief motivational feedback interventions were associated with reduced alcohol use or negative consequences (LaChance, 2004, unpublished doctoral dissertation, University of Colorado) [63,71,75–77].

Research conducted in the 2 years since publication of the Larimer and Cronce review [30] supports the effectiveness of BMI for reducing alcohol consumption as well as the use of other drugs. Werch et al. [78] employed a one-time intervention based on the Behavior Image Model. In this model, images depicting healthy behaviors are shown to subjects via computer during a 25-minute consultation. Fitness specialists use these images to help students formulate goals for improving health and well-being. The images help students envision healthier futures. Those in the intervention group exhibited lower levels of alcohol and marijuana use relative to controls when assessed three months post-intervention.

Similarly, LaBrie et al. [79] reported a single session BMI tailored to address reasons for drinking among first year college women succeeded in reducing consumption. Data from a 10-week follow up revealed that, relative to controls, intervention participants consumed fewer drinks per week, exhibited lower levels of peak consumption and experienced fewer alcohol-related consequences.

In their review of computer-based interventions for college drinking, Elliott and colleagues [80] found strong support for the effectiveness of such approaches, particularly when compared to control groups receiving assessments only. The authors identified 17 randomized controlled trials of computerized interventions. Outcomes, including reductions in consumption and alcohol-related problems, were roughly similar to those found in assessments of in-person brief motivational interviewing and were superior to no treatment. Interestingly, it appears that the length of computerized interventions and the depth of involvement required by subjects do not necessarily extend the benefits of such programs beyond the benefits of initial personalized feedback, particularly when the feedback is gender specific.

Butler and Correia [81] directly compared the effectiveness of in-person and computerized BMI. Despite the fact that students only spent 11 minutes on average reviewing computerized feedback – only $\frac{1}{4}$ the time spent receiving feedback in the face-to-face condition – levels of consumption were lower in both groups 4 weeks later compared to controls, and no differences between the two feedback conditions were observed.

Early research supports the use of computerized BMI to deter heavy drinking during specific events. For instance, Neighbors et al. [82] evaluated the utility of an Internet-based intervention aimed at reducing alcohol consumption by students celebrating their 21st birthdays. Relative to those in the control group, subjects in the intervention group were estimated to reach lower peak BAC during their birthday celebrations. The impact was particularly large for subjects who intended to drink heavily during their 21st birthdays. The findings provide support for the use of web-based intervention strategies to reduce levels of consumption during specific events associated with overindulgence.

It appears that the effectiveness of event-specific BMI could depend upon the means by which the feedback is provided. Lewis *et al.* [83] did not observe reductions in 21st birthday drinking levels or the incidence of alcohol-related consequences associated with such consumption when feedback was provided in the form of a physical card. The reason for the discrepancy between the effectiveness of web-based and mailed feedback is not clear, but the findings provide additional support for the value of web-based interventions.

Two recent reports suggest that the effectiveness of BMI for mandated students might be confounded by a naturally occurring post-sanction reduction in drinking. White *et al.* [84] divided sanctioned college students into two groups – one receiving feedback at baseline and during a 2-month follow-up and the other receiving feedback only during the 2-month follow-up. Both groups exhibited decreases in consumption during the 2-month window between baseline and follow-up and no differences were detected between the groups on any measures. The authors interpret this finding as suggesting either the incident leading to the sanction, the act of being sanctioned, or both, trigger reductions in consumption and that BMI might make a smaller contribution in these cases than previously assumed.

A related study provides additional support for a natural reduction in alcohol consumption as a result of being reprimanded for an infraction. Morgan *et al.* [85] measured self-reported drinking levels in sanctioned college students during the one month period leading up to the infraction and the one month period prior to their mandated intake assessment at the Rutgers University Alcohol and Other Drugs Assistance Program for College Students. Significant reductions in alcohol use were observed during the month prior to intake relative to the month prior to the infraction. The authors conclude that the reduction must be related to the infraction itself (personal re-appraisal of drinking habits, negative affect associated with the infraction, etc.). The greater the severity of the infraction, the greater the reduction in drinking levels, suggesting that the act of getting into trouble and being sanctioned is sufficient to trigger reduced consumption in many students.

A natural reduction in drinking following alcohol-related sanctions could help explain the findings of a recent study by Carey and colleagues [86]. The researchers assigned college students sanctioned for violating campus alcohol policies to two groups – one receiving in-person feedback in the form of BMI and the other completing a CD-ROM based alcohol education program. Students were followed up 1 month, 6 months and 12 months after the intervention. No significant differences between the two intervention groups were noted in any of the dependant measures, perhaps due to a sanction-related decrease in consumption.

Individual-level interventions

In a separate review, Carey *et al.* [87] conducted a meta-analysis of 62 randomized controlled studies of individual-level interventions to reduce college student drinking between 1985 and 2007 with 13 750 participants and 98 intervention conditions. Short-term (4–13-week post-intervention) follow-up showed intervention participants reduced their quantity and drinking frequency of heavy drinking and alcohol-related problems. At intermediate follow-up (14–26 weeks post-intervention), participants reduced the quantity of alcohol consumed and frequency of heavy drinking. At long-term follow-up (27–195 weeks post-intervention), frequency of drinking days and alcohol-related problems were reduced. They concluded that their findings demonstrate clearly that individually oriented alcohol risk reduction interventions of various forms reliably reduce quantity and frequency of drinking by college students. A second and equally important finding is that alcohol risk reduction interventions succeed in reducing alcohol-related problems reported by college drinkers.

Intervention characteristics influenced problem outcomes. Interventions delivered to individuals rather than groups and interventions that used motivational interviewing, provided feedback on expectancies or motives, normative comparison, and included decisional balance exercises (e.g. exercises that engage subjects in exploring the pros and cons of particular decisions) were more successful at reducing alcohol-related problems than a range of comparison conditions. In contrast, interventions that used skills training or expectancy challenge components were less successful at reducing alcohol-related problems relative to control conditions.

They also reported that effect size magnitude regarding drinking diminished over time. In contrast, reduction in alcohol-related problems took longer to emerge but continued in long-term follow-up.

Parent initiatives. Ichiyama *et al.* used an experimental design to test the effects of sending parents a 45-page handbook for *Talking with College Students About Alcohol*. Parents in the comparison group received a brochure detailing university alcohol policies and consequences of alcohol policy violations [88].

Of 347 parents in the intervention group, 72% evaluated the handbook and 83% said they had read most or all of it. Students whose parents reviewed the handbook who did not drink prior to college were less likely to start drinking and those already drinking were less likely to show growth in drinking over the freshman year. This latter finding resulted from effects on female students, not males.

Student assistance program. Amaro *et al.* tested a Student Assistance Program in a randomized experimental study of students sanctioned for alcohol or drug violations. The University Assistance Program reduced 90-day weekday alcohol consumption and number of alcohol-related consequences. Total alcohol consumption and weekend consumption were not affected [89].

Environmental interventions: legal drinking age of 21. The most powerful environmental intervention to reduce drinking among college students is the minimum drinking age of 21. In 1984, when 17 states had a legal drinking age of 21, the US Congress passed legislation that would withhold highway construction fund for states that did not make it illegal to sell alcohol to people younger than age 21. By 1988, all states adopted the law [90].

In all 50 states and the District of Columbia, it is illegal for a person under 21 to possess alcohol, to furnish it to a person under 21, or to use a fake ID to obtain alcohol. However, there are some important exceptions. In 24 states, persons under 21 can possess alcohol with parental or guardian consent and/or presence. Parents can legally furnish alcohol to their children under 21 in 31 states. Only 31 states and the District of Columbia explicitly prohibit consumption by a person under 21, and in 47 states, people under 21 can serve alcohol [91].

In August 2008, a group of 130 college presidents called for debate about whether the drinking age should be lowered to age 18. Some suggested, after receiving education about safe drinking levels, 18 year olds should be given drinking licenses that would be rescinded if their drinking posed dangers to themselves or others. Given this widely publicized

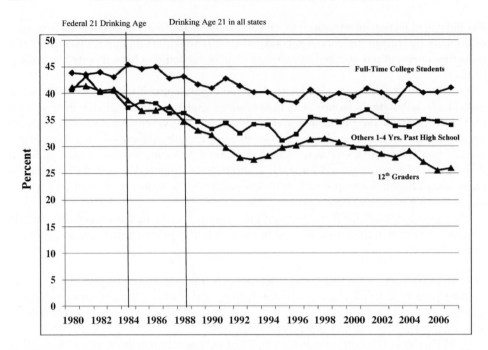

Figure 15.2 *Alcohol: trends in 2-week prevalence of five or more drinks in a row among college students vs. others 1–4 years beyond high school. Source: Monitoring the Future, 2007.*

challenge to the legal drinking age of 21, it is worth reviewing evidence on the topic. Figure 15.2 examines Monitoring the Future data on trends in the frequency of binge drinking from 1982 to 2007 (5+ drinks on an occasion). Monitoring the Future is a yearly assessment of the attitudes, behaviors and values of nearly 50 000 eighth, tenth and twelfth graders. According to the survey data [92], binge drinking among high school seniors dropped from 40% to just over 25%. Among persons 1–4 years past high school, the declines were less, from 40% to just under 35%. Little change was seen among full-time college students. Figure 15.3 examines trends in alcohol-related traffic fatalities among persons 18–20 targeted by the drinking age changes and those 21–24 not targeted. Both groups experienced proportional declines, but the declines were greater in the 18–20 year age group than in the 21–24 year group (60% vs. 44%). An examination of the percentage of fatal crash deaths in each age group that involved alcohol reveals a similar pattern of results (Figure 15.4). Analyses of trends in fatal crash deaths over the same time period involving drivers 18–20 vs. 21–24 who had positive blood alcohol levels also reveals a similar pattern (data available on request).

A review of 49 studies of the legal drinking age changes revealed that in the 1970s and 1980s, when many states lowered the drinking age, alcohol-related traffic crashes among people younger than 21 decreased 16%. In contrast, when states increased the legal drinking age to 21, alcohol-related crashes among people younger than 21 decreased 16% [93]. Wagenaar and Toomey [94] reviewed 48 studies of the effects of drinking age changes on drinking and 57 studies on traffic crashes. They concluded that increases in the legal age of alcohol purchase and consumption have been the most successful interventions to date in reducing drinking and alcohol-related crashes among persons under 21. One national study of laws raising the drinking age to 21 indicated that persons who grew up in states with a

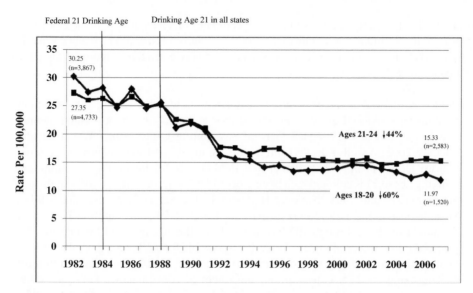

Figure 15.3 *Alcohol-related traffic fatalities, rate per 100 000, ages 18–20 vs. 21–24, United States, 1982–2007. Source: US Fatality Analysis Reporting System, 2009; US Census Bureau, 2009.*

drinking age of 21, relative to those with lower drinking ages, drank less when they were younger than 21, but also when they were ages 21–25 [95]. Conversely, college students who were high school seniors in states with a minimum drinking age of 18 drank more in college than counterparts who were high school seniors with a drinking age of 21 [95]. The National

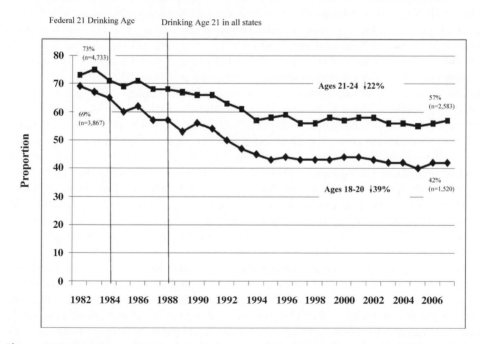

Figure 15.4 *Proportion of fatal crash deaths in the united states that were alcohol-related, ages 18–20 vs. 21–24, 1982–2007. Source: US Fatality Analysis Reporting System, 2009.*

Highway Traffic Safety Administration [97] estimates that a legal drinking age of 21 saves 700–1000 lives annually and more than 25,000 lives have been saved by the law since 1976 [96]. In 2004, the National Academy of Sciences [25] reviewed the literature on age 21 laws and concluded:

> ...[A] substantial body of scientific evidence shows that raising the minimum drinking age reduced alcohol-related crashes and fatalities among young people (Cook and Tauchen, 1984; US General Accounting Office, 1987; Wagenaar and Toomey, 2002) as well as deaths from suicide, homicide, and nonvehicle unintentional injuries (Jones *et al.*, 1992; Parker and Rebbun, 1995). Increasing the minimum drinking age to 21 is credited with having saved 18,220 lives on the nation's highways between 1975 and 1998 (National Highway Traffic Safety Administration, 1998). Voas, Tippetts, and Fell (1999), using data from all 50 states and the District of Columbia for 1982 through 1997, concluded that the enactment of the uniform 21-year-old minimum drinking age law was responsible for a 19 percent net decrease in fatal crashes involving young drivers who had been drinking, after controlling for driving exposure, beer consumption, enactment of zero tolerance laws, and other relevant changes in the laws during that time. These findings reinforce the decision by Congress to act in 1984. In short, current national policy rests on the view, supported by substantial evidence, that delaying drinking reduces problem drinking and its consequences. The nation's legislators and public health leaders have reached the nearly uniform judgment that the benefits of setting it at 21 far exceed the costs of doing so [25].

Several additional analyses of the age 21 law have appeared since the reviews by Shults *et al.* [93], Wagenaar and Toomey [94], and the National Academy of Sciences [25]. Ponicki *et al.* [97] reviewed the impact of the minimum legal drinking age (MLDA) and beer taxes using a panel of 48 US states over the period 1975–2001. The analysis showed that either MLDA or increases in beer taxes in isolation led to fewer youth fatalities. The analysis controlled analytically for real income per capita; seat belt laws; 0.08% BAC limits; zero tolerance laws; keg registration laws; the proportion of the population who were Catholic, Mormon, Southern Baptist, or other religions; the proportion who were white; hotel employees per 100,000; hospital beds per 100,000; and the proportion of the population living in metropolitan areas. The study found the strength of the legal drinking age impact was influenced by the level of tax on beer. An MLDA increase to 21 resulted in an 11% decline in fatalities among persons under 21 if beer taxes are 25% below their mean level, 0.09% if beer taxes are at the mean level, and 6% if beer taxes are 25% above the mean.

Males [98] compared states that raised the drinking age to 21 between 1975 and 2005 with those with a legal drinking age throughout the period. He examined night fatal crashes involving 18–20-year-olds, day fatal crashes, other unintentional injury deaths, homicides, and suicides.

Three groupings of states were compared to the 21 states with age 21 throughout. Night fatal crashes (likely to involve alcohol) declined 11.9% on average in 20 states that raised the drinking age from 18 to 21, whereas day fatal crashes (unlikely to involve alcohol) remained unchanged. In states with legal drinking of beer and wine at age 18 that adopted the age 21 law (10 states plus the District of Columbia), night fatal crashes involving 18–20-year-olds declined 1%, while day fatal crashes, unlikely to involve alcohol, increased 10.1%. In states with former drinking ages of 19 or 20 that raised the age to 21 (eight states), night fatal crashes declined 8.8% more than day fatal crashes, which declined 5.8%.

In states that raised the drinking age from 18 to 20, other unintentional injury deaths declined 1.7%, suicides 7%, and homicides 0.5%. In states raising the drinking age from 19 or 20 to 21, non-traffic unintentional injury deaths among 18–20-year-olds increased 3.9%, suicides declined 8.9%, while homicides increased 17.2%. In the 10 states plus the District of Columbia that formerly had legal beer and wine at 18, unintentional non-traffic injuries increased 47%, suicides 143.7%, and homicides 185%.

It should be noted that the comparison of night traffic deaths (known to more frequently involve alcohol) to day fatal crashes (less likely to involve alcohol) revealed results consistent with the large body of research on the topic already cited above. The night (alcohol) crashes decline among 18–20-year-old drivers relative to day fatal crashes. Among 21–24-year-olds in those same states, night-time fatal crashes actually increased slightly.

The new findings in Males' study were that homicides and suicides increased among 18–20-year-olds after drinking age increases to 21, particularly in states that had previously allowed drinking of beer and wine at age 18. It is not known whether those homicide and suicide increases involved individuals who had been drinking or not since states do not routinely test homicide and suicide deaths for alcohol. Interpretation of Males' results, however, should take into consideration that enactment dates for MLDA 21 used in Males' calculations were off by 4 years in six states, 3 years in eight states, 2 years in seven states, and 1 year in 11 states. All the misclassification considered post-law years as pre-law years.

Miron and Tetelbaum [99] found significant declines in traffic fatalities among persons under 21 in states that changed the MLDA to 21 prior to the 1984 federal mandate to raise the drinking age to 21. However, when the analyses examined only states that raised the drinking age after the federal legislation, the MLDA increases were not associated with significant declines in traffic deaths. Miron and Tetelbaum's analyses controlled for whether states had a seat belt law, the legal blood alcohol limit, beer taxes, and vehicle miles traveled.

In their discussion, Miron and Tetelbaum emphasized the many improvements in vehicle design that have occurred during the 1960s and suggest these improvements, rather than the drinking age, was probably responsible for fatality declines that have been attributable to the drinking age. Of note, Miron and Tetelbaum examined all traffic deaths collectively regardless of whether they were known to be alcohol-related or not.

Yet, analyses of alcohol-related traffic deaths among 16–20-year-olds relative to other traffic fatalities in the same age group during the time period 1982–2007 reveal that alcohol-related fatalities involving 16–20-year-olds declined 62% while those that did not involve alcohol actually increased 22% (see Figure 15.5). After adjusting for changes in the population that age, alcohol-related traffic fatalities among persons ages 16–20 declined 64% while those that did not involve alcohol increased 17%. A similar pattern is seen for the number of drivers 16–20 in fatal crashes over the same time period. The number of drinking drivers 16–20 in fatal crashes declined 70% per population from 1982–2007 while the number of drivers that age in fatal crashes who had not been drinking alcohol increased 36%.

Fell, in two separate analyses [90,100], made the following distinction between being a drinking driver in fatal crashes vs. not being a drinking driver in fatal crashes. In his first analysis [100], he examined fatal crash data from 1982–1990 and monitored the rates of drinking to non-drinking drivers in fatal crashes. He compared states that adopted age 21

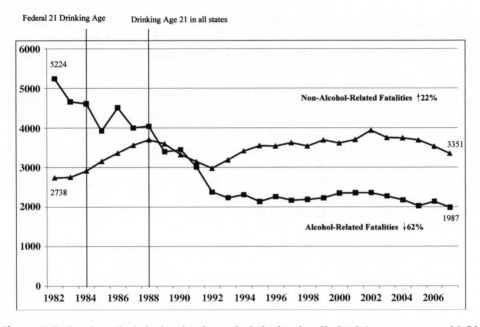

Figure 15.5 *Trends in alcohol related and non alcohol related traffic fatalities, persons ages 16–20, United States, 1982–2007. Source: US Fatality Analysis Reporting System, 2009.*

laws between 1982 and 1990 to those with age 21 laws throughout. His analyses controlled for state employment rates, state vehicle miles traveled, percent of the population living in urban areas, percent of drivers age 25+ alcohol positive in fatal crashes, administrative license revocation, 0.10% and 0.08% BAC limits, primary and secondary seat belt laws, and region of the country. That analysis for adoption of a minimum legal drinking age associated with an 11% reduction in the ratio of drinking to non-drinking drivers under 21 in fatal crashes.

In his 2009 paper [90], Fell examined trends in the ratio of drinking to non-drinking drivers in fatal crashes in each state annually from 1982–2004 (unlike Miron's analyses). This analysis controlled for zero tolerance laws, graduated license night restrictions, and use/lose laws that target drivers under 21, and could influence their involvement in alcohol-related crashes. Fell also controlled for 0.10% and 0.08% BAC *per se* legal limits, mandatory seat belt laws, per capita beer consumption, unemployment rates, vehicle miles traveled, frequency of sobriety checkpoints, number of licensed drivers, ratio of drinking to non-drinking drivers age 26+ in fatal crashes.

Fell's findings are quite informative. Adoption of the minimum legal drinking age of 21 was associated with a 16% decline in the ratio of drinking to non-drinking drivers in fatal crashes under 21 even after controlling for all the other factors listed above. Of note, other laws targeting drivers under 21 alcohol independently predicted lower involvement of drinking drivers in fatal crashes. Use/lose laws and zero tolerance laws were each associated with 5% declines. Further, laws aimed at adult drivers also independently contributed to declines in the ratio of drinking to non-drinking drivers in fatal crashes: 0.08% laws were independently associated with an 8% decline, 0.10% laws a 7% decline, administrative license revocation a 5% decline, and seat-belt laws a 3% decline.

Thus, the preponderance of evidence suggests that raising the drinking age to 21 reduced alcohol involvement of drivers under 21 in fatal crashes and that other laws aimed at drivers under 21 can reduce alcohol involvement of drivers under 21 in alcohol-related fatal crashes.

Zero tolerance laws[2]

Zero tolerance laws, which made it illegal in every state for persons under 21 to drive after any drinking, have also contributed to declines in alcohol-related traffic deaths among people younger than 21. A comparison of the first eight states to adopt zero tolerance laws with nearby states without such laws revealed a 21% greater decline in zero tolerance law states in the proportion of fatal crashes among drivers younger than 21 that were of the type most likely to involve alcohol (i.e. single-vehicle fatal crashes at night [101]. Wagenaar [102] found that, in the first 30 states to adopt zero tolerance laws relative to the rest of the nation, there was a 19% decline in the proportion of people younger than 21 who drove after any drinking and a 23% decline in the proportion who drove after having five or more drinks.

Voas *et al.* [103] examined the effects of zero tolerance laws and the minimum legal drinking age of 21 on the ratio of drinking to non-drinking drivers less than age 21 in fatal crashes from 1982–1997 in a national analysis controlling for state/urban composition, number of licensed drivers, vehicle and roadway features, state per capita alcohol consumption, 0.10% *per se* BAC laws, 0.08% *per se* BAC laws, administrative license revocation, safety belt laws, and unemployment. Zero tolerance laws were associated with a 24% decline and minimum legal drinking age of 21 with a 19% decline in the ratio of alcohol- to non-alcohol-involved drivers in fatal crashes.

Liang and Huang [104] examined data from the Harvard School of Public Health College Alcohol Surveys in 1993, 1995, and 1997. In 1993, less than 8% of the sample was in a zero tolerance law state. By 1997, 84% were covered by zero tolerance laws, and by 1999, all were covered. The study analytically controlled for respondent high school drinking history, including binge drinking, gender, race/ethnicity, marital status, religion, fraternity/sorority membership, type of campus attended (e.g. women's college, black college, community college, large or small private school, or large or small public college), 0.08% BAC laws, 0.10% BAC laws, fake ID laws, laws making it illegal to sell alcohol to minors, keg registration (in which the identity of the individual renting the keg is recorded), child endangerment laws, happy hour, responsible server training laws, mandatory fines for driving while intoxicated (DWI), mandatory fines, and mandatory prison and mandatory license actions. After zero tolerance laws, there was a 5% drinking and 2% binge drinking reduction and a 4.9% reduction in drinking and driving among drinkers.

The Fell [90] study also showed that laws found to reduce driving after drinking among adult populations, such as 0.08% BAC laws and administrative license laws can affect not only alcohol-related crash involvement of adult drivers but also those under 21. An earlier review by Shults [93] of 19 studies of states lowering legal blood alcohol limits for persons ages 21 and older reported that this law cut alcohol-related fatalities on average by 7% and concluded there is strong evidence in favor of having such a change.

Unfortunately, despite their demonstrated benefits, legal drinking age and zero tolerance laws generally have not been vigorously enforced [105]. Young drivers are substantially under-represented in the DWI arrest population relative to their contribution to the alcohol

---

[2] The zero tolerance laws we are reviewing here refer to illegality of persons under 21 driving after any drinking. This is different than residence hall zero tolerance policies (one drink and you are out).

crash problem [106,107]. Younger drivers may be more likely to drink at locations where DWI enforcement resources are less likely to be deployed. Young drivers are also more likely to be missed by police at sobriety checkpoints [108]. Stepped-up enforcement of alcohol purchase laws aimed at sellers and buyers can be effective [106,109,110] if resources are made available for this purpose. Enforcement of zero tolerance laws is hindered in some states because their implied consent laws require either an arrest for DWI or probable cause for a DWI arrest. Thus, in practice, zero tolerance laws are often not enforced independently of DWI. In states such as New Mexico, where this situation exists, most teenagers are unaware there is a zero tolerance law [111].

Price of alcohol. The National Academy of Sciences [25] reviewed the literature on price of alcohol and alcohol-related problems and recommended that Congress and state legislators raise excise taxes to reduce underage alcohol consumption and to raise additional revenues to reduce underage drinking problems.

With rare exceptions [112,113] research since the early 1980s generally has concluded that increases in the price of alcohol beverages lead to reductions in drinking and heavy drinking, as well as reductions in the adverse consequences of alcohol use and abuse [114]. Higher alcohol prices have also been found to reduce alcohol-related problems such as motor vehicle fatalities [25,115–117], robberies, rapes, cirrhosis deaths [118–124], sexually transmitted diseases [125], domestic violence [126], and child abuse [127,128]. Among moderate drinkers, investigators have estimated that a 1% price increase results in a 1.19% decrease in consumption [129]. Younger, heavier drinkers tend to be more affected by price than older, heavier drinkers [112,116,118,130–133], perhaps because younger drinkers have less discretionary income. Laixuthai and Chaloupka [120], Grossman *et al.* [122], and Coate and Grossman [123] all found increasing the price of alcohol reduces the percent of youths who drink infrequently and produces even greater percentage declines in youths who drink frequently.

Research taking into account the addictive nature of alcohol shows that the long-term price elasticity is well above short-term elasticity [126]. Kenkel [116] reported a 10% increase in the price of alcohol would reduce DWI 7% among men and 8% among women, and among persons under 21 this action would produce a 13% decrease among men and a 21% decrease among women.

Toomey *et al.* [134] recently updated an earlier review [133] that Toomey and Wagenaar conducted on environmental policies to reduce college drinking. They found that, consistent with previous studies, several recent studies found higher prices are associated with lower levels of alcohol use [129–133,135–138]. Other recent studies, however, found mixed results depending on beverage type [139–141] or little effect [142].

Toomey *et al.* [132] identified two studies that evaluated the effects of alcohol prices specifically on college student drinking. Both were cross-sectional, national surveys. Environments where alcohol was cheap and more accessible were linked with heavy college student drinking [141]. Williams *et al.* [143] found increasing the prices of alcohol was associated with reductions in heavy and moderate drinking by college students. Kuo *et al.* [144] found lower prices and promotion were associated with higher rates of heavy alcohol use on college campuses.

Excise taxes. Excise taxes on alcohol can affect price. Recent studies on raising alcohol taxes identified by Toomey *et al.* [132] showed mixed results [144–157]. One study [163] found higher beer taxes associated with slightly higher rates of alcohol consumption among college students.

Most recently, Wagenaar *et al.* [158] conducted an extensive review of 112 studies of alcohol tax or price effects containing 1003 estimates of the tax/price-consumption relationship. Meta-analytical results documented the highly significant relationships between alcohol tax or price measures for beer, wine, spirits, and total alcohol. Price and tax was found to effect heavy drinking significantly, but the magnitude of effect was smaller than effects on overall drinking. Thus, a large literature establishes that beverage alcohol prices are related inversely to drinking, and the effects are large compared to other policies and programs.

Other environmental interventions. Alcohol outlet density has been associated with alcohol-related problems both in cross-sectional and prospective studies, and reducing outlet density may, in turn, reduce drinking-related problems [159,160]. Wechsler [161] found students who attend colleges in states with more restrictions on underage drinking, high volume consumption and sales of alcohol beverages and which devote more resources to enforce drunk-driving laws report less drinking and driving. Laws in these states included prohibitions against using a false age identification, restrictions on attempting to buy or consume for those under the drinking age, enforcement of a clerk age minimum and maintenance of minimum-mandatory postings of warning signs in retail outlets to potential underage buyers. Laws pertaining to volume alcohol sales were keg registration, a statewide 0.08 g/dl *per se* BAC law and restrictions on happy hours, open container laws, beer sold in pitchers, billboards, and advertising. The availability of large volumes of alcohol (24–30-can cases of beer, kegs, and small kegs know as party balls), low sales prices, and frequent promotions and advertisements at both on- and off-premise establishments were also associated with higher binge drinking rates on the college campuses [162].

Cohen *et al.* [163] reported that keg registration is negatively correlated with traffic fatality rate. Fell *et al.* [90] did not replicate this result.

Responsible beverage service and dram shop laws
Alcohol purchase surveys indicate that 40–90% of outlets will sell alcohol to underage people. Responsible beverage service (RBS) is a training and monitoring approach designed to help minimize the chances that underage drinkers can purchase alcohol, as well as minimizing sales of alcohol to intoxicated persons. RBS standards require all servers to be above age 21 years, to not sell alcohol to individuals who are under-age, to check identification and verify age, to train managers to identify false credentials, and to monitor drinks consumed by patrons. Lang *et al.* [164] and Saltz and Stanghetta [165] found little effect of RBS on car crashes. Others [166,167] found that RBS can reduce car crashes. Shults *et al.* [93] found that server training programs were effective in reducing car crashes if they involved face-to-face instruction and strong management support. Dram shop laws, which enable injured individuals to recover damages from the retailer who sold alcohol to the individual causing the injury, have been estimated to reduce traffic fatalities among underage drinkers by 3–4% [168].

Hingson *et al.* [22] recently reviewed interventions to reduce alcohol-related injuries. In addition to level blood alcohol limits such as 0.08% *per se* laws for adults and zero tolerance laws for drivers under 21, they found research supporting the effectiveness of lower legal blood alcohol limits for convicted offenders [169]. Impoundment of vehicles or license plates of previously convicted DWI offenders [170,171], ignition inter-locks [172], and publicized sobriety checkpoints are highly effective enforcement interventions [93,173,174].

Elder *et al.* [175] found a median decrease in injury crashes of 10% in their systematic review of the effectiveness of some mass media educational campaigns. The effects were similar for messages focused on legal consequences and on health consequences. They concluded that carefully planned, well-executed media campaigns that attain adequate audience exposure and are implemented in conjunction with other ongoing prevention activities are effective in reducing alcohol-impaired driving and alcohol-related crashes. Additional support for media effects comes from a study demonstrating alcohol advertising has a direct link to alcohol consumption among underage drinkers [176].

Comprehensive community interventions. Several carefully conducted community-based initiatives have had particular success in reducing drinking- and/or alcohol-related problems among young people [177]. These programs typically coordinate efforts of:

- City officials from multiple departments of city government, school, health, police, alcohol beverage control, and so on.

- Concerned private citizens and their organizations; students; parents; and merchants who sell alcohol.

Often multiple intervention strategies are incorporated into the programs, including school-based programs involving students, peer leaders, and parents; media advocacy; community organizing and mobilization; environmental policy change to reduce alcohol availability to youth; and heightened enforcement of laws regulating sales and distribution of alcohol and laws to reduce alcohol-related traffic injuries and deaths.

Four comprehensive community programs in particular have shown reduction in alcohol problems among college-age youth:

- Communities Mobilizing for Change Program [109,110] – A community organizing program aimed at reducing the flow of alcohol to youth from illegal sales by retail establishments and from the provision of alcohol to youth by adults in the community

- Community Trials Program [178] – Helps communities form coalitions aimed at reducing illegal sales of alcohol to youth, implementing RBS and decreasing drunk driving offenses by increasing awareness of consequences.

- Saving Lives Program [179] – Community based program aimed at reducing drunk driving and related consequences through media campaigns, police training, high school peer-led education, college prevention programs, increased alcohol outlet surveillance, and other measures.

- Fighting Back Program [180] – Community-wide approach to addressing substance use by involving business, health care, the public school system, local government, law enforcement, community groups, local media, and others.

Two programs [178,179] focused on publicized police enforcement of drinking driver laws and alcohol service laws, and one [179] targeted risky motorist behaviors – such as speeding, running red lights, failing to wear safety belts, and yielding to pedestrians in crosswalks – engaged in disproportionally by drinking drivers.

Relative to the comparison communities, the Communities Mobilizing for Change communities achieved a 17% increase in outlets checking the age identification of youthful-appearing alcohol purchasers, a 24% decline in sales by bars and restaurants to potential underage purchasers, a 25% decrease in the proportion of 18–20-year-olds seeking to buy alcohol, a 17% decline in the proportion of older teens who provided alcohol to younger teens, and a 7% decrease in the percentage of respondents younger than 21 who drank in the previous 30 days [109]. Further, drinking and driving arrests declined significantly among 18–20-year-olds, and disorderly conduct violators declined among 15–17-year-olds [110]. In the Community Trials Program, single-vehicle crashes at night, a measure of alcohol-related crashes, declined 11% more in program than in comparison communities. Alcohol-related trauma visits to emergency departments declined 43% [178]. In the Saving Lives Program [179] the proportion of drivers younger than 20 who reported in telephone surveys driving after drinking declined from 19% to 9% over the course of the program. The proportion of vehicles observed speeding through use of radar was cut in half, and there was a 7% increase in safety belt use. Minimal change in these outcomes occurred in comparison areas. Fatal crashes declined from 178 during the five preprogram years to 120 during the five program years, a 25% greater reduction than in the rest of Massachusetts. Fatal crashes involving alcohol declined 42%, and the number of fatally injured drivers with positive BACs declined 47%, relative to the rest of Massachusetts. Visible injuries per 100 crashes declined 5% more in Saving Lives cities than in the rest of the state during the program period. The fatal crash declines were greater in all six program cities relative to comparison areas, particularly among drivers ages 15–25.

Five Fighting Back communities that combined environmental interventions to reduce availability of alcohol with interventions to increase substance abuse treatment use observed over a 20% decline in alcohol-related fatal crashes during ten program years related to the 10 preprogram years and relative to companion comparison community drawn from the same states [180].

Efforts to reduce alcohol availability included:

- Compliance check surveys to monitor underage access to alcohol over time
- Responsible beverage service training
- Ordinances to prohibit public consumption or beverage sales
- Closing of liquor stores
- Monitoring problematic outlets and advertising.

Initiatives to expand treatment included:

- Increasing publicly funded treatment
- Establishment of referral or expanded treatment and after-care programs
- Initiating hospital emergency department screening and referral
- Establishing drug courts
- Opening of new treatment and after-care facilities.

Communities varied somewhat in the initiatives that they pursued, but most of the five communities pursued most of the activities described above.

Two recent studies took this comprehensive community intervention model and applied it to different geographic entities. Treno *et al.* [181] selected two neighborhoods in Sacramento for intervention, one for intervention and the other for comparison. Project interventions included a mobilization component to support the overall project, a community-awareness component, a responsible beverage server component, and an intoxicated-patron law enforcement component. They reported significant reductions in assaults as reported by police, aggregate emergency medical services (EMS), EMS outcomes, EMS assaults, and EMS motor vehicle accidents.

Wagenaar *et al.* [182] compared 10 intervention states with 40 other states. In the intervention states, coalitions were formed to change the policy and normative environment regarding youth access to alcohol. The coalitions achieved significant increases in media coverage on underage drinking, alcohol pricing, taxes, social-host liability, and alcohol policies restricting youth access to alcohol through social channels.

The intervention states achieved significant declines in drinking in the past 12 months, consumption of five or more drinks on an occasion in the past 2 weeks, among twelfth graders getting drunk in the past month for eighth and twelfth graders and the number of times a respondent drove a car in the past two weeks after drinking. Reductions in alcohol-related fatal crash involvement by drivers under 21 fell just below statistical significance.

Five investigators have now explored elements of the comprehensive community organizing model as a method for reducing drinking or alcohol-related harms specifically among college students. Clapp *et al.* [183] adopted some of the Community Trials [184] interventions to a college setting. At an experimental university, there was a marked increase in driving under the influence enforcement coupled with a media campaign. The prevention campaign featured driving under the influence (DUI) checkpoints, media coverage, and a student-designed social marketing campaign designed to increase student perception of risk of arrest for DUI. DUI checkpoints were operated jointly by campus and local city police. Telephone surveys of randomly selected students revealed significant declines in self-reported DUI from pre- to post-test.

McCartt *et al.* [184] studied a comprehensive community program focusing on underage drinking and drinking and driving among 16–24-year-olds in Huntington, West Virginia, home of Marshall University (enrollment 18,000 students). Morgantown, West Virginia, home to West Virginia University, with 40,000 students, was selected for comparison. During late winter 2006 and spring 2007, local, university, and state enforcement agencies increased enforcement of drunken and driving laws, including zero tolerance laws, through low-manpower sobriety checkpoints, saturation patrols, and stepped-up DUI directed patrols. The state Alcohol Beverage Control Administration, with assistance from local and state law enforcement agencies, increased enforcement of the minimum legal drinking age laws. This included enforcement of laws aimed at servers/sellers and underage persons, including use of fake identifications.

A multi-media campaign included paid and earned print and broadcast media. Intensive publishing of the campaign also occurred on the Marshall campus. Roadside surveys of night-time drivers conducted alcohol breath tests during the fall of 2006, spring of 2007, and fall of 2007. Compliance check survey of underage alcohol purchase attempts produced declines in successful buy attempts, from 43% to 18% in the intervention city. Little change occurred in the comparison city. Reductions in BACs at the roadside surveys in the intervention city showed marked declines in the proportions of 16–20-, 21–24-, and 25+ -year-old operators at 0.02%, 0.05%, and 0.08%. Little change was found in the comparison city.

Saltz *et al.* examined a college community partnership at Western Washington University and another Washington state university. Police patrols focused on off-campus student parties, and compliance check surveys were used to restrict sales of alcohol to minors. Public forums bought community residents, students, and police together for dialogues about disruptive parties and other neighborhood issues. The college also offered alcohol-free late night activities. Significant restrictions in the prevalence of heavy drinking (5 or more consecutive drinks) were observed at the two intervention colleges [185].

Wood *et al.* evaluated the Common Ground Program, a University of Rhode Island/community partnership featuring increased driving while intoxicated and minimum legal drinking age enforcement, a media campaign, and a safe risks program. While the program resulted in increased student awareness of alcohol control measures and a greater perceived likelihood of apprehension for underage drinking as well as a reduction in police reported alcohol-related incidents, no changes were observed or reported alcohol use or alcohol-impaired driving by college students [186].

15.7 Conclusions

The percentage of 18–24-year-olds in college and not in college who binge drink and drive under the influence of alcohol has increased significantly since 1999. Rates of alcohol-related injury deaths per 100,000 in this age group have not changed significantly during this time period. Alcohol-related traffic deaths per 100,000 declined slightly (3%), and alcohol-related non-traffic deaths, excluding poisoning, also declined slightly (2%). Poisoning deaths where alcohol may be present, however, have increased. It should be noted, though, that our estimates on poisoning deaths assume the percentage of poisoning deaths that involve alcohol has remained constant during this period. Alcohol testing is not done on all poisoning deaths, and we are not certain whether this assumption is correct.

It is ironic that binge drinking and driving under the influence of alcohol continue to rise and unintentional injuries attributable to alcohol have not declined during a period of time when there has been a considerable expansion of the scientific literature and knowledge base regarding how to reduce drinking and related harms among college students.

There is now a sizable scientific literature that demonstrates individually-oriented approaches like screening and brief motivational interventions can reduce drinking not only among students who voluntarily seek out these programs but also among those mandated to receive counseling because of alcohol-related disciplinary actions.

Unfortunately, these interventions are not reaching a sizeable portion of college students with problematic drinking practices. Although nearly 20% of college students meet *DSM-IV* alcohol dependence or abuse criteria, less than 5% of them have sought counseling or treatment [19]. An important challenge is to sufficiently expand screening and counseling so that these effective individually-oriented interventions can achieve general population-level effects. Establishing alcohol screening and brief intervention as a routine part of student health service encounters and use of the internet and mail back screening and advice might help remedy this situation.

Also, a variety of environmental policy interventions that reduce availability of alcohol and deter driving while impaired by alcohol have been shown to be effective in reducing drinking and driving and alcohol-related crash involvement of college students.

These policies must, however, be implemented and enforced at the community level. Research evidence now indicates colleges and universities can reduce harmful drinking and drinking and driving through the use of comprehensive cooperative college/community multi-component approaches that include heightened enforcement of the legal drinking age and other laws aimed to reduce drinking and driving.

A strong hypothesis is that intervention at multiple levels targeting: (1) individual students through screening and counseling; (2) family before and during college years; (3) colleges; (4) state and community environmental policies; and (5) multi-component college/community programs, will be more effective than single level interventions. Careful systematic testing of this hypothesis is a pressing research priority.

But clearly colleges by themselves cannot resolve the alcohol problems of all persons of college age. For every 18–24-year-old college student, two 18–24-year-olds are not in college. Further, many college students develop problematic drinking habits before they enter college. Analyses of the national College Alcohol Survey indicates the younger college students were when they first drank to intoxication, the greater the likelihood while they were in college that they experienced alcohol dependence, rode with drinking drivers, drove after drinking, were injured under the influence of alcohol, and had unplanned and unprotected sex after drinking [187,188]. Hence community conditions and the availability of alcohol to persons under 21 contributes to college drinking problems. Further, many of the problems experienced as a result of excessive college student alcohol consumption affect people other than the college drinkers themselves.

Consequently, colleges and surrounding communities need to work together implementing multi-faceted programs at various levels of intervention. Collectively, they need to involve multiple departments of city government as well as concerned private citizens and organizations and multiple sectors of the college community, presidents, deans, other administrators, campus security, residence counselors, health service providers, alumni, faculty, and students if they want to most effectively reduce harmful drinking and the myriad of health and social problems linked to harmful drinking.

References

1. Wechsler, H., Davenport, A., Dowdall, G. *et al.* (1994) Health and behavioral consequences of binge drinking in college: a national survey of students at 140 campuses. *Journal of the American Medical Association*, **272**(21), 1672–1677.
2. Wechsler, H., Dowdall, G.W., Maenner, G. *et al.* (1998) Changes in binge drinking and related problems among American college students between 1993 and 1997: results of the Harvard School of Public Health College Alcohol Study. *Journal of American College Health*, **47**(2), 57–68.
3. Wechsler, H., Lee, J.E., Kuo, M.C. *et al.* (2000) College binge drinking in the 1990s: a continuing problem – results of the Harvard School of Public Health 1999 College Alcohol Study. *Journal of American College Health*, **48**(5), 199–210.
4. Hingson, R., Heeren, T., Winter, M. *et al.* (2005) Magnitude of alcohol-related mortality and morbidity among US college students ages 18–24: changes from 1998 to 2001. *Annual Review of Public Health*, **26**, 259–279.
5. Centers for Disease Control and Prevention (2009) Web-Based Injury Statistics Query and Reporting System (WISQARS) Available at, http://www.cdc.gov/injury/wisqars/index.html/, Accessed April 8, 2009.
6. Smith, G.S., Branas, C.C. and Miller, T.R. (1999) Fatal nontraffic injuries involving alcohol: a metaanalysis. *Annals of Emergency Medicine*, **33**(6), 659–668.

7. National Highway Traffic Safety Administration (2002) *Transitioning to Multiple Imputation: A New Method to Estimate Missing Blood Alcohol Concentration Values in FARS*, US Department of Transportation, Washington, DC., DOT HS 809-403.

8. National Highway, Traffic Safety Administration (2002) *Traffic Safety Facts, 2002*, US Department of Transportation, Washington, DC, DOT HHS 809-470.

9. U.S. Census Bureau (2001) Integrated Post Secondary Education Data System, Fall Enrollment, 1999. Available at, http://www.census.gov/population/socdemo/school/p20-533/tab09.pdf. Accessed 8 April 2009.

10. National Center for Education Statistics (2000) *Digest of Education Statistics, 1999*, Department of Education, Washington, DC, NCES 2000-031.

11. National Center for Education Statistics (2004) *Digest of Education Statistics, 2003*, Department of Education, Washington, DC, NCES 2005-025.

12. National Center for Education Statistics (2007) *Digest of Education Statistics, 2006*, Department of Education, Washington, DC, NCES 2007-017.

13. Centers for Disease Control and Prevention (2009) Web-Based Injury Statistics Query and Reporting System (WISQARS). Available at http://www.cdc.gov/injury/wisqars/index.html/. Accessed 14 April 2009.

14. Substance Abuse and Mental Health Services Administration (2000) *Summary of Findings of the 1999 National Household Survey on Drug Abuse*, Substance Abuse and Mental Health Services Administration, Rockville, MD, DHHS Publication No. SMA 003466.

15. Substance Abuse and Mental Health Services Administration (2002) *Results from the 2001 National Household Survey on Drug Abuse: Volume 1. Summary of National Findings*, Substance Abuse and Mental Health Services Administration, Rockville, MD, DHHS Publication No. SMA 02-3758.

16. Substance Abuse and Mental Health Services Administration (2006) *Results from the 2005 National Survey on Drug Use and Health: National Findings*, Substance Abuse and Mental Health Services Administration, Rockville, MD, DHHS Publication No. SMA 06-4194.

17. Hingson, R. and Zha, W. (2009) Magnitude of and trends in alcohol-related mortality and morbidity among US college students ages 18–24, 1998–2005. *Journal of Studies on Alcohol and Drugs*, (Suppl. 16), 12–20.

18. Substance Abuse and Mental Health Services Administration (2009) *The National Survey on Drug Use and Health Report: Nonmedical use of Adderall® among Full-Time College Students*, Department of Health and Human Services, Bethesda, MD, Available at http://www.oas.samhsa.gov/2k9/adderall/adderall.pdf.

19. National Institute on Alcohol Abuse and Alcoholism (2007) *What Colleges Need to Know Now: an update on College Drinking Research*, Department of Health and Human Services, Bethesda, MD, NIH Publ. No. 07-5010.

20. Johnston, L., O'Malley, P. and Bachman, J. (2000) *Monitoring the Future: National Survey Results on Drug use, 1975–1999, Volume II: College Students and Adults Ages 19–40*, National Institute on Drug Abuse, Bethesda, MD, NIH Publ. No. 00-480.

21. Johnston, L., O'Malley, P. and Bachman, J. (2001) *Monitoring the Future: National Survey Results on Drug use, 1975–1999, Volume II: College Students and Adults Ages 19–40*, National Institute on Drug Abuse, Bethesda, MD, NIH Publ. No. 02-5107.

22. Hingson, R., Swahn, M. and Sleet, D. (2007) Interventions to prevent alcohol-related injuries, in *Handbook of Injury and Violence Prevention* (eds L. Doll, S. Bonzo, D. Sleet and J. Mercy), Springer Science + Business Media, LLC, New York, NY, pp. 295–310.

23. Sober Truth on Preventing (STOP) (2006) Underage Drinking Act. Publ L No. 109-422, US Statutes at Large 120, 2890–2899.

24. Office of the Surgeon General (2007) *The Surgeon General's call to action to prevent and reduce underage drinking*, Department of Health and Human Services, Rockville, MD.

25. National Research Council Institute of Medicine of the National Academies (2004) *Reducing Underage Drinking: a Collective Responsibility*, The National Academies Press, Washington, DC.

26. Klein, T. (1986) *Methods for Estimating Posterior BAC Distribution for Persons Involved in Fatal Crashes*, National Highway Traffic Safety Administration, Washington, DC., DOT HS 807-904.

27. National Institute on Alcohol Abuse and Alcoholism (2002) *A Call to Action: Changing the Culture of Drinking at U.S. Colleges*, Department of Health and Human Services, Bethesda, MD, NIH Publ. No. 02-5010.

28. Goldman, M., Boyd, G. and Faden, V. (2002) College drinking: what is it and what to do about it? A review of the state of the science. *Journal of Studies on Alcohol*, (Suppl. 14), 1–250.

29. Lake, P. (2002) *Keynote Address*, College Alcohol Summit, Pennsylvania Liquor Control Board, Harrisburg, PA.

30. Larimer, M.E. and Conce, J.M. (2007) Identification, prevention, and treatment revisited: individual-focused college drinking prevention strategies 1999–2006. *Addictive Behaviors*, **32**, 2439–2468.

31. Larimer, M.E. and Cronce, J.M. (2002) Identification, prevention and treatment: a review of individual-focused strategies to reduce problematic alcohol consumption by college students. *Journal of Studies on Alcohol*, **14**, 148–163.

32. Lysaught, E.M., Wodarski, J.S. and Parris, H. (2003) A comparison of an assessment/information-based group versus an assessment-only group: an investigation of drinking reduction with young adults. *Journal of Human Behavior in the Social Environment*, **8**(4), 23–43.

33. Neighbors, C., Spieker, C.J., Oster-Aaland, L. *et al.* (2005) Celebration intoxication: an evaluation of 21st birthday alcohol consumption. *Journal of American College Health*, **54** (2), 76–80.

34. Smith, B.H., Bogle, K.E., Talbott, L. *et al.* (2006) A randomized study of four cards designed to prevent problems during college students' 21st birthday celebrations. *Journal of Studies on Alcohol*, **67**(4), 607–615.

35. Collins, S.E., Carey, K.B. and Sliwinski, M.J. (2002) Mailed personalized normative feedback as a brief intervention for at-risk college drinkers. *Journal of Studies on Alcohol*, **63**(5), 559–567.

36. Keillor, R.M., Perkins, W.B. and Horan, J.J. (1999) Effects of videotaped expectancy challenges on alcohol consumption of adjudicated students. *Journal of Cognitive Psychotherapy: An International Quarterly*, **13**(3), 179–187.

37. Murphy, J.G., Duchnick, J.J., Vuchinich, R.E. *et al.* (2001) Relative efficacy of a brief motivational intervention for college student drinkers. *Psychology of Addictive Behaviors*, **15**, 373–379.

38. Neal, D.J. and Carey, K.B. (2004) Developing discrepancy within self-regulation theory: use of personalized normative feedback and personal strivings with heavy-drinking college students. *Addictive Behaviors*, **29**(2), 281–297.

39. Kypri, K., Saunders, J.B., Williams, S.M. *et al.* (2004) Web-based screening and brief intervention for hazardous drinking: a double-blind randomized controlled trial. *Addiction*, **99**(11), 1410–1417.

40. Sharmer, L. (2001) Evaluation of alcohol education programs on attitude, knowledge, and self-reported behavior of college students. *Evaluation & The health Professions*, **24**(3), 336–357.

41. Smith, B.H. (2004) A randomized study of a peer-led, small group social norming intervention designed to reduce drinking among college students. *Journal of Alcohol and Drug Education*, **47** (3), 67–75.

42. Stamper, G.A., Smith, B.H., Gant, R. *et al.* (2004) Replicated findings of an evaluation of a brief intervention designed to prevent high-risk drinking among first-year college students: implications for social norming theory. *Journal of Alcohol and Drug Education*, **48**(2), 53–72.

43. McNally, A.M. and Palfai, T.P. (2003) Brief group alcohol interventions with college students: examining motivational components. *Journal of Drug Education*, **33**(2), 159–176.

44. Peeler, C.M., Far, J., Miller, J. *et al.* (2000) An analysis of the effects of a program to reduce heavy drinking among college students. *Journal of Alcohol and Drug Education*, **45**(2), 39–54.

45. Walters, S.T., Vader, A.M. and Harris, T.R. (2007) A controlled trial of web-based feedback for heavy drinking college students. *Prevention Science*, **8**(1), 83–88.

46. Neighbors, C., Larimer, M.E. and Lewis, M.A. (2004) Targeting misperceptions of descriptive drinking norms: efficacy of a computer-delivered personalized normative feedback intervention. *Journal of Consulting and Clinical Psychology*, **72**(3), 434–447.

47. Neighbors, C., Lewis, M.A., Bergstrom, R.L. *et al.* (2006) Being controlled by normative influences: self-determination as a moderator of a normative feedback alcohol intervention. *Health Psychology*, **25**(5), 571–579.

48. Deci, E. and Ryan, R. (1985) *Intrinsic Motivation and Self-Determination in Human Behavior*, Plenum, New York, NY.

49. Deci, E. and Ryan, R.M. (1985) The general causality orientations scale: self-determination in personality. *Journal of Research in Personality*, **19**(2), 109–134.

50. Lewis, M.A. and Neighbors, C. (2006) Who is the typical college student? Implications for personalized normative feedback interventions. *Addictive Behaviors*, **31**(11), 2120–2126.

51. Turner, J., Perkins, H.W. and Bauerle, J. (2008) Declining negative consequences related to alcohol misuse among students exposed to a social norms marketing intervention on a college campus. *Journal of American College Health*, **57**(1), 85–93.

52. DeJong, W., Schneider, S.K., Towvim, L.G. *et al.* (2006) A multisite randomized trial of social norms marketing campaigns to reduce college student drinking. *Journal of Studies on Alcohol and Drugs*, **67**, 868–879.

53. DeJong, W., Schneider, S.K., Towvim, L.G. *et al.* (2009) A multisite randomized trial of social norms marketing campaigns to reduce college student drinking: a replication failure. *Substance Abuse*, **30**, 127–140.

54. LaBrie, J.W., Hummer, J.F., Neighbors, C. *et al.* (2008) Live interactive group-specific normative feedback reduces misperceptions and drinking in college students: a randomized cluster trial. *Psychology of Addictive Behaviors*, **22**(1), 141–148.

55. Labrie, J.W., Hummer, J.F., Huchting, K.K. *et al.* (2009) A brief live interactive normative group intervention using wireless keypads to reduce drinking and alcohol consequences in college student athletes. *Drug and Alcohol Review*, **28**(1), 40–47.

56. Musher-Eizenman, D.R. and Kulick, A.D. (2003) An alcohol expectancy-challenge prevention program for at-risk college women. *Psychology of Addictive Behaviors*, **17**(2), 163–166.

57. Wiers, R.W. and Kummeling, R.H. (2004) An experimental test of an alcohol expectancy challenge in mixed gender groups of young heavy drinkers. *Addictive Behaviors*, **29**(1), 215–220.

58. Wiers, R.W., van de Luitgaarden, J., van den Wildenberg, E. *et al.* (2005) Challenging implicit and explicit alcohol-related cognitions in young heavy drinkers. *Addiction*, **100**(6), 806–819.

59. Greenwald, A.G., Nosek, B.A. and Banaji, M.R. (2003) Understanding and using the implicit association test: I. an improved scoring algorithm. *Journal of Personality and Social Psychology*, **85**(2), 197–216.

60. Wiers, R.W., Wood, M.D., Darkes, J. *et al.* (2003) Changing expectancies: cognitive mechanisms and context effects. *Alcoholism: Clinical and Experimental Research*, **27**(2), 186–197.

61. Corbin, W.R., McNair, L.D. and Carter, J.A. (2001) Evaluation of a treatment-appropriate cognitive intervention for challenging alcohol outcome expectancies. *Addictive Behaviors*, **26**(4), 475–488.

62. Lau-Barraco, C. and Dunn, M.E. (2008) Evaluation of a single-session expectancy challenge intervention to reduce alcohol use among college students. *Psychology of Addictive Behaviors*, **22**(2), 168–175.

63. Borsari, B. and Carey, K.B. (2005) Two brief alcohol interventions for mandated college students. *Psychology of Addictive Behaviors*, **19**(3), 296–302.

64. McNally, A.M., Palfai, T.P. and Kahler, C.W. (2005) Motivational interventions for heavy drinking college students: examining the role of discrepancy-related psychological processes. *Psychology of Addictive Behaviors*, **19**(1), 79–87.

65. McCambridge, J. and Strang, J. (2004) The efficacy of single-session motivational interviewing in reducing drug consumption and perceptions of drug-related risk and harm among young people: results from a multi-site cluster randomized trial. *Addiction*, **99**(1), 39–52.

66. McCambridge, J. and Strang, J. (2005) Deterioration over time in effect of Motivational Interviewing in reducing drug consumption and related risk among young people. *Addiction*, **100**(4), 470–478.

67. Carey, K.B., Carey, M.P., Maisto, S.A. *et al.* (2006) Brief motivational interventions for heavy college drinkers: a randomized controlled trial. *Journal of Consulting and Clinical Psychology*, **74**(5), 943–954.

68. Murphy, J.G., Benson, T.A., Vuchinich, R.E. *et al.* (2004) A comparison of personalized feedback for college student drinkers delivered with and without a motivational interview. *Journal of Studies on Alcohol*, **65**(2), 200–203.

69. White, H.R. (2006) Reduction of alcohol-related harm on United States college campuses: the use of personal feedback interventions. *International Journal of Drug Policy*, **17**(4), 310–319.

70. Schaus, J., Sole, M., McCoy, T. *et al.* (2009) Alcohol screening and brief intervention in a college student health center: a randomized controlled trial. *Journal of Studies on Alcohol and Drugs*, (Suppl. 16), 131–141.

71. White, H.R., Morgan, T.J., Pugh, L.A. *et al.* (2006) Evaluating two brief substance-use interventions for mandated college students. *Journal of Studies on Alcohol*, **67**(2), 309–317.

72. Chiauzzi, E., Green, T.C., Lord, S. *et al.* (2005) My student body: a high-risk drinking prevention web site for college students. *Journal of American College Health*, **53**(6), 263–274.

73. Saunders, J.B., Kypri, K., Walters, S.T. *et al.* (2004) Approaches to brief intervention for hazardous drinking in young people. *Alcoholism: Clinical and Experimental Research*, **28**(2), 322–329.

74. Larimer, M.E., Lee, C.M., Kilmer, J.R. *et al.* (2007) Personalized mailed feedback for college drinking prevention: a randomized clinical trial. *Journal of Consulting and Clinical Psychology*, **75**(2), 285–293.

75. Barnett, N.P., Tevyaw, T.O., Fromme, K. *et al.* (2004) Brief alcohol interventions with mandated or adjudicated college students. *Alcoholism: Clinical and Experimental Research*, **28**(6), 966–975.

76. Barnett, N.P., Murphy, J.G., Colby, S.M. *et al.* (2007) Efficacy of counselor vs. computer-delivered intervention with mandated college students. *Addictive Behaviors*, **32**(11), 2529–2548.

77. Fromme, K. and Corbin, W. (2004) Prevention of heavy drinking and associated negative consequences among mandated and voluntary college students. *Journal of Consulting and Clinical Psychology*, **72**(6), 1038–1049.

78. Werch, C.E., Moore, M.J., Bian, H. *et al.* (2008) Efficacy of a brief image-based multiple-behavior intervention for college students. *Annals of Behavioral Medicine*, **36**(2), 149–157.

79. LaBrie, J.W., Huchting, K., Tawalbeh, S. *et al.* (2008) A randomized motivational enhancement prevention group reduces drinking and alcohol consequences in first-year college women. *Psychology of Addictive Behaviors*, **22**(1), 149–155.

80. Elliott, J.C., Carey, K.B. and Bolles, J.R. (2008) Computer-based interventions for college drinking: a qualitative review. *Addictive Behaviors*, **33**(8), 994–1005.

81. Butler, L.H. and Correia, C.J. (2009) Brief alcohol intervention with college student drinkers: face-to-face versus computerized feedback. *Psychology of Addictive Behaviors*, **23**(1), 163–167.

82. Neighbors, C., Lee, C.M., Lewis, M.A. *et al.* (2009) Internet-based personalized feedback to reduce 21st-birthday drinking: a randomized controlled trial of an event-specific prevention intervention. *Journal of Consulting and Clinical Psychology*, **77**(1), 51–63.

83. Lewis, M.A., Neighbors, C., Lee, C.M. *et al.* (2008) 21st birthday celebratory drinking: evaluation of a personalized normative feedback card intervention. *Psychology of Addictive Behaviors*, **22**(2), 176–185.

84. White, H.R., Mun, E.Y. and Morgan, T.J. (2008) Do brief personalized feedback interventions work for mandated students or is it just getting caught that works? *Psychology of Addictive Behaviors*, **22**(1), 107–116.

85. Morgan, T.J., White, H.R. and Mun, E.Y. (2008) Changes in drinking before a mandated brief intervention with college students. *Journal of Studies on Alcohol and Drugs*, **69**(2), 286–290.

86. Carey, K.B., Henson, J.M., Carey, M.P. *et al.* (2009) Computer versus in-person intervention for students violating campus alcohol policy. *Journal of Consulting and Clinical Psychology*, **77**(1), 74–87.

87. Carey, K.B., Scott-Sheldon, L.A.J., Carey, M.P. *et al.* (2007) Individual-level interventions to reduce college student drinking: a meta-analytic review. *Addictive Behaviors*, **32**, 2469–2494.

88. Ichiyama, M.A., Fairlie, A.M., Wood, M.D. *et al.* (2009) A randomized trial of a parent-based intervention on drinking behavior among incoming college freshmen. *Journal of Studies on Alcohol and Drugs*, (Suppl. 16), 67–76.

89. Amaro, H., Ahl, M., Matsumoto, A. *et al.* (2009) Trial of the University Assistance Program for alcohol use among mandated students. *Journal of Studies on Alcohol and Drugs*, (Suppl. 16), 45–56.

90. Fell, J., Fisher, D.A., Voas, R.B. *et al.* (2009) The impact of underage drinking laws on alcohol-related fatal crashes of young drivers. *Alcoholism: Clinical and Experimental Research*, **33**(7), 1–12.

91. National Institute on Alcohol Abuse and Alcoholism (2009) Alcohol Policy Information System. Available at http://www.alcoholpolicy.niaaa.nih.gov/. Accessed March 3, 2009.

92. National Institute on Drug Abuse (2008) *Monitoring the Future: National Survey Results on Drug use, 1975–2007: Volume 1: Secondary School Students*, U.S. Department of Health and Human Services, Bethesda, MD, Available at http://www.monitoringthefuture.org/pubs/monographs/vol1_2007.pdf.

93. Shults, R.A., Elder, R.W., Sleet, D.A. *et al.* (2001) Reviews of evidence regarding interventions to reduce alcohol-impaired driving. *American Journal of Preventive Medicine*, **21**(4), 66–88.

94. Wagenaar, A.C. and Toomey, T.L. (2002) Effects of minimum drinking age laws: review and analyses of the literature from 1960 to 2000. *Journal of Studies on Alcohol*, 206–225.

95. O'Malley, P.M. and Wagenaar, A.C. (1991) Effects of minimum drinking age laws on alcohol-use, related behaviors and traffic crash involvement among American youth, 1976–1987. *Journal of Studies on Alcohol*, **52**(5), 478–491.

96. National Highway and Traffic Safety Administration (2003) *Traffic Safety Facts, 2002*, National Highway Traffic Safety Administration, Washington, DC, DOT HS 809-6061.

97. Ponicki, W.R., Gruenewald, P.J. and LaScala, E.A. (2007) Joint impacts of minimum legal drinking age and beer taxes on US youth traffic fatalities, 1975 to 2001. *Alcoholism: Clinical and Experimental Research*, **31**(5), 804–813.

98. Males, M. (2008) Should California reconsider its legal drinking age? *California Journal of Health Promotion*, **6**(2), 1–11.

99. Miron, J.A. and Tetelbaum, E. (2009) Does the minimum legal drinking age save lives? *Economic Inquiry*, **47**(2), 317–336.

100. Fell, J.C., Fisher, D.A., Voas, R.B. *et al.* (2008) The relationship of underage drinking laws to reductions in drinking drivers in fatal crashes in the United States. *Accident Analysis and Prevention*, **40**(4), 1430–1440.

101. Hingson, R., Heeren, T. and Winter, M. (1994) Lower legal blood-alcohol limits for young drivers. *Public Health Reports*, **109**(6), 738–744.

102. Wagenaar, A.C., O'Malley, P.M. and LaFond, C. (2001) Lowered legal blood alcohol limits for young drivers: effects on drinking, driving, and driving-after-drinking behaviors in 30 states. *American Journal of Public Health*, **91**(5), 801–804.

103. Voas, R.B., Tippetts, A.S. and Fell, J. (2000) The relationship of alcohol safety laws to drinking drivers in fatal crashes. *Accident Analysis and Prevention*, **32**(4), 483–492.

104. Liang, L. and Huang, J.D. (2008) Go out or stay in? The effects of zero tolerance laws on alcohol use and drinking and driving patterns among college students. *Health Economics*, **17**(11), 1261–1275.

105. Jones, R. and Lacey, J. (2001) *Alcohol and Highway Safety 2001: a Review of the State of Knowledge*, National Highway Traffic Safety Administration, Washington, DC, Report No. DOT HS-809-383.

106. Preusser, D., Ulmer, R. and Preusser, C. (1992) *Obstacles to Enforcement of Youthful (under 21) Impaired Driving*, National Highway Traffic Safety Administration, Washington, DC, DOT HS 807-878.

107. Voas, R. and Williams, A. (1986) Age difference of arrested and crash-involved drinking drivers. *Journal of Studies on Alcohol*, **47**, 244–248.

108. Wells, J.K., Greene, M.A., Foss, R.D. *et al.* (1997) Drinking drivers missed at sobriety checkpoints. *Journal of Studies on Alcohol*, **58**(5), 513–517.

109. Wagenaar, A.C., Murray, D.M. and Toomey, T.L. (2000) Communities Mobilizing for Change on Alcohol (CMCA), effects of a randomized trial on arrests and traffic crashes. *Addiction*, **95**(2), 209–217.

110. Wagenaar, A.C., Murray, D.M., Gehan, J.P. *et al.* (2000) Communities mobilizing for change on alcohol: outcomes from a randomized community trial. *Journal of Studies on Alcohol*, **61**(1), 85–94.

111. Ferguson, S.A. and Williams, A.F. (2002) Awareness of zero tolerance laws in three states. *Journal of Safety Research*, **33**(3), 293–299.

112. Chaloupka, F.J. and Wechsler, H. (1996) Binge drinking in college: the impact of price, availability, and alcohol control policies. *Contemporary Economic Policy*, **14**(4), 112–124.

113. Dee, T.S. (1999) State alcohol policies, teen drinking and traffic fatalities. *Journal of Public Economics*, **72**(2), 289–315.

114. Chaloupka, F.J., Grossman, M. and Saffer, H. (2002) The effects of price on alcohol consumption and alcohol-related problems. *Alcohol Research & Health*, **26**(1), 22–33.

115. Dee, T. and Evans, W.N. (2001) Teens and traffic safety, in *Risky behavior among Youth: An Economic Perspective* (ed. J. Gruber), University of Chicago Press, Chicago, IL, pp. 121–165.

116. Kenkel, D.S. (1993) Drinking, driving, and deterrence: the effectiveness and social costs of alternative policies. *Journal of Law & Economics*, **36**(2), 877–913.

117. Saffer, H. and Grossman, M. (1987) Beer taxes, the legal drinking age, and youth motor-vehicle fatalities. *Journal of Legal Studies*, **16**(2), 351–374.

118. Sutton, M. and Godfrey, C. (1995) A grouped data regression approach to estimating economic and social influences on individual drinking behavior. *Health Economics*, **4**(3), 237–247.

119. Cook, P. and Moore, M. (1993) Economic perspectives on reducing alcohol-related violence, in *Alcohol and Interpersonal Violence: Fostering Multidisciplinary Perspectives* (ed. S. Martin), National Institute on Alcohol Abuse and Alcoholism, Rockville, MD, NIH Publication No. 93-3496: 193-212.

120. Laixuthai, A. and Chaloupka, F.J. (1993) Youth alcohol use and public policy. *Contemporary Policy Issues*, **11**(4), 70–81.

121. Cook, P.J. and Tauchen, G. (1982) The effect of liquor taxes son heavy drinking. *Bell Journal of Economics*, **13**(2), 379–390.

122. Grossman, M., Coate, D. and Anluck, G. (1997) Price sensitivity of alcoholic beverages in the United States, in *Control Issues in Alcohol Abuse Prevention: Strategies for States and Communities* (eds M. Moore and D. Gerstein), JAI Press, Greenwich, CT, pp. 169–198.

123. Coate, D. and Grossman, M. (1988) Effects of alcoholic beverage prices and legal drinking ages on youth alcohol use. *Journal of Law & Economics*, **31**(1), 145–171.

124. Ruhm, C.J. (1996) Alcohol policies and highway vehicle fatalities. *Journal of Health Economics*, **15**(4), 435–454.

125. Chesson, H., Harrison, P. and Kassler, W.J. (2000) Sex under the influence: the effect of alcohol policy on sexually transmitted disease rates in the United States. *Journal of Law & Economics*, **43**(1), 215–238.

126. Grossman, M., Chaloupka, F.J. and Sirtalan, I. (1998) An empirical analysis of alcohol addiction: results from the monitoring the future panels. *Economic Inquiry*, **36**(1), 39–48.

127. Markowitz, S. and Grossman, M. (1998) Alcohol regulation and domestic violence towards children. *Contemporary Economic Policy*, **16**(3), 309–320.

128. Markowitz, S. and Grossman, M. (2000) The effects of beer taxes on physical child abuse. *Journal of Health Economics*, **19**(2), 271–282.

129. Manning, W.G., Blumberg, L. and Moulton, L.H. (1995) The demand for alcohol: the differential response to price. *Journal of Health Economics*, **14**(2), 123–148.

130. Cameron, L. and Williams, J. (2001) Cannabis, alcohol and cigarettes: substitutes or complements? *Economic Record*, **77**(236), 19–34.

131. Farrell, S., Manning, W.G. and Finch, M.D. (2003) Alcohol dependence and the price of alcoholic beverages. *Journal of Health Economics*, **22**(1), 117–147.

132. Toomey, T.L., Lenk, K.M. and Wagenaar, A.C. (2007) Environmental policies to reduce college drinking: an update of research findings. *Journal of Studies on Alcohol and Drugs*, **68**(2), 208–219.

133. Godfrey, C. (1997) Can tax be used to minimize harm? A health economist's perspective, in *Alcohol: Minimizing the Harm: What works?* (eds M. Plant, E. Single and T. Stockwell), Free Association Books, London, UK, pp. 29–42.

134. Toomey, T.L. and Wagenaar, A.C. (2002) Environmental policies to reduce college drinking: options and research findings. *Journal of Studies on Alcohol*, (Suppl. 14), 193–205.

135. Angulo, A.M., Gil, J.M. and Gracia, A. (2001) The demand for alcoholic beverages in Spain. *Agricultural Economics*, **26**(1), 71–83.

136. French, M.T., Browntaylor, D. and Bluthenthal, R.N. (2006) Price elasticity of demand for malt liquor beer: findings from a US pilot study. *Social Science & Medicine*, **62**(9), 2101–2111.

137. Heeb, J.L., Gmel, G., Zurbrugg, C. *et al.* (2003) Changes in alcohol consumption following a reduction in the price of spirits: a natural experiment in Switzerland. *Addiction*, **98**(10), 1433–1446.

138. Kuo, M., Heeb, J.L., Gmel, G. *et al.* (2003) Does price matter? The effect of decreased price on spirits consumption in Switzerland. *Alcoholism: Clinical and Experimental Research*, **27**(4), 720–725.

139. Gius, M.P. (2005) An estimate of the effects of age, taxes, and other socioeconomic variables on the alcoholic beverage demand of young adults. *Social Science Journal*, **42**(1), 13–24.

140. Gruenewald, P.J., Ponicki, W.R., Holder, H.D. *et al.* (2006) Alcohol prices, beverage quality, and the demand for alcohol: Quality substitutions and price elasticities. *Alcoholism: Clinical and Experimental Research*, **30**(1), 96–105.

141. Zhang, J.F. and Casswell, S. (1999) The effects of real price and a change in the distribution system on alcohol consumption. *Drug and Alcohol Review*, **18**(4), 371–378.

142. Brinkley, G.L. (1999) The causal relationship between socioeconomic factors and alcohol consumption: a Granger-causality time series analysis, 1950–1993. *Journal of Studies on Alcohol*, **60**(6), 759–768.

143. Williams, J., Chaloupka, F.J. and Wechsler, H. (2005) Are there differential effects of price and policy on college students' drinking intensity? *Contemporary Economic Policy*, **23**(1), 78–90.

144. Kuo, M., Wechsler, H., Greenberg, P. *et al.* (2003) The marketing of alcohol to college students: the role of low prices and special promotions. *American Journal of Preventive Medicine*, **25**(3), 204–211.

145. Bishai, D.M., Mercer, D. and Tapales, A. (2005) Can government policies help adolescents avoid risky behavior? *Preventive Medicine*, **40**(2), 197–202.

146. Markowitz, S. (2005) Alcohol, drugs and violent crime. *International Review of Law and Economics*, **25**, 20–44.

147. Dave, D. and Kaestner, R. (2002) Alcohol taxes and labor market outcomes. *Journal of Health Economics*, **21**(3), 357–371.

148. Dee, T.S. and Evans, W.N. (2003) Teen drinking and educational attainment: evidence from two-sample instrumental variables estimates. *Journal of Labor Economics*, **21**(1), 178–209.

149. DiNardo, J. and Lemieux, T. (2001) Alcohol, marijuana, and American youth: the unintended consequences of government regulation. *Journal of Health Economics*, **20**(6), 991–1010.

150. Gius, M. (2002) The effect of taxes on alcohol consumption: an individual level analysis with a correction for aggregate public policy variables. *Pennsylvania Economic Review*, **11**, 79–93.

151. Markowitz, S., Chatterji, P. and Kaestner, R. (2003) Estimating the impact of alcohol policies on youth suicides. *Journal of Mental Health Policy and Economics*, **6**(1), 37–46.

152. Mast, B.D., Benson, B.L. and Rasmussen, D.W. (1999) Beer taxation and alcohol-related traffic fatalities. *Southern Economic Journal*, **66**(2), 214–249.

153. Mohler-Kuo, M., Rehm, J., Heeb, J.L. *et al.* (2004) Decreased taxation, spirits consumption and alcohol-related problems in Switzerland. *Journal of Studies on Alcohol*, **65**(2), 266–273.

154. Sen, B. (2003) Can beer taxes affect teen pregnancy? Evidence based on teen abortion rates and birth rates. *Southern Economic Journal*, **70**(2), 328–343.

155. Xie, X., Mann, R.E. and Smart, R.G. (2000) The direct and indirect relationships between alcohol prevention measures and alcoholic liver cirrhosis mortality. *Journal of Studies on Alcohol*, **61**(4), 499–506.

156. Young, D.J. and Bielinska-Kwapisz, A. (2006) Alcohol prices, consumption, and traffic fatalities. *Southern Economic Journal*, **72**(3), 690–703.

157. Williams, J., Liccardo Pacula, R., Chaloupka, F.J. *et al.* (2004) Alcohol and marijuana use among college students: economic complements or substitutes? *Health Economics*, **13**(9), 825–843.

158. Wagenaar, A.C., Salois, M.J. and Komro, K.A. (2009) Effects of beverage alcohol price and tax levels on drinking: a meta-analysis of 1003 estimates from 112 studies. *Addiction*, **104**(2), 179–190.

159. Treno, A.J., Ponicki, W.R., Remer, L.G. *et al.* (2008) Alcohol outlets, youth drinking, and self reported ease of access to alcohol: a constraints and opportunities approach. *Alcoholism: Clinical and Experimental Research*, **32**(8), 1372–1379.

160. Treno, A.J., Johnson, F.W., Remer, L.G. *et al.* (2007) The impact of outlet densities on alcohol-related crashes: a spatial panel approach. *Accident Analysis & Prevention*, **39**, 894–901.

161. Wechsler, H., Lee, J.E., Nelson, T.F. *et al.* (2002) Underage college students' drinking behavior, access to alcohol, and the influence of deterrence policies. Findings from the Harvard School of Public Health College Alcohol Study. *Journal of American College Health*, **50**(5), 223–236.

162. Weitzman, E.R., Nelson, T.F. and Wechsler, H. (2003) Taking up binge drinking in college: the influences of person, social group, and environment. *Journal of Adolescent Health*, **32**(1), 26–35.

163. Cohen, D.A., Ghosh-Dastidar, B., Scribner, R. *et al.* (2006) Alcohol outlets, gonorrhea, and the Los Angeles civil unrest: a longitudinal analysis. *Social Science & Medicine*, **62**(12), 3062–3071.

164. Lang, E., Stockwell, T., Rydon, P. *et al.* (1998) Can training bar staff in responsible serving practices reduce alcohol-related harm? *Drug and Alcohol Review*, **17**(1), 39–50.

165. Saltz, R.F. and Stanghetta, P. (1997) A community-wide Responsible Beverage Service program in three communities: early findings. *Addiction*, **92**, (Suppl 2), S237–S249.

166. Forster, J.L., McGovern, P.G., Wagenaar, A.C. *et al.* (1994) The ability of young people to purchase alcohol without age identification in northeastern Minnesota, USA. *Addiction*, **89**(6), 699–705.

167. Grube, J.W. (1997) Preventing sales of alcohol to minors: results from a community trial. *Addiction*, **92**, (Suppl 2), S251–S260.

168. Chaloupka, F.J., Saffer, H. and Grossman, M. (1993) Alcohol-control policies and motor-vehicle fatalities. *Journal of Legal Studies*, **22**(1), 161–186.

169. Hingson, R., Heeren, T. and Winter, M. (1998) Effects of Maine's 0.05% legal blood alcohol level for drivers with DWI convictions. *Public Health Reports*, **113**(5), 440–446.

170. Voas, R.B., Tippetts, A.S. and Taylor, E. (1997) Temporary vehicle immobilization: evaluation of a program in Ohio. *Accident Analysis and Prevention*, **29**(5), 635–642.

171. Voas, R.B., Tippetts, A.S. and Taylor, E. (1998) Temporary vehicle impoundment in Ohio: a replication and confirmation. *Accident Analysis and Prevention*, **30**(5), 651–655.

172. Beck, K.H., Rauch, W.J., Baker, E.A. *et al.* (1999) Effects of ignition interlock license restrictions on drivers with multiple alcohol offenses: a randomized trial in Maryland. *American Journal of Public Health*, **89**(11), 1696–1700.

173. Elder, R.W., Shults, R.A. *et al.* (2002) Effectiveness of sobriety checkpoints for reducing alcohol-involved crashes. *Traffic Injury Prevention*, **3**(4), 266–274.

174. Fell, J.C., Lacey, J.H. and Voas, R.B. (2004) Sobriety checkpoints: evidence of effectiveness is strong, but use is limited. *Traffic Injury Prevention*, **5**(3), 220–227.

175. Elder, R.W., Shults, R.A., Sleet, D.A. *et al.* (2004) Effectiveness of mass media campaigns for reducing drinking and driving and alcohol-involved crashes: a systematic review. *American Journal of Preventive Medicine*, **27**(1), 57–65.

176. Snyder, L.B., Milici, F.F., Slater, M. *et al.* (2006) Effects of alcohol advertising exposure on drinking among youth. *Archives of Pediatrics & Adolescent Medicine*, **160**(1), 18–24.

177. Hingson, R.W. and Howland, J. (2002) Comprehensive community interventions to promote health: implications for college-age drinking problems. *Journal of Studies on Alcohol*, (Suppl. 14), 226–240.

178. Holder, H.D., Gruenewald, P.J., Ponicki, W.R. *et al.* (2000) Effect of community-based interventions on high-risk drinking and alcohol-related injuries. *Journal of the American Medical Association*, **284**(18), 2341–2347.

179. Hingson, R., McGovern, T., Howland, J. *et al.* (1996) Reducing alcohol-impaired driving in Massachusetts: The Saving Lives Program. *American Journal of Public Health*, **86**(6), 791–797.

180. Hingson, R.W., Zakocs, R.C., Heeren, T. *et al.* (2005) Effects on alcohol related fatal crashes of a community based initiative to increase substance abuse treatment and reduce alcohol availability. *Injury Prevention*, **11**(2), 84–90.

181. Treno, A.J., Gruenewald, P.J., Lee, J.P. *et al.* (2007) The Sacramento Neighborhood Alcohol Prevention Project: outcomes from a community prevention trial. *Journal of Studies on Alcohol and Drugs*, **68**(2), 197–207.

182. Wagenaar, A.C., Erickson, D.J., Harwood, E.M. *et al.* (2006) Effects of state coalitions to reduce underage drinking: a national evaluation. *American Journal of Preventive Medicine*, **31**(4), 307–315.

183. Clapp, J.D., Johnson, M., Voas, R.B. *et al.* (2005) Reducing DUI among US college students: results of an environmental prevention trial. *Addiction*, **100**(3), 327–334.

184. McCartt, A.T., Hellinga, L.A. and Wells, J.K. (2009) Effects of a college community campaign on drinking and driving with a strong enforcement component. *Traffic Injury Prevention*, **10**(2), 141–147.

185. Saltz, R.F., Welker, L.R., Paschall, M.J. *et al.* (2009) Evaluating a comprehensive campus-community prevention intervention to reduce alcohol-related problems in a college population. *Journal of Studies on Alcohol and Drugs*, (Suppl. 16), 21–27.

186. Wood, M.D., DeJong, W., Fairlie, A.M. *et al.* (2009) Common Ground: an investigation of environmental management alcohol prevention initiatives in a college community. *Journal of Studies on Alcohol and Drugs*, (Suppl. 16), 96–105.

187. Hingson, R., Heeren, T., Zakocs, R. *et al.* (2003) Age of first intoxication, heavy drinking, driving after drinking and risk of unintentional injury among U.S. college students. *Journal of Studies on Alcohol*, **64**, 23–31.

188. Hingson, R., Heeren, T., Winter, M. *et al.* (2003) Early age of first drunkenness as a factor in college students' unplanned and unprotected sex due to drinking. *Pediatrics*, **111**(1), 34–41.

16 Conducting Research in College and University Counseling Centers

Chris Brownson

Counseling and Mental Health Center, Department of Educational Psychology, The University of Texas at Austin, Austin, TX, USA

16.1 Introduction

The preceding chapters of this book outline the many unique factors involved in college student mental health and firmly establish the role of college mental health providers as specialists in this field. As with any specialty, research is a defining cornerstone that helps establish what is unique, identify the competencies for its professionals, and advance the knowledge within the area that leads to best and promising practices to serve the population. While it is important for university counseling centers to engage in research, it can also be challenging because of the high service demands of these environments. Assessment and evaluation have become more common in counseling centers over the past two decades, but the majority of staff members in college counseling centers still engage in little or no scholarly research or writing [1]. Additionally, despite the high value explicitly placed upon conducting both applied and theoretical research by the International Association of Counseling Centers, these activities are currently ranked lowest among counseling center priorities [1].

Student services departments, such as university and college counseling centers, now emphasize student learning outcomes and retention as a means of demonstrating added value to the institution's academic mission. Research is therefore important for the ultimate success of counseling centers. The ability to measure outcomes, accurately assess and demonstrate need, and identify changing trends is a critical component of justifying and maintaining current resources and establishing enhanced funding and support in order to meet the needs of today's students. These data provide a solid foundation upon which to base proposals for increased funding for new positions and programs. As university budgets tighten further in challenging economic times, counseling centers will need to empirically demonstrate both the needs of students and the efficacy of counseling services

A special thanks to Adryon Burton Denmark for her help with this chapter.

---

and programs in order to justify continued and increased resource allocation to mental health services. Furthermore, outcome research is a fundamental part of knowing where and how to efficiently use available resources. Counseling centers must engage in research programs in order to identify emerging areas for which staff might require additional training, develop and evaluate new treatment practices and prevention-oriented initiatives, and emerge as leaders in high-quality mental health care.

16.1.1 Research and Professional Development

In addition to these practical considerations for the importance of research in enhancing counseling center services, an opportunity also exists for counseling center professionals to contribute to the broader field of mental health in unique and meaningful ways. College and university campuses are ideal venues in which to examine the impact of individual, group, and especially public mental health interventions. Outside of the lab, counseling centers are well positioned to conduct research within a defined and relatively easy to reach population in an environment where service provision, mental health promotion, and prevention are generally valued.

Because counseling centers serve not only those students who seek psychological services but also the entire student body, the contained nature of most college and university campuses contributes to an ideal environment in which to create, incubate, establish, and assess population-based mental health interventions. A majority of US colleges and universities provide students with free access to on-campus mental health care [2] and therefore have the potential to collect data on rates and reasons for utilization, diagnostic trends, and treatment outcomes. Innovative programs such as the integration of behavioral health care with traditional medical health care services can be developed and evaluated with relative ease and efficiency at college health centers [3], and the models thus generated can then be generalized to a national health care system. The college health model, which implements universal access and focuses on developing best intervention and prevention practices with an emphasis on interdisciplinary collaboration, has long been promoted as a useful model for guiding population-based health approaches and new directions in a US national healthcare system [4–6].

16.1.2 Challenges to Conducting Research

Although there are many opportunities for university and college counseling centers to conduct research and numerous benefits for doing so, there are also considerable challenges. The greatest challenge for most counseling centers is the high demand for services in the context of limited resources, particularly time and money. In previous chapters it has been mentioned frequently that counseling centers have seen a growing demand for services and increasing severity of student pathology over the past several years. As a result, the counseling center staff is often stretched thin and over-taxed. An increasing demand combined with static or shrinking budgets force counseling center directors to make difficult decisions about what roles their centers can serve, and research efforts can suffer as a result. Traditionally the summer semester was a slower time for counseling centers and therefore provided an ideal opportunity to conduct research, but some have had to reduce staff during the summer in order to provide resources for the longer semesters. Others have been so busy keeping up with service demand in the long semesters that the summer must be used for projects that used to be completed during the regular course of the academic year. Cooper and Archer [1] surveyed counseling center directors and found that lack of time was the most frequently cited reason for not engaging in research, followed by lack of financial support.

A second major challenge to conducting research in counseling centers is that students are often flooded with requests to participate in various surveys. Whether they are being surveyed about their customer satisfaction by the multitude of units that they interact with on campus, they are being solicited by campus researchers, or they are being contacted by any of a host of national surveys, students are at high risk for developing survey fatigue [7]. Some national surveys are actually re-emphasizing paper and pencil options because response rates from e-mail requests are decreasing. Survey researchers would behoove themselves to work more closely together, possibly shortening their surveys while adding items of interest from other researchers to reduce survey fatigue and increase response rates. Also, when looking to randomly survey the university or college student population, using sampling without replacement across all research projects or other techniques that are centrally coordinated by an office of Student Information Services or the Registrar can help to reduce the number of surveys that any given student receives each year.

Another challenge can be obtaining support and approval from university administration, particularly for a topic that might be considered sensitive, as many mental health issues are. Cooper and Archer [2] found that less than 20% of surveyed counseling centers reported moderate or strong institutional support for staff writing and research, compared with over 70% reporting moderate or strong support for attending continuing education workshops. Some administrators view research as a luxury that cannot be afforded in light of the need for service provision and believe that emphasizing research would place an undue burden on their staff and clinical system. It is important to note that there is truth in this perspective, particularly for smaller institutions and understaffed counseling centers. Even without staff and budget pressures, counseling centers are sometimes viewed by administration as solely offices of service and support rather than also part of the academic enterprise of the university. Unfortunately, this view leads to the loss of great opportunities for collaborative research, accessible participant pools, excellent training opportunities for graduate students, interns, and residents, and an environment ripe for practical application of research.

All of these challenges and encumbrances to conducting university and college mental health research illustrate the need to consider the many options available to campus counseling centers for engaging in research. Even in the face of these challenges, choosing the right type of research participation allows for collecting valuable data and contributing to the field within the practical constraints that exist for each campus. What follows are some options to consider for different types of research.

16.2 Types of Research in University and College Counseling Centers

The good news about research in counseling centers is that there is a plethora of choices when considering a program of research. Setting goals for the collection and use of research data, broadly defined, is an important first step. Looking at data that the center currently collects or could easily collect in the course of providing clinical services or prevention programs to students can be a simple starting point. Counseling center staff typically use assessment and evaluation methods to document outcomes or demonstrate accountability, whereas the use of formal research methodology to meet goals such as enhancing understanding of student needs, attitudes and behaviors is less common [1]. Outcome based research, topic-specific research, broad surveys of non-clinical student populations, and clinician/director-based surveys are all options, and are discussed below.

16.2.1 Data Collected from Counseling Center Clients

Most counseling centers collect some type of intake data about client concerns [8,9]. Data collection commonly occurs in the form of self-report problem checklists or scaled symptom inventories. Problem checklists offer some advantages since they:

- are quick and easy for clients to complete

- can be scored efficiently by clinicians

- may help clients to endorse sensitive items that they might not readily report in an interview

- may prepare clients for the intake interview by bringing their attention to specific symptoms.

However, checklists typically fail to assess other important client factors such as problem-solving styles, readiness for change, or level of interference with overall functioning [10].

16.2.2 Center-Specific Data and Intake Instruments

Many counseling centers develop their own problem checklists or inventories; these tend to be derived rationally rather than empirically, and they are frequently perceived as being of great clinical utility but less useful for research purposes since they are not standardized [9]. Nevertheless, this data can provide a great start to a center's research efforts. If the same data has been collected for multiple years, it can indicate changing demographics, presenting concerns, and/or mental health severity of a center's clients, for example. In addition to client self-report inventories, therapist case notes can also be used for research. Random chart review, although time consuming, can yield data on client self-report, assessment of functioning, risk, and some of the more qualitative aspects of psychotherapy. Chart reviews can also offer valuable data about clinician assessment and documentation, an under-researched area in the field of college mental health. Combining quality improvement efforts and peer review with the aim of publishable research would make useful contributions to improving the quality of care for students.

16.2.3 General Intake Instruments

Counseling centers may also draw upon a wide array of established and validated problem rating scales and intake instruments that are not specifically designed for the college student. Although not intended to be a comprehensive list, following are some of the more commonly used instruments:

The Behavioral Health Measure-20 (BHM-20; [11]), is based on the phase model of behavioral health change and assesses progress in the areas of

- *well-being* (distress, life satisfaction, motivation)

- *psychological symptoms* (depression, anxiety, panic disorder, mood swings associated with bipolar disorder, eating disorder, alcohol/drug abuse, suicidal tendencies, risk of violence)

- *life functioning* (work/school, intimate relationships, social relationships, life enjoyment)

- *positive psychology* with the Personal Effectiveness Scale.

The Outcome Questionnaire-45 (OQ-45; [12]) is a standardized outcome and tracking instrument designed to measure change in client distress levels across therapy sessions and following termination [13]. Although the developers of the OQ-45 proposed a three-factor structure of Symptom Distress, Interpersonal Problems, and Social Role Dysfunction, confirmatory factor analysis in at least one study has failed to support the proposed structure [14]. The OQ-45 is often used as a general measure of client distress and to assess the effectiveness of psychotherapy over time [15,16].

Measures such as the Symptom Checklist-90-Revised and the Brief Symptom Inventory (SCL-90-R; BSI; [17]), are commonly administered during intake and may be used to assess therapeutic outcomes [18]. These inventories use Likert-type rating scales to assess presenting concerns and self-reported level of distress in various problem areas. Both the SCL-90-R and the BSI, which is a 53-item abbreviated version that correlates highly with the longer SCL-90-R, assess the degree to which clients were distressed by various problems in the past week across nine factors: somatization, obsessive-compulsive, interpersonal sensitivity, depression, anxiety, hostility, phobic anxiety, paranoid ideation, and psychoticism.

Additionally, counseling centers often use specific screening instruments to assess presenting problems and psychotherapy outcomes, such as the Beck Depression Inventory (BDI-II; [19]), Beck Anxiety Inventory (BAI; [20]) or the Patient Health Questionnaire-9 (PHQ-9; [21]), which screens for depression. Established symptom inventories, whether general or specific, have the advantages of being empirically validated, free (like the PHQ-9) or relatively inexpensive, and easily administered and scored. However, they are not specific to college student mental health, and therefore do not collect information about areas that may be of special concern to college students such as learning problems or academic difficulties.

16.2.4 University and College Student Specific Intake Instruments

Some counseling centers prefer to use intake instruments that directly address college student concerns. Also, with the proliferation of electronic health record management systems (EHRs) for health and counseling centers, university and college specific assessment instruments are more commonly being integrated into these EHRs. This practice facilitates the consistency of data collection, makes the data easier to use and analyze, and aides in the development of data pooling and multi-site studies. These systems have the potential to generate comprehensive, nationally representative data while reducing the testing burden of individual sites and students.

The Counseling Center Assessment of Psychological Symptoms (CCAPS; [22]) is a 70-item assessment and outcome instrument developed by Counseling and Psychological Services at the University of Michigan. The CCAPS uses rating scales to assess college student mental health problems within the previous 2 weeks and includes nine subscales that measure

- depression

- eating issues

- substance use

- general anxiety

- hostility

- social role anxiety

- family of origin issues

- academic stress

- spirituality.

In addition, five freestanding items inquire about dissociative symptoms, cultural/ethnic identity, violent thoughts, and history of abuse.

The Kansas State Problem Identification Rating Scale (K-PIRS; [10]) is a 50-item client concern inventory designed to provide information on both academic and clinical problems reported by counseling center clients in addition to level of interference with functioning, and self-reported readiness to change. The K-PIRS collects basic demographic variables and identifies client concerns at intake across seven clinical factors:

- mood difficulties

- learning problems

- food concerns

- interpersonal conflict

- career uncertainties

- self-harm indicators

- substance/addiction issues.

When used with K-PIRS Form-B, behavior change over time can be assessed as a means of examining therapeutic efficacy.

The first edition of the Standardized Data Set (SDS-I; [41] 2007) is distributed by the Center for the Study of Collegiate Mental Health (CSCMH) at Penn State University for the purposes of standardized data collection, de-identified national data-pooling, and aggregate reporting (see Box 16.1). This inventory represents a set of collaboratively defined data standards for use by college and university counseling centers. The SDS-I was initially derived from the intake materials of more than 50 counseling centers and then refined via

---

Box 16.1   Center for the Study of Collegiate Mental Health

The Center for the Study of Collegiate Mental Health (CSCMH), directed by Ben Locke, PhD, is a national mental health informatics initiative for college and university counseling centers. Penn State University Counseling and Psychological Services developed this collaboration in partnership with Titanium Software. Using automated processes to aggregate de-identified raw data from a national network of counseling centers, CSCMH will provide routine reports of the state of college mental health for providers, administrators, and the public. Currently, participating counseling centers must use Titanium Schedule and integrate the Standardized Data Set, 1st edition (SDS-I) and, optionally, the Counseling Center Assessment of Psychological Symptoms (CCAPS) into their intake procedures. Findings from the 2009 pilot study were presented at the CSCMH conference in April 2009 [41]. Further information is available online at http://www.sa.psu.edu/caps/research_center.shtml.

---

feedback from over 100 counseling centers and guidance from the CSCMH Advisory Board. The SDS-I is flexibly structured with a range of optional and required items, and with the expectation that counseling centers may add additional questions specific to their institution, center, services, or preferences. The SDS-I serves primarily to standardize the type of information that counseling centers gather about clients such as their demographics, activities, and mental health history.

16.2.5 Outcome-Based Research

Outcome-based research provides tremendous value to individual centers and to the larger field. Most of the aforementioned instruments can be used in a pre-post test design to measure treatment outcomes. With the technological advancements that some EHRs offer, historical difficulties of outcome-based research with college students such as frequent moves, changing contact information, and inconsistent therapy attendance are lessened. Outcome-based research conducted at single institutions is difficult to generalize to other centers for comparison purposes because of the differences in clinical systems, scope of care, student concerns, frequency of visits, and a variety of other differences between centers. However, single institution outcome-based research has tremendous utility to the institution, as it is an excellent way to measure the efficacy of the treatment and systems offered at the institution. Individual institution outcome-based research, which is often unpublished, is likely the largest body of research currently undertaken by counseling centers.

16.2.6 Multi-Center Outcome Research

Multi-center outcome-based research can be more complicated to conduct, but often yields more generalizable information for all participating centers. Especially when measuring infrequently occurring phenomena within a population, having a larger, multi-center data set is important to be able to do robust analyses that yield meaningful results. Either an individual or a team must be primarily responsible for implementing this research, which entails a significant amount of work, but participating in this type of study can be quite easy and cost effective, depending on how the study is set up and conducted. Coordinating research between centers requires using the same data collection systems, coordinating a standardized collection schedule, holding many variables constant in analysis, and submitting identical applications to all participating campus internal review boards when necessary.

Another benefit of multi-site outcome-based research is that it generates campus-level data as well as aggregate data from all sites. But, issues of counseling center anonymity need to be discussed in advance, so that all centers are in agreement about the use of the data since some centers might be concerned about data that present an unfavorable comparison to their peer institutions. This is a legitimate concern, since many factors such as student demographics, unique aspects of a clinical system, duration between sessions, level of training of the clinical staff, center funding, staff to student ratios, and myriad other variables influence treatment outcomes. Having an agreement ahead of time about use of comparison data is crucial in making all centers comfortable with participation.

An example of multi-center outcome based research is the first four studies of the National Research Consortium of Counseling Centers in Higher Education (see Box 16.2). In 1991 it implemented its first study, the "Nature and severity of college students" counseling concerns', which was a survey of students seeking counseling services. The primary goal was to establish baseline measures of the severity of students' concerns in order to assess variations in types and severity of presenting problems over the next several years. Students were administered the Counseling Concerns Survey, which was composed of the following instruments: a 42-item Presenting Problems List [23] constructed from lists submitted by 12-member centers, the BSI; [17]), and an 18-item list of

---

Box 16.2   The National Research Consortium of Counseling Centers in Higher Education

The National Research Consortium of Counseling Centers in Higher Education, housed at the University of Texas at Austin's Counseling and Mental Health Center, conducts large scale, national research studies on the mental health issues of college students. The Research Consortium was founded in 1990 under the leadership of David Drum, PhD and Augustine Barón, PsyD, and is currently directed by Chris Brownson, PhD. Participation in the Research Consortium is open to any US institution of higher education, and membership in the Research Consortium changes for each study. The Research Consortium has completed five different studies since its inception, with two studies focusing on clinical student populations, two studies using non-clinical student populations, and one study which sampled the entire student population. The Research Consortium allows individual college counseling centers to participate in research collection with relative ease, and generates campus-level data in addition to national data sets examining various topics of interest to college counseling centers. Manuscripts and further information can be obtained online at http://cmhc.utexas.edu/researchconsortium.html.

family experiences involving various family history, characteristics, and demographic information. Students seeking services at the counseling centers involved in the consortium were surveyed over the course of 12 months, resulting in data from some 3,000 clients from 32 centers. A subsequent study in 1994 used the same Counseling Concerns Survey to assess the mental health concerns of students who had not sought counseling in order to compare data from the clinical sample in the first project to the non-clinical sample of the second project. Each center recruited a diverse sample from students who had not sought counseling at the time of contact, resulting in some 2,500 participants from 28 campuses.

Building on the first two projects, The Research Consortium implemented a psychotherapy process and outcome study to investigate the impact of counseling services on the mental health concerns of college students. Students were recruited for the study during the 1997–1998 school year when they came to the counseling centers for their initial appointment. Clients completed the Counseling Concerns Survey described above and the University of Rhode Island Change Scale (URICA; [24]) before the first session and completed the OQ-45 [12] before each subsequent individual therapy session. Participating counseling centers were also encouraged to have both the client and the therapist complete the Working Alliance Inventory (WAI; [25]) before the start of the fourth session of therapy. Six weeks after the date of termination, the student was mailed the OQ-45 and the Service Satisfaction Scale-30 [26] as follow-up measures. Information about therapist experience and training was collected and therapist theoretical orientation was obtained using Coan's [27] Theoretical Orientation Survey. Data were obtained on 4,500 clients and 241 therapists across 42 centers.

In order to continue establishing a database which includes both clinical and non-clinical samples, the fourth Research Consortium project concentrated on recruiting students who had not sought counseling at the time they were surveyed. They were asked to fill out the same Counseling Concerns Survey booklet that was used in Project 3. Such sampling helped to determine differences in mental health concerns experienced by students who seek counseling versus those who do not avail themselves of such services. This fourth sampling allowed the comparing and contrasting of students' mental health concerns over a 12-year time span (i.e. across the previous three samples). Data were obtained on 1,500 students at 15 colleges and universities. Monographs and publications on the outcomes of these studies can be found at http://cmhc.utexas.edu/researchconsortium.html. All Research Consortium databases are available to researchers upon approval of an application that can be found at the above link. This is another opportunity to engage in research without having to undergo the laborious task of data collection.

16.2.7 Topic-Specific Research

Counseling centers can also engage in research that focuses on one or more topic areas of student mental health. Unlike the analysis of intake instruments or the use of those instruments for outcome-based research, topic-specific research deeply explores a certain symptomatic or diagnostic domain. Data collection may be accomplished in a variety of ways and may either use counseling center client data or random sampling of an institution's student population. Counseling centers can embark upon their own topic-specific research either through a focused analysis of their intake data, through measures that they have devised, or through other available measures. There are also various options for participation in national topic-specific programs and studies. Counseling centers that participate in this type of research are typically entitled to analyzed campus-level data, an analysis of comparisons of the specific campus to the national data, and the use of the institution's local dataset for further analysis.

Participation in topic-specific research that is being conducted nationally varies in the amount of time and resources required from each participating counseling center. Participation fees can also vary greatly depending on the amount of training necessary, the administrative cost of the study, and whether the organization running the study subsidizes its cost. The following are examples of recent and/or ongoing topic-specific research related to college mental health. This list is not meant to be exhaustive.

The Harvard School of Public Health College Alcohol Study (CAS; [28]) conducted four national surveys involving over 14,000 students at 120 four-year colleges between 1993 and 2001. In addition, participating colleges for which students reported heavy alcohol use were resurveyed in 2005. The CAS was designed to provide the first nationally representative picture of alcohol use among college students and to describe the drinking behavior of this high-risk group. In 1994, the first report of the CAS was published, launching a decade of research and debate about college-student drinking behavior. The CAS examined key issues in college alcohol abuse, including heavy drinking on college campuses, the role of fraternities, sororities, and athletic teams, the relationship of state and college alcohol policies to drinking patterns, and the impact of easy access to affordable alcohol. The study also examined other high-risk behaviors among college students including tobacco and illicit drug use, unsafe sex, violence, and other behavioral, social, and health problems confronting today's American college students [28]. Further information regarding the CAS and related publications can be found online at http://www.hsph.harvard.edu/cas/About/index.html.

The National College Depression Partnership (NCDP; [29]) is a national healthcare quality improvement project focused on demonstrating improved depression care and outcomes at college and university health and counseling centers. This project builds upon and expands the College Breakthrough Series for Depression (CBS-D) coordinated by New York University in 2006. The CBS-D is a depression-focused adaptation of The Institute for Health Care Improvement Breakthrough Series model for healthcare improvement. The initiative implements depression screening for students who visit the student health center or counseling center. Seven colleges and universities participated in the pilot and over 71,000 students in primary care were administered the PHQ-9 to screen for the presence of depression and to assess and monitor the severity of symptoms during treatment [29]. The stated goals of the NCDP are to:

- increase student access to effective treatments through a collaborative model for depression treatment, with particular attention to students who traditionally underutilize mental health services

- improve identification and treatment of depression and track patient outcomes across the broader health service, including health and counseling centers

- facilitate better coordinated care in order to expand the safety net for at risk students

- apply methods that optimize existing resources via dissemination of real-world strategies for systematic depression care in college health and counseling centers.

Further information about the NCDP and related publications can be found online at http://www.nyu.edu/ncdp/.

The National Research Consortium of Counseling Centers in Higher Education's (see Box 16.2 above) fifth project, "The nature of suicidal crises in college students", was an in-depth exploration of college and university students' experiences of suicidal thoughts and behaviors. This was the organization's first foray into topic-specific research. Using an 89-item, web-based survey, the study collected both qualitative and quantitative information to increase understanding of the decisions, behaviors, attitudes, feelings, and beliefs of students during a suicidal crisis. This survey gathered information on previous mental health history, lifetime and 12-month data on suicidal ideation and attempts, emotional mood states during the suicidal crisis, help-seeking behavior, who students told about the crisis, events coincidental to their suicidal thinking, and their attributions for why they considered suicide. The study included over 26,000 participants from 70 colleges and universities [30].

16.2.8 Broad Surveys of Non-Clinical Student Populations

In order to understand the mental health concerns that impact students, counseling centers must expand their scope of research beyond the centers' client population to include the general student body. University and college counseling centers not only have an obligation to their student clients, but also a mission that extends beyond the walls of their center. By studying non-clients, counseling centers can better understand the broader mental health needs of the student body, learn why students in need hesitate to seek help, and develop prevention programs targeting populations at-risk for various psychological issues. Many students will never become clients and might not need the individual, group, or psychiatric clinical services available, so counseling centers should explore population-based inter-ventions that apply a public health model to mental health. In order to assess the needs of the population and develop the appropriate interventions, data about the population must be known. Ironically, college students, particularly those in introductory psychology classes, provide an available and convenient sample and are therefore arguably over-represented in general academic psychological research [31–34]. However, much of this research is not necessarily intended to explore college student functioning, nor is it conducted by experts in college mental health. Research of this type may therefore neglect variables that are unique to the college student experience in an attempt to generalize the knowledge gained to the larger population. Below are some of the more common large-scale surveys that are designed specifically for a college student population.

The American College Health Association's National College Health Assessment (ACHA-NCHA; [35] 2009) is a research survey that has collected data about students' health habits, behaviors and perceptions biannually since the spring of 2000. The survey has also included several general items related to mental health and substance abuse. The ACHA-NCHA includes 2- and 4-year institutions of higher education and has cumulative survey responses from over 500,000 students. Participating institutions choose the sample size, target population, and time period for administration, and receive campus-level data. The survey takes about 30 minutes to complete and can be administered in both paper and web-based formats. An updated version of the survey, the ACHA-NCHA II, was released in August of 2008 with a number of new and modified items to capture sleep behaviors, self-injury, and the use or abuse of prescription drugs in addition to an increased number of mental health issues [35]. Further information and related data reports can be obtained online at http://www.acha-ncha.org.

The Healthy Minds Study (HMS; [36] 2009) is an annual, national survey that explores a variety of mental health issues among college students. The survey was initiated by Daniel Eisenberg and implemented through a partnership between the University of Michigan School Of Public Health, the University of Michigan Comprehensive Depression Center, and the Center for Student Studies in Ann Arbor. After the 2005 launch of the pilot study, 13 colleges and universities across the country participated in the 2007 HMS and 15 participated in the 2009 HMS. In addition to generating a national pool of data to inform broadly applicable, evidence-based guidelines for improving student mental health, HMS provides school-specific data to participating institutions about mental health topics including the disease burden of depression, anxiety, and other mental health issues; the unmet need for mental health treatment; barriers to receiving treatment; and attitudes about mental health. Further information and related publications can be obtained online at http://www.healthymindsstudy.net.

The National College Health Risk Behavior Survey (NCHRBS; [37] 1995) was conducted in 1995 among undergraduate students at 2- and 4-year colleges and universities. The survey monitored the self-reported prevalence of behaviors that contribute to health and social problems among young adults in the United States, including tobacco use, unhealthy eating behaviors, inadequate physical activity, alcohol and other drug use, unsafe sexual behaviors, and behaviors that may result in intended or unintended injuries. The NCHRBS questionnaire was developed by the Centers for Disease Control and Prevention (CDC) in collaboration with representatives from universities, national organizations, and federal agencies. The survey was conducted through the mail and questionnaires were received from 4,609 students. The data collected was intended to aid college health and education officials in improving health policies and programs designed to reduce risks associated with the leading causes of mortality and morbidity among college students [37]. A follow-up to this original study is currently under development by the CDC. Further information on the NCHRBS 1995 can be obtained at http://www.cdc.gov/mmwr/preview/mmwrhtml/00049859.htm.

16.2.9 Surveys of Mental Health Providers

While it is important to understand the mental health needs of the college student population and the experiences and treatment outcomes for students who seek help at their school's counseling center, there is also a need to conduct survey research regarding the practices and perceptions of those who provide mental health services on college campuses. Centers that elect to complete these surveys also receive access to national data so that they can compare their campus data to national trends. Some more sophisticated surveys also allow respondents to compare their responses to subsets of national data, such as groupings based on school size. Highlighted below are three national surveys of counseling center directors that provide valuable insight into the current state of college mental health and university and college counseling centers.

The mission of the Association for University and College Counseling Center Directors (AUCCCD) is "to assist counseling center directors in providing effective leadership and management of their centers in accord with the professional principles and standards of Psychology, Counseling, and Higher Education. AUCCCD promotes the awareness of college student mental health through research, education, and training provided to members, professional organizations, and the public with special attention to issues of diversity and multiculturalism" [38]. In 2006, AUCCCD developed and administered the Annual Survey to its membership as a way to increase understanding of those factors critical to the functioning of university and college counseling centers. Topics include staffing issues, director and staff demographics, mental health issues on campus, utilization rates, clinical data, and myriad other issues related to the provision of college mental health services at university and college counseling centers. Results are available at www.aucccd. org.

Maryland's Online Trend Analysis of College and University Counseling Centers began as the Maryland Databank for Counseling Center Directors, founded by Dr Thomas Mayo Magoon in 1964. The Maryland Databank collected national survey data from US and Canadian colleges and universities, and was the first on-going attempt to gather institutional benchmarks in order to define and shape the delivery of counseling and psychological services on college and university campuses. In 2006 the Databank survey was discontinued, and the University of Maryland Trend Analysis of College and University Counseling Centers was created under the directorship of Dr Vivian Boyd. In contrast to the historical Maryland Databank, only a select number of counseling centers are invited to participate in the trend analysis, and each annual survey covers only one selected topic. Additionally, the data collection process has been institutionalized and so does not depend on any one individual to continue the survey. The Maryland Trend Analysis completed its second annual data collection in January of 2008. (V. Boyd, personal communication, 23 April 2009).

The National Survey of Counseling Center Directors (NSCCD) is an annual survey implemented by Robert Gallagher of the University of Pittsburgh. Since 1981, the survey has gathered data about budget trends, current concerns, innovative programming, and administrative, ethical and clinical issues, provided by the administrative heads of college and university counseling centers in the United States and Canada. The goal of the survey is to monitor trends in college counseling centers and to provide counseling center directors with access to data, opinions, and solutions from their colleagues in the field [39]. Additional information can be found at www.iacsinc.org.

16.3 Practical Aspects of Conducting Research in Counseling Centers

Throughout this chapter we have discussed practical considerations in conducting research in counseling centers. Of course, there is no "right way" to do this. Cooper and Archer [1] discuss recommendations for ways that counseling centers can develop a more comprehensive research agenda, including discussing research priorities and research findings during staff meetings as well as actively disseminating project findings to enhance appreciation for counseling center research among both the staff and the larger campus community. But in deciding what direction to take, centers must also consider their available resources of time, money, and staff. Centers must carefully consider their goals for research, which might include generating campus-level data to identify areas of student need, answering a specific question to help develop an intervention, evaluating services for quality improvement, justifying the quality of services to administration or funding sources,

---

Box 16.3   Steps for initiating a research project [40]

1. Pose a question that is both important and answerable.

2. Read the existing literature on the topic and review any recent articles that have asked similar questions.

3. If necessary, reformulate your question so that it can replicate and extend previous work, and will lead to a study that is feasible, interesting, novel, ethical, and relevant.

4. Determine who or what will be the subjects of research, and how they will be sampled.

5. Select outcome and predictor variables, and instruments with which to measure those variables. An ideal instrument is appropriate, objective, sensitive, and specific.

6. Consider collaborating with a statistician early in the process – she or he can contribute to the study design and assist with determining how large the sample must be and how the data will be analyzed.

7. Remember that most research projects start small. Projects often progress from single patient experiences and basic descriptive designs to complex analytic or experimental research endeavors requiring funding and collaboration.

---

or making a contribution to the larger field of college mental health. Centers must also consider the very real issue of administrator support in establishing a course of research. In general, the more specific the research goal and the more circumscribed the investigation, the greater the likelihood of receiving helpful data and avoiding burdening staff.

Of course, having a staff member who is knowledgeable about research methods and data analysis is helpful in establishing a course of research for a counseling center. Clinicians who are contemplating becoming involved with research may perceive their own lack of technical research skills as a barrier. Pato's (1999) recommendations for initiating a research project (see Box 16.3) may be helpful in overcoming clinicians' hesitancy about research [40]. Appointing a research coordinator allows this responsibility to fall to an interested and qualified staff member who can lead the center's efforts.

16.3.1 Campus Collaborations

Counseling centers should also consider what natural collaborations exist on campus that could aid in the pursuit and execution of research projects. For example, there may be faculty members in multiple departments who share an interest in college student mental health. Graduate students in clinical or counseling psychology, social work, sociology, anthropology, and psychiatry residents are often eager to be involved in research. Some centers hire graduate research assistants specifically to help the center reach their research and data analysis goals. Doctoral or master's students working on their dissertations or theses might also be natural collaborators. Defining research goals for the center enables the center to be more proactive in seeking these collaborations. Faculty and graduate students are often looking for involvement in defined projects, and the opportunity to partner with a college mental health content expert makes collaborating with the counseling center more attractive. This is particularly true because, depending on the project, data collection within this well-defined and easily accessible population can be a relatively painless endeavor when compared to some of the challenging data collection issues that researchers typically face.

Before establishing these collaborations, centers should consider the criteria by which the merit of research proposals will be judged. Many centers are approached with research ideas from faculty and graduate students because of the relatively easy access to a clinical population. But collaborations set precedent, and this requires forethought. Counseling center staff should decide whether collaborations will be restricted to a particular group, such as current or former trainees, and whether to consider research projects that further the goals of the college or university faculty member or graduate students, but do not contribute to the center's research goals. Additional questions to be decided include issues of client privacy and care, such as whether non-counseling center mental health professionals will be allowed to intervene with student clients, whether wait list controls or comparison of treatments for student clients will be allowed, and how to ensure client privacy, especially if some of the researchers are graduate assistants. Thinking through some of these issues in advance will help counseling center staff be clear and judicious about the types of collaborations that will be considered.

16.3.2 Ethical Considerations for Research at Counseling Centers

As with all research involving human subjects, consulting with your campus Institutional Review Board (IRB) is a must. Not all projects, especially relatively benign surveys, need full board review, but most research does require an application to the IRB. If you are unsure, it is appropriate to call the IRB to consult about whether an application is necessary. Participation in the IRB application process can be a significant learning experience for graduate students.

Another ethical consideration in research is the protection of your student clients. Any research project sponsored by your center should be voluntary, and should not be a requirement for treatment. Also, any research sponsored by the center should be vetted for student client safety and privacy, and it should be ensured by the center that any interventions used in the research are not harmful to students. Although this is the purview of any university IRB, an extra obligation is placed on counseling center research since the potential participants are not just research subjects, but also the center's clients.

16.4 Future Directions and Conclusion

As with most professional endeavors, conducting research in counseling centers is best accomplished with the support of colleagues, continuing education and professional development, and affiliation in professional organizations. Creating a national professional organization which exclusively serves counseling center research coordinators and other interested professionals would help facilitate collaboration, identify best practices as well as growth areas, educate newer professionals about counseling center research, and support and encourage those who do this important work. Committees exist in some professional organizations to try to fulfill this role, but they have not enjoyed the consistency and broad participation that characterizes other role-specific professional organizations within the profession of college mental health.

Research in counseling centers is at a critical juncture. On the one hand, the proliferation of electronic health records that incorporate intake data, the current emphasis on program evaluation and student learning outcomes, and the national data collection programs of numerous professional, public, governmental, and private organizations have lead to an increase in research opportunities that has helped further define the field of college mental health. At the same time, tighter budgets, increasing service demand, and greater client severity is forcing a difficult balancing act between the service delivery mission of college counseling centers and the ability to do research, which can sometimes be seen as an unnecessary luxury.

However, research is not a luxury, but rather a necessity. Counseling centers operate in a unique environment in the field of mental health, and understanding the unique qualities of that environment is fundamental to the development of best practices necessary to serve the mental health needs of college students. Conducting research in some form should be part of the mission of every counseling center, and such endeavors have the added benefit of strengthening professional identity and career development. Program evaluation initiatives, participation in national surveys, site-specific research efforts, and the contribution of data into decision-making, practice, and resource allocation are vital to the intellectual and clinical growth of a college mental health service. Finally, conducting research is a vital contribution to the field of college mental health.

References

1. Cooper, S.E. and Archer, J.A.J. (2002) Evaluation and research in college counseling center contexts. *Journal of College Counseling*, **5**(1), 50–59.
2. Cooper, S.E., Benton, S.A., Benton, S.L. and Phillips, J.C. (2008) Evidence-based practice in psychology among college counseling center clinicians. *Journal of College Student Psychotherapy*, **22**(4), 28–50.
3. Westheimer, J.M., Steinley-Bumgamer, M. and Brownson, C. (2008) Primary care providers' perceptions of and experiences with an integrated healthcare model. *Journal of American College Health*, **57**(1), 101–108.
4. American College Health Association (2009 March 16) College health and national healthcare reform. Retrieved March 31, 2009 from http://www.acha.org/HealthCareReform2009.cfm.
5. Carmona, R. (2008 June) Keynote address delivered at the opening general session of the Amercian College Health Association 2008 Annual Meeting, Orlando, Florida.
6. Larson, E.A., Barger, B. and Cahoon, S.N. (1969) College mental health programs: A paradigm for comprehensive community mental health centers. *Community Mental Health Journal*, **5**(6), 461–467.
7. Porter, S.R., Whitcomb, M.E. and Weitzer, W.H. (2004) Multiple surveys of students and survey fatigue. In Porter, S.R. ed., *Overcoming Survey Research Problems: New Directions for Institutional Research*, (Vol. **121**), Jossey-Bass, San Francisco.
8. Heppner, P.P., Kivlighan, D.M., Good, G.E., Roehlke, H.J., Hills, H.I. and Ashby, J.S. (1994) Presenting problems of university counseling center clients: A snapshot and multivariate classification scheme. *Journal of Counseling Psychology*, **41**(3), 315–324.
9. Zalaquett, C.P. and McManus, P.W. (1996) A university counseling center problem checklist: a factor analysis. *Journal of College Student Development*, **37**(6), 692–697.

10. Robertson, J.M. (2006) K-State problem identification rating scales for college students. *Measurement & Evaluation in Counseling & Development*, **39**(3), 141–160.

11. Kopta, S.M. and Lowry, J.L. (2002) Psychometric evaluation of the Behavioral Health Questionnaire-20: A brief instrument for assessing global mental health and the three phases of psychotherapy outcome. *Psychotherapy Research*, **12**, 413–426.

12. Lambert, M.J., Burlingame, G.M., Umphress, V., Hansen, N.B., Vermeersch, D.A., Clouse, G.C. and Yanchar, S.C. (1996) The reliability and validity of the Outcome Questionnaire. *Clinical Psychology and Psychotherapy*, **3**, 249–258.

13. Vermeersch, D.A., Whipple, J.L., Lambert, M.J., Hawkins, E.J., Burchfield, C.M. and Okiishi, J. C. (2004) Outcome Questionnaire: Is it sensitive to changes in counseling center clients? *Journal of Counseling Psychology*, **51**(1), 38–49.

14. Mueller, R.M., Lambert, M.J. and Burlingame, G.M. (1998) Construct validity of the Outcome Questionnaire: A confirmatory factor analysis. *Journal of Personality Assessment*, **70**(2), 248–262.

15. Beretvas, S.N., Kearney, L.K. and Barón, A. (2003) A shortened form of the outcome questionnaire: A validation of scores across ethnic groups. Published on-line by The Counseling & Mental Health Center at The University of Texas at Austin. Retrieved on 26 May 2009 from http://cmhc. utexas.edu/rc_project3.html.

16. Kadera, S.W., Lambert, M.J. and Andrews, A.A. (1996) How much therapy is really enough? A session-by-session analysis of the psychotherapy dose-effect relationship. *Journal of Psychotherapy Practice & Research*, **5**(2), 132–151.

17. Derogatis, L.R. and Lazarus, L. (1994) SCL-90–R, Brief Symptom Inventory, and matching clinical rating scales, in *The Use of Psychological Testing for Treatment Planning and Outcome Assessment* (ed. M.E. Maruish), Lawrence Erlbaum Associates, Inc., Hillsdale, NJ, pp. 217–248.

18. Froyd, J.E., Lambert, M.J. and Froyd, J.D. (1996) A review of practices of psychotherapy outcome measurement. *Journal of Mental Health*, **5**(1), 11–15.

19. Beck, A.T., Steer, R.A. and Brown, G. (1996) *Beck Depression Inventory: Manual*, 2nd edn, Psychological Corporation, San Antonio.

20. Beck, A.T., Epstein, N., Brown, G. and Steer, R.A. (1988) An inventory for measuring clinical anxiety: Psychometric properties. *Journal of Consulting and Clinical Psychology*, **56**(6), 893–897.

21. Kroenke, K. and Spitzer, R.L. (2002) The PHQ-9: A new depression diagnostic and severity measure. *Psychiatric Annals*, **32**(9), 509–515.

22. Sevig, T.D. and Soet, J.E. (2006) Mental health issues facing a diverse sample of college students: Results from the College Student Mental Health Survey. *NASPA Journal* **43**(3), 410–431.

23. Draper, M.R., Jennings, J. and Baron, A. (2003) Factor analysis and concurrent validity of a university counseling center presenting problems checklist. A research report of the Research Consortium of Counseling and Psychological Services in Higher Education. http://cmhc. utexas.edu/pdf/FactorAnalysis.pdf.

24. McConnaughy, E.A., Prochaska, J.O. and Velicer, W.F. (1983) Stages of change in psychotherapy: Measurement and sample profiles. *Psychotherapy: Theory, Research & Practice*, **20** (3), 368–375.

25. Horvath, A.O. and Greenberg, L.S. (1989) Development and validation of the Working Alliance Inventory. *Journal of Counseling Psychology*, **36**, 223–233.

26. Greenfield, T.K. and Attkisson, C.C. (1999) The UCSF Client Satisfaction Scales: II. The Service Satisfaction Scale-30. In *The Use of Psychological Testing for Treatment Planning and Outcomes Assessment*, 2nd edn.. pp. 1347–1367. Mahwah, NJ US: Lawrence Erlbaum Associates Publishers.

27. Coan, R.W. (1979) *Psychologists: Personal and Theoretical Pathways*, Irvington, New York.

28. Harvard School of Public Health (2005) College Alcohol Study: About CAS. Retrieved 17 April 2009 from http://www.hsph.harvard.edu/cas/About/index.html.

29. National College Depression Partnership (2009) Retrieved May 5, 2009 from http://www.nyu.edu/shc/about/college_depression_partnership.htm.
30. Drum, D.J., Brownson, C., Burton Denmark, A. and Smith, S. (2009) New data on the nature of suicidal crises in college students: Shifting the paradigm. *Professional Psychology: Research and Practice*, **40**(3), 213–222.
31. Higbee, K.L., Millard, R.J. and Folkman, J. R. (1982) Social psychology research during the 1970s: Predominance of experimentation and college students. *Personality and Social Psychology Bulletin*, **8**(1), 180–183.
32. Miller, A. (1981) A survey of introductory psychology subject pool practices among leading universities. *Teaching of Psychology*, **8**(4), 211–213.
33. Sieber, J.E. and Saks, M.J. (1989) A census of subject pool characteristics and policies. *American Psychologist*, **44**(7), 1053–1061.
34. Stevens, C.D. and Ash, R.A. (2001) The conscientiousness of students in subject pools: Implications for "laboratory" research. *Journal of Research in Personality*, **35**(1), 91–97.
35. American College Health Association (2009) ACHA-NCHA-II. Retrieved 5 May 2009, from http://www.acha-ncha.org/ACHA-NCHAII_announcement.html.
36. Healthy Minds Study (2009) Retrieved 17 April 2009, from http://www.healthymindsstudy.net/.
37. Centers for Disease Control and Prevention (1995) Youth risk behavior surveillance: National college health risk behavior survey. *MMWR Surveillance Summaries*, **46**(SS-6), 1–54, Retrieved 17 April 2009, from http://www.cdc.gov/mmwr/preview/mmwrhtml/00049859.htm.
38. Association for University and College Counseling Center Directors (2009) About AUCCCD. Retrieved 5 May 2009, from http://www.aucccd.org/?page=about.
39. Gallagher, R.P. (2006) *National Survey of Counseling Center Directors*, Arlington, VA.
40. Pato, M. (1999) Generating and implementing research ideas. In J. Kay, E. Silberman and L. Pessar (Eds.), *Handbook of Psychiatric Education and Faculty Development*. Washington, DC: American Psychiatric Publishing, Inc., pp. 181–193.
41. Locke, B., Hayes, J., Crane, A., Schendel, C., Castonguay, L., Boswell, J., McAleavey, A., and Nelson, D. (2009) Center for the Study of Collegiate Mental Health (CSCMH) 2009 pilot study executive summary. Retrieved 5 May 2009, from the Penn State University Counseling and Psychological Services web site http://www.sa.psu.edu/caps/research_center.shtml.

17 International Perspectives: College Mental Health in the United Kingdom

Mark Phippen

Cambridge University Counselling Service, Cambridge, UK

17.1 Introduction

The main issues concerning student mental health being faced in US colleges and universities are also seen in the United Kingdom. Yet there are sufficient differences of style in the way that counselling has developed in UK universities, that the casual observer may be distracted by these differences and miss the considerable parallels. This chapter describes these parallels and differences and further describes the counselling and support services available in UK universities, before addressing the big issues regarding student mental health that are facing counsellors working in UK higher education. The chapter also includes a section on the experience of international students who come to the United Kingdom to study and may require mental health services.

17.1.1 A Brief `US–UK Dictionary'

It has been said that the United Kingdom and the United States are 'two nations separated by a common language'.[1] We use all the same words, but to mean something slightly different. In order that we are not divided by differences in language, here are a few of the likely confusions that are relevant to this chapter:

In this chapter I will be using UK spelling and terminology throughout (Table 17.1).

17.2 Setting the Scene

First we must set the scene as some of the practices that are taken for granted in the US are handled differently in the United Kingdom. The reasons for this are best understood by a very brief look back to the roots of counselling in UK universities.

---

[1] Quote attributed to George Bernard Shaw.

Mental Health Care in the College Community   Edited by Jerald Kay and Victor Schwartz
© 2010 John Wiley & Sons, Ltd.

Table 17.1	US–UK dictionary
American English	**UK English – typical terminology**
College or University (an educational institution)	Also College or University (but only universities have degree-awarding powers)
2-year College	Further Education College (approximate equivalent); they do not award degrees
College (i.e. an academic department within a University, for example College of Engineering)	Faculty or School (e.g. of Engineering)
President (i.e. most senior person in the University)	Vice Chancellor (usually; universities do have a 'Chancellor' but this is a ceremonial role only')
Administration (i.e. senior people in the University)	Management or Senior Management
Professor (generic title for lecturers)	Lecturer or Tutor (A professor is the most senior level of academic staff, and the title 'professor' is not used generally for lecturers)
Faculty (i.e. people)	Lecturers or Academic Staff
Staff	Administration (i.e. clerical employees) ('staff' means any employee, including academic staff)
Student Life, Student Affairs	Student Services (most commonly)
Counselor, therapist	Counsellor (different spelling), psychotherapist, or therapist
Counseling Center	Counselling Service
Licensure	Accreditation or Registration (approximate equivalents)
Practicum (unpaid trainee position)	Placement
Students don't go to 'school' …	… they go to college or university, or 'uni' (only children go to school!)

17.2.1 A Brief History

The oldest universities in the United Kingdom were founded over 800 years ago, but it is only relatively recently that higher (degree level) education was available to a large section of the population. In the mid-1900s less than 10% of the population earned a degree, whereas about 40% now go to university. Access to university is based on school pupils gaining sufficiently high grades at Advanced-level examinations, usually taken at age 18, though universities vary considerably in the grades required for admission.

Virtually all universities are state funded, so there is no public/private divide, though most students have to pay fees to attend. The UK government currently sets a limit to these fees for UK citizens (this applies in England and Wales, while Scottish students pay no fees to attend Scottish universities), so there is little variation in the costs of attending different universities. However, universities can set their own fees for international students. Most degree courses last 3 years (though typically 4 years in Scottish universities).

With the foundation of the National Health Service (NHS) in 1948, all UK citizens had access to medical and mental health treatment free at the point of use. Although many universities had a medical centre for their students, these were normally a part of the NHS provision based on campus. While the NHS did offer psychiatric and psychological support for those with serious mental health problems, it did not offer counselling or support for those with developmental, emotional or relatively minor psychological problems.

Counselling services in universities first appeared in the late 1960s and by the late 1970s it became fairly common for a university to have a counselling service. There were several roots to this growth, but the most influential was the work of US psychologist Carl Rogers and his approach of 'client-centred counselling' (more often termed 'person-centred therapy' in recent decades). This established counselling in universities as an educational and developmental process, eschewing the medical and behavioural psychology models that were more typical at that time within UK health services. It was this stance that kept the counselling and psychology professions largely distinct in the United Kingdom; counsellors were, by and large, humanistic in their approach, and were clear that they were not psychologists, who were at that time commonly working in medical or research settings and using behavioural models. Thus counsellor training grew up separately from that of psychologists. University counselling services employed counsellors, and only rarely psychologists.

In more recent years, these distinctions have been much eroded. For example, psychologists in the UK now work in many approaches, and in 1994 the British Psychological Society formed a Division of Counselling Psychology, and today there is a much broader array of counselling approaches represented amongst counsellors working in universities. However, it is still the case that it is uncommon for university counselling services to employ psychologists.

17.2.2 Counsellor Training and Professional Bodies

The very different nature of counsellor training in the United Kingdom causes much confusion in the United States, and can lead those in the United States to wrongly assume that those working in UK counselling services are poorly trained. Moreover, in the United Kingdom the term 'counsellor' is generally used to encompass counsellors, psychotherapists and cognitive therapists – who in the United States would normally be termed 'therapists'.

Counselling and psychotherapy are currently unregulated professions in the United Kingdom; that is, anyone can call himself or herself a counsellor or psychotherapist, though this situation is likely to change in the next few years. But this also means that, historically, training courses for counsellors and therapists have grown up in an unregulated manner, many outside universities, and range from a brief introductory course to professional level courses taking several years. Moreover, the titles of counselling qualifications are not consistent, but can be generalized as indicated in follows (Table 17.2).

Table 17.2	Levels of counsellor training in the UK	
Typical name of qualification	**Rough description**
Certificate	Introductory course in counselling skills, suitable either for related professionals (e.g. social workers, teachers, clergy) to gain some counselling skills, or for a more focused study of a specific area of counselling work, for example bereavement counselling
Diploma	Basic level of therapeutic counselling qualification. Probably takes two years part-time
Postgraduate diploma	Professional level qualification – the main qualification for professional counsellors. These courses focus on both counselling theory, typically from a particular therapeutic approach, and counselling practice; their prime aim is to train able practitioners rather than theoreticians or researchers. The courses are almost always part-time and last several years, including placements, to gain this qualification.
Masters and doctorates	... in counselling have not existed in the UK until recent years, and those that do are often research degrees rather than practitioner qualifications. This means that very few therapists working in educational settings have a doctorate.

In response to this confusing situation, the main professional bodies for counsellors and therapists developed their own standards for professional practice in the 1970s and 1980s. The UK Council for Psychotherapy[2] (UKCP), originally a professional organization for analytic and psychodynamic psychotherapists, formed its own training bodies offering professional level training, and 'registered' those who had successfully completed these courses. And the British Association for Counselling and Psychotherapy[3] (BACP), originally an organization primarily made up of humanistic and person-centred counsellors, developed an accreditation scheme for counsellors who had completed courses meeting professional standards, and who had been in supervised practice for at least three years and met ongoing standards of professional practice.

17.2.3 Setting Standards for Professional Counselling Practice

The BACP's professional and ethical standards are set out in its 'Ethical Framework',[4] and all BACP accredited counsellors need to subscribe to this. There is also a BACP Complaints Procedure that a client can use to address malpractice, and counsellors can ultimately lose their accreditation and BACP membership if a complaint is upheld, although this does not preclude them from practising as an unaccredited counsellor.

One of the requirements of accreditation is that counsellors are in regular ongoing clinical supervision for at least one and a half hours per month. This is a requirement for as long as a counsellor is practising, not just for counsellors in training, and offers counsellors an opportunity to consider the overall scope of their current work and in particular to think about their difficult cases. Clinical supervision is provided by experienced counsellors, psychotherapists, or sometimes psychiatrists with psychotherapy training, and who ideally have specialist supervision training. This supervision has to be paid for by the counsellor, but most counsellors working in university settings will have this fee paid by their institution.

Thus setting of standards of practice and handling complaints is currently dealt with entirely by the professional bodies, rather than involving government legislation. Hence counsellors in the United Kingdom, when faced with difficult cases or ethical dilemmas will routinely speak with their supervisor or refer to their codes of ethics, but the idea of seeking legal advice would be highly unusual or considered in extreme situations only.

Thus the terms 'UKCP Registered' or 'BACP Accredited' became hallmarks of professional-level work, and are the closest equivalent to licensure in the United States. More recently a third body, the British Association for Behavioural and Cognitive Psychotherapies[5] (BABCP) has also developed an accreditation scheme of a similar standing for cognitive behavioural psychotherapists. (It is possible to be member of any of these organizations without being accredited.) Whilst universities are not legally obliged to employ accredited counsellors, it is usual practice for them to require at least eligibility for accreditation when hiring counsellors.

In 2008 BACP had approximately 30 000 members, UKCP 6500 members, and BABCP 5500 members,[6] though not all these are accredited/registered. Although there are other

---

[2] UK Council for Psychotherapy (UKCP): www.psychotherapy.org.uk
[3] British Association for Counselling and Psychotherapy: www.bacp.co.uk
[4] BACP Ethical Framework: www.bacp.co.uk/ethical_framework
[5] British Association for Behavioural and Cognitive Psychotherapies: www.babcp.com.
[6] All membership figures quoted by BACP in June 2008.

Table 17.3	US–UK equivalent counselling organizations
US organization	**UK organization – approximate equivalents**
American Counseling Association	British Association for Counselling and Psychotherapy
American College Counseling Association	Association for University and College Counselling
Association for University and College Counseling Center Directors	Heads of University Counselling Services

smaller professional bodies for counselling in the United Kingdom, the majority of counsellors employed in universities will be a member of one of these three organizations, and most commonly of BACP.

17.2.4 Organizational Equivalents

BACP has several Divisions for members from different areas of therapeutic counselling, and is alone in having one specifically for counsellors working in further and higher education, the 'Association for University and College Counselling'[7] (AUCC), to which the great majority of counsellors working in universities and colleges belong. A subsection of AUCC is the 'Heads of University Counselling Services'[8] (HUCS). Approximate equivalents to the US professional bodies are included in (Table 17.3):

Note that, while in the United States the AUCCCD is a free-standing organization, in the United Kingdom HUCS comes within the BACP umbrella as part of the AUCC. However, it is often perceived that much of the power within BACP has come from its members working in educational settings, and a disproportionate number of the Chairs (Presidents) of BACP have previously been Chairs of AUCC or HUCS.

17.3 Support Systems in UK Universities – Student Services

Whereas in the United States the overarching structure for supporting students tends to be 'Student Affairs' or 'Student Life', in the United Kingdom this is typically called 'Student Services' and is likely to comprise medical, counselling, careers and disability services as well as support for faith groups. A learning support unit, accommodation service (i.e. housing) and sports service may also be included. In some universities the various student services are co-located in a 'one-stop shop', which is likely to have a centralized reception area for all services, whereas in other institutions the services will have their own separate locations.

17.3.1 Brief Outline of Common Support Services

Here is a brief summary of the most common support services for students in UK universities. Counselling is described separately below in more detail (Table 17.4).

---

[7] Association for University & College Counselling: www.aucc.uk.com
[8] Heads of University Counselling Services: www.hucs.org

Table 17.4	Typical support services within UK universities
Accommodation (i.e. housing)	Whilst most universities offer housing to some of their students, often in residence blocks, there is likely to be an Accommodation Office which also helps students to find housing in the locality.
Careers	Careers Services help students to both discover suitable career areas as well as to locate and apply to vacancies of interest.
Counselling	This is described in more detail in the text.
Disability	Students with disabilities, including physical, mental health and learning difficulties can access a Disability Service, ideally at the application stage, so that information about accessibility and ongoing support can be given.
Faith issues	Most universities will have some form of faith support, typically in the shape of a Chaplaincy or multi-faith centre. Clergy and religious leaders of various faiths will offer both specific faith-based activities, as well as general pastoral support to anyone who seeks it.
International	International students make up a sizable minority of many university populations and an International Office will help students from outside the UK with visa enquiries (where relevant) and will usually be involved with orientation and some ongoing support. (There is more about the experience of international students in the UK in the last section of this chapter.)
Medical	Not all universities have on-campus medical facilities. Reorganizations and changes in NHS funding models have meant that many university health centres have closed down as students can access the general NHS provision in the locality.
Sports	University sporting clubs and facilities are sometimes included within Student Services
Student Union	All universities will have a Student Union, which is commonly run by sabbatical student officers (usually recently graduated students elected to paid work full-time for a year). They tend to run social events and sometimes offer advice to students on practical and welfare issues.

17.3.2 Counselling Services

The very great majority of UK universities have a counselling service of some form. They will be professionally staffed with therapists, often representing several different counselling approaches, with the most common being person-centred, psychodynamic and integrative; cognitive behavioural psychotherapists may also be included in the team; currently they are a small but growing group.

Here are some key statistics about university counselling in the United Kingdom:[9]

- The ratio of counsellors to students varies widely, with the best staffed counselling services having a ratio better than 1 : 2000, but the average is about 1 : 4000

- The most common presenting problems are depression, anxiety, academic problems and relationship problems.

- About two-thirds of services operate a waiting list system, with these services having an average waiting time of 1–2 weeks for a student to be seen, though this may be longer at the busiest times of year.

---

[9] All information drawn from AUCC Annual Survey of Student Counselling Services, using the most recent data available, mainly from 2006–2007.

- The percentage of students who use a counselling service in any year varies widely between universities, but 3%–6% is the typical range. (NB this is governed more by levels of counselling resources than by the degree of student need!)

- Students are typically seen about five times each on average, though over 60% of services do not impose a session limit.

- About one third of services feel vulnerable in some way, for example to reductions in resources or staffing, or having to work more briefly then they feel is appropriate.

Although the counsellor to student ratio probably seems poor compared to US averages, it should be said that UK counselling services tend to have a narrower sphere of activity – that is for the most part to undertake one-to-one counselling with students who request counselling. Some services offer a group or workshop programme, but except in a few universities, this is not usually done on a large scale. Mandated referrals are rare and are generally discouraged by counsellors. Outreach and preventative work tends to be relatively small scale and undertaken where time and resources allow, although counsellors do see this work as being important.

Although there is sometimes a visiting psychiatrist in the service, the counselling service would not include any role in monitoring students' medications, which would be undertaken by the medical centre, or more often, by the student's General Practitioner (GP; part of the NHS; this is described in greater detail below).

17.3.3 Liaison Between Services

Liaison and cross referral arrangements between services tend to vary considerably depending on the particular line-management structures in place and the physical location of the services, but counselling services will tend to have particularly close working relationships with both the medical and the disability services.

17.4 Student Mental Health – A Growing Issue

For years counsellors working in further and higher education have reported a growth in the severity and complexity of the problems that students present at counselling services. Much of this reporting is impressionistic and anecdotal, but the commonly held notion is that, 20 years ago, students would present with straightforward life-change and developmental issues such as:

- Homesickness

- Relationship problems, for example boy- or girlfriend difficulties

- Anxiety about examinations (test anxiety)

- whereas nowadays, the presentations will commonly include:

- Long-standing disordered eating

- Personality disorders

- Self-harming behaviour of one kind or another.

It is fair to say that, because there is little longitudinal 'hard' evidence to back up this perception, some researchers are unconvinced that there is such a dramatic change [1]. However, counsellors working in the field tend to have little doubt on the matter and would point to the following factors to explain the phenomenon.

The `widening participation' agenda

Over recent decades the UK government has greatly increased the percentage of the population who attend further or higher education, and it has also encouraged universities to accept potentially able students from sections of society who have traditionally never considered staying in education beyond high school. In the 1960s about one in ten school leavers went on to university; now that figure is over 40% and rising. This has been a very welcome initiative, but it has meant that the student population now much more closely reflects the general UK population, including the general range of health and mental health issues in the general population. It also includes many more students who are the first generation in their families to attend university, so many come with a limited idea of the challenges they will be confronting.

A more complex world

Most would accept that over the last generation the 'world' students inhabit has become much more complex and the traditional support systems fewer.

- In the United Kingdom the affinity between the majority of students and alcohol is not new; the legal drinking age is 18, but many people are drinking well before this age. In recent years there has been a national trend, not just amongst students, to consuming larger amounts of alcohol and in particular to binge drinking.

- Similarly, the existence of 'recreational' drugs on campus is not new, but the acceptance of their use and the strength of the substances available have grown, as has the evidence of a link with resulting mental health problems for some users.

- Young people face choices about their sexual behaviour at seemingly ever-younger ages and many students are in sexual relationships.

- Meanwhile there has been a growth in eating disorders, not just amongst students. But as the media has highlighted both the 'ideals' of appearing slim, as well as the growing incidence of anorexia, bulimia and other patterns of disordered eating, this has been reflected amongst the student population, perhaps particularly amongst those who are highly competitive perfectionists.

- Alongside these changes, in the last decade or so, the means of funding higher education has changed substantially, with the majority of students paying significant course fees and coping with levels of student debt that were unheard of in the United Kingdom until quite recently.

To exacerbate matters further, the sources of support and security available to students have tended to diminish and any sense of stability has been undermined by trends such as the greater incidence of family breakdown. The Children's Society, a respected national charity in the United Kingdom, has recently published a report on the changing lives of young people [2], which supports these impressions.

It should also be noted that university counselling services in the United Kingdom rarely have a major role in relation to students whose primary problems are alcohol or drug addiction. In part this is because relatively few such students present at counselling services seeking help (and mandated referral is very unusual), and partly because these are areas of work which are seen as requiring specialist training which most counsellors working in this setting will not have. However, there are specialist drug and alcohol agencies in most parts of the country to which students can turn or be referred.

Academic changes

In the last 20 years or so the staff:student ratios at most universities have deteriorated considerably and an increasing proportion of academic staff have part-time contracts. Meanwhile the pressure on many academics to publish has increased. Taken together, these changes have greatly eroded the amount of time academic staff have to fulfil the traditional role of being a 'tutor' – that is a member of academic staff who knows a group of students, follows and advises on their academic progress, and is also available to offer friendly support over personal or emotional issues. This role has never been conceived of as being a therapist, rather as a friendly and supportive 'first port of call' in difficulty. Although the title of 'tutor' still exists in most universities, there is frequently little real relationship there, and students and tutors often do not even know each other by sight; only in the most competitive universities does the role still have significance.

Over the same period most universities have changed from offering 3-year courses in which a cohort of students would, by and large, remain as one group, to having a modularized semester system of course delivery, in which students will probably only work under the same lecturers and alongside the same peer-group for a matter of weeks. Whilst this offers greater flexibility and choice, it also tends to result in a reduced sense of cohesion amongst student cohorts and a greater risk of isolation. In some universities it is not uncommon for students to feel that there is no one who knows them personally over any period of time, or who would notice if they were struggling in some way.

Moreover, higher education has tended to become a much more competitive environment, where students feel a strong need to get a good CV (résumé) in order to get the job they want. University is less often about discovering who you are or 'having a good time', and has become a much more serious endeavour upon which one's future depends.

17.4.1 The Evidence and Universities' Response

In 2003 the Royal College of Psychiatry, the professional body for psychiatrists in the United Kingdom, looked at the evidence for the growth in mental health problems amongst students and produced a very influential report on 'The Mental Health of Students in Higher Education' [3]. Its conclusions and recommendations are summarized on its web site as:

1. The number of students presenting with symptoms of mental ill health has increased in recent years, as has the number of students presenting with more severe mental health problems. Drug and alcohol misuse is a serious and growing concern.

2. Students report increased mental health symptoms compared with age-matched controls, but there is no evidence to confirm that students are more likely to suffer mental illness.

3. Higher education is associated with significant stressors, including the emotional demands of transition from home and school to the less structured environment of college, independent study and examinations, and financial pressures. While stress is not pathological in itself, these factors may contribute to the higher rate of emotional symptomatology amongst students.

4. Mental health problems in students may be seriously disruptive to their education and emotional development.

5. Students in higher education are at no higher risk of suicide than the general population, and may be at lower risk.

6. The increased numbers of students seeking help with mental health problems may reflect:

   • The increasing numbers of students entering higher education;

   • The progressive approximation of the characteristics of the student population to the general population;

   • The increasing willingness of young people to seek help for a range of emotional and mental health problems.

7. University counselling services are the primary mental health care option for many students, and should be resourced accordingly.

8. Nationally agreed policies should be developed to ensure continuity of mental health care between the student's home area and the university, and to preclude conflicts between home and college NHS providers about funding.

9. Local networks should be developed to ensure shared policies and co-operation between colleges, primary care services, mental health services, and other relevant agencies [3].

One recommendation in particular, though, was double-edged. Recognizing that university counselling services were 'primary mental health care' facilities and 'should be resourced accordingly' created the expectation but not the funding, as there was no suggestion that NHS mental health funding should be used to fund university counselling. However, university counselling services warmly welcomed this report, and in many cases were able to use it to successfully argue for increased resources from their institution.

Various other developments in university counselling followed the publication of this report.

• University authorities have generally accepted that the growth in mental health problems amongst their student populations is something that they have to respond to in some way; this was not simply a matter of complaining counsellors!

- 'Universities UK' (the national body for university Vice Chancellors) together with the Standing Conference of Principals (now called GuildHE),[10] set up a 'Committee for the Promotion of Mental Well-Being in Higher Education', which has continued to highlight the issue to senior people in universities nationally.

- University counselling services have made a greater effort to build useful and workable links with local NHS mental health services, though it is reasonable to say that the outcome of these efforts has been patchy, that is, it has resulted in an effective working partnership in some areas, while in others it has stalled or met with no interest.

- And perhaps most significantly, there has been a rapid growth in the number of universities employing specialist 'mental health advisors'.

This last point is worth expanding upon. Whilst the titles for Mental Health Advisor posts, their location within the university and the precise nature of their roles vary, the common thread is uni-versities' desire to respond to the growing mental health problems amongst the student population. Mental Health Advisors tend to have either a mental health nursing or social worker background, or are sometimes clinical psychologists, and their roles often include some of the following:

- Liaison with prospective students who declare a mental health disability prior to university admission, to establish their requirements and advise of appropriate funding under the Disabled Students Allowance

- Assessment and case support to students with emerging mental health difficulties

- Liaison with appropriate university staff and tutors on these students' behalf

- Referral of such students to and liaison with relevant support services in the university

- Developing links with local NHS mental health services in order to facilitate referrals to these services

- Coordination of 'mentors' engaged (and usually funded by the Disabled Students Allowance) to provide support to students with specific issues such as Asperger's syndrome.

- Work with the counselling service and others to help in the containment of student crises involving mental health issues

- Contribute to the development of university policies, procedures and good practice in relation to students with mental health problems.

- And in some cases to be involved in maintaining a 'risk register' of students whose mental health might result in harm to themselves or to others – though this is an area fraught with

---

[10] GuildHE web site: www.guildhe.ac.uk

practical, ethical and legal constraints, and many universities are only recently beginning to grapple with this issue.

Although the numbers of students with serious mental health disorders may be relatively small, they can require significant support and a 2008 survey[11] by 'Universities UK' showed that 79% of universities now have such a post, a considerable rise since their previous survey on the subject.

One of the rather practical but important issues that universities face in employing such personnel is where they will be located, and there is no consensus amongst universities on this point. In some, the Mental Health Advisor will be part of the university's Health Centre where one exists, but more often they are located either within the disability service or the counselling service. The advantages for their being within disability include the legal responsibilities that lie upon institutions in regard to supporting students with disabilities (which include many mental health conditions), but the disadvantage to the counselling service is that the responsibility and funding for supporting these students is split, and a number of counselling services have found their funding static while additional resources have been put into mental health workers within disability services.

17.4.2 UK Disability Legislation and Mental Health

The main legislation in the UK relating to discrimination on the grounds of disability is the Disability Discrimination Act (DDA), 1995, revised in 2006. A Disability Rights Commission booklet[12] describes the intention of the legislation as being to:

- Prohibit discrimination and harassment against disabled people

- Ensure that 'reasonable adjustments' are put in place for disabled people

- Ensure full and equal participation in learning and public life.

and goes on to say that the Act has a very broad definition of a disability, including:

- Physical or sensory impairments

- Mental health difficulties, such as depression

- Specific learning difficulties, such as dyslexia

- Health conditions, such as Alzheimer's, human immunodeficiency virus, epilepsy, arthritis and cancer.

The impairment must have:

- A substantial, adverse effect on a person's ability to carry out normal day-to-day activities

- Lasted for at least 12 months, or be likely to last for 12 months or more.

---

[11] "Universities UK" is the national organisation for UK university Vice Chancellors. This figure comes from their 2008 survey on mental health provision, not yet published; quoted from a personal communication.
[12] Disability Rights Commission (2007) Understanding the Disability Discrimination Act, available from: http:// 83.137.212.42/sitearchive/drc/library/publications/education/understanding_the_disability_d.html

It is clear that people with a long-standing mental health condition are covered by the Act, meaning that universities and colleges have a duty to make 'reasonable adjustments' to ensure that these students may participate without a 'substantial disadvantage' compared with other students. Moreover, institutions have a responsibility under the DDA, not just to respond when a student declares that they have a disability, but also to promote disability equality.

Amongst other things, this means that institutions offer opportunities for students to declare a disability prior to arrival at the start of their course. Where a student does declare a disability under the terms of the DDA the institution is deemed then to know about the disability and the student can reasonably expect that relevant people on their course will know about their disability and have considered what implications there are, if any, and have considered what adjustments might need to be made.

Students can also inform the institution about a disability at any later stage on their course, but they cannot expect adjustments to have been made if they have a disability they have not declared. (It is worth noting that, due to confidentiality rules within counselling services, it is accepted for practical purposes that a student telling a counsellor about a disability is not deemed to have told the institution, unless they also ask the counsellor to do so.)

The DDA applies equally to all students, including international students studying in the United Kingdom. However, while UK students may apply for Disabled Students Allowance, which is a state benefit, to help fund special equipment or support they may need, this is not open to international students. This leaves institutions in a difficult financial position, as they are required under the DDA to make reasonable adjustments for all disabled students including international students.

This legal responsibility to support students with mental health difficulties falling within the scope of the Act is very much to be welcomed, but can lead to some confusion within a university or college over where responsibility for support for mental health issues lies: does a student with a mental health problem go to the college's disability service, or to the counselling service? In practice, the answer is likely to be both, as disability services are good at supporting students to access the support they need, but the counselling service is likely to be high on the list of places where such support is delivered.

17.4.3 The Impact of the NHS on University Counselling Services

The existence of NHS in the United Kingdom has a considerable impact on the nature of the work conducted by counselling services in universities and colleges. Counselling services do not get directly involved with medical or psychiatric diagnoses or prescribe clients' medications, as they are not staffed with medically qualified personnel, and these tasks are handled by the health services. However, it is necessary for there to be good liaison and referral routes between the counselling and health services, and counsellors will be very alert to the signs of potential mental ill health in the students they see.

Whilst the NHS system has many strengths, it has also historically had some weaknesses, including long waiting times for some referrals and some kinds of treatment. Although the government has increased NHS funding in recent years with the aim of reducing waiting times, problems remain and some of these relate specifically to providing services to students.

NHS services work on the assumption that a person is resident in one area, that is where they are registered with their GP; moreover they do not record the fact that someone is a student. Of course, it is common for students to spend a part of the year living in their college or university, and the rest of the year elsewhere, perhaps at the parental home. This can result in unhelpful scenarios, such as a student being referred by their GP to a specialist (say, psychiatrist), and by the time they are notified of this appointment they are back home and unaware that they are missing the appointment, only to later find that their referral has been cancelled and the process has to start again. Although GPs can refer to specialists in other parts of the country, this tends to be rather 'hit or miss' as the GP is likely to be most familiar with the specialists and services in their own locality. And again, the timescales may well mean that the student is by then back at university!

There is further information about students accessing NHS services in the final section of this chapter, written for international students who are studying in the United Kingdom. However, the next two sections outline the growing impact on university counselling which has come from the National Institute for Health and Clinical Excellence (NICE), a government-sponsored organization, and from the NHS 'Improving Access to Psychological Therapies' initiative. Furthermore, at the time of writing, the registration of the counselling profession is about to have a significant impact.

The influence of nice

Just as health systems which are primarily funded by patients' health insurance may be influenced by what insurers are prepared to pay for, in the United Kingdom NICE advises the NHS on what treatments and medications are considered to be both clinically and cost effective.

NICE is a government-sponsored but independent organization charged with examining the clinical and research evidence (particularly from randomized controlled trials) of the effectiveness of treatments, and the guidelines they produce are a major factor in determining the treatments and medications that are used throughout the NHS. Whilst their guidelines are mainly concerned with physical health conditions, mental health and talking therapies are increasingly included. NICE Guidelines are public documents, and can be accessed from their web site.[13]

Many mental health conditions, including common problems such as anxiety and depression are covered by NICE Guidelines. These tend to recommend a combination of medication and talking therapy. NICE has therefore looked at the research evidence for the effectiveness of various forms of talking therapy, and in the main recommends cognitive behavioural therapy (CBT), saying that there is insufficient evidence (i.e. insufficient research) for the use of most other therapeutic approaches to be recommended.

Although university counselling services are not a part of the NHS (as they are funded by the universities out of student fees), and are not bound by NICE Guidelines, these are inevitably having an impact here too. While it is still the case that the majority of counsellors working in colleges and universities are person-centred, psychodynamic or integrative in approach, the majority of referrals to university counselling services from GPs now suggest students are offered CBT. This mismatch is leading to a degree of tension: counsellors who are very experienced in working with students are clear about the effectiveness of their work, but are not employed or funded in a manner to enable them to undertake significant research to prove their effectiveness. Moreover, they can resent referrals from GPs who recommend

---

[13] NICE Guidelines can be downloaded from their web site: www.nice.org.uk/Guidance/Topic.

only CBT, without their actually knowing much about the variety of therapeutic approaches available. While university counselling services are sometimes now employing CBT therapists, these are currently a small minority of the therapists employed.

`Improving access to psychological therapies'

There is another level to this area of tension.

With government support and additional funding, the NHS is in the process of reorganizing its mental health services. One significant new venture is called Improving Access to Psychological Therapies (IAPT), which is intended to offer readily accessible help to those who have common mild to moderate psychological problems, such as anxiety and depression. The principle is to offer a 'stepped care' approach, with people receiving the minimum intervention necessary to treat their symptoms. Thus, following initial assessment, a person may be given self-help strategies, or offered guided self-help or computerized CBT, and only if they need more support will they receive either short-term or longer-term CBT (or a very limited range of other therapeutic interventions, eye movement desensitization and reprocessing including or interpersonal therapy). The scheme is described fully on its web site.[14]

Hence the IAPT scheme is employing and training staff to offer 'low intensity' and 'high intensity' support. The 'low intensity workers' will have a very basic training and a manualized approach, with only the 'high intensity workers' being fully experienced and accredited (mainly cognitive behavioural) therapists.

The roll-out of IAPT in the United Kingdom is happening during the 2008–2011 period and at the time of writing (2009) it is rather early to say what impact this will really have. However, the current general view of the IAPT scheme amongst counsellors working in educational settings may be summarized by the following:

- The increase in psychological help offered by the NHS is to be welcomed.

- While the stepped care, low/high intensity approach sounds fine as a plan, there is some scepticism that it will work quite as smoothly in real life.

- There is worry that the very basic level of training that low-intensity workers are receiving will not be sufficient for them to offer a professional service.

- There is a degree of anger that the scheme focuses so heavily on offering CBT as the treatment of choice.

The coming registration of counsellors in the united kingdom

As already mentioned, counselling in the United Kingdom has grown up in a rather haphazard manner and has developed ethical and professional standards via several professional bodies, who have also instituted accreditation schemes for those meeting these standards. Following a lengthy push by the British Association for Counselling and Psychotherapy for the government to regulate counselling, this has now been accepted and a decision taken that counselling will come under the Health Professions Council (HPC). The HPC currently regulates about a dozen professions allied to medicine,

---

[14] Improving Access to Psychological Therapies web site: www.iapt.nhs.uk

including dieticians, occupational therapists, podiatrists, physiotherapists and speech therapists.

However, the decision for the counselling profession to be regulated by the HPC has caused some division amongst counsellors. There are those who welcome the state recognition and protection of the title that will follow, but there are others who feel strongly that this will remove the scope for counsellors to reflect thoughtfully on their work, and replace it with a bureaucratic and rigidly systematized approach, and moreover will medicalize a process that is (in the main) about personal fulfilment and well being, maintaining satisfying relationships and personal direction, which are not medical issues.

The final outcome of this regulatory process is not yet known – it is expected to take effect in 2010 or 2011. Counsellors working in universities will almost certainly in practice need to be on the HPC register; this is an issue that is being followed with interest, as well as some concern.

17.5 The Experience of International Students in the United Kingdom

We now turn to the question of study abroad and look briefly at the experience and support available to students who come to the United Kingdom to study.

Studying abroad is a great way for students to further their education as well as their experience of the world, as well as helping them to get to know and understand themselves better. While some particularly adventurous students may want to trek in a jungle or go to remote corners of the Earth, most will feel reassured to have the relative security of an educational institution to go to, confident that there will be help with sorting out the practicalities of housing, and so on and the structure of an educational programme. However, most students will underestimate how much the regular routines and familiarity with their home and college environment, and their friends and family matter; they tend to take these for granted. But even in the safe surroundings of a college or university in another country, once these familiar places and people are taken away, most people will be surprised at how unsettled they feel, at least to start with. Not knowing anyone, or understanding the expectations of the new university, or how the phone system and banks work, or the value of things in a different currency – all these are likely to lead even the most confident student to feel initially uneasy.

This section of the chapter is not a full exploration of the pros and cons of studying abroad, but does mention some of the issues that international students may face in coming to the United Kingdom, and in particular, highlights the issues and support available to students who experience some level of mental health difficulty whilst here.

17.5.1 Culture Shock Applies

Although some think of the United Kingdom as the '51st State', most visitors find it more different from the United States than they expect. Although we speak the 'same' language, do most of the same things and watch many of the same TV programmes, there are a host of subtle and not so subtle differences that can leave the visiting student puzzled. Before they come, it is worth their while reading up on 'culture shock', because to some extent this is likely to apply.

Here are a few of the differences students may find within the academic environment:

- Academic teaching styles can be very different, particularly at the most competitive UK universities, which tend to have a much less structured programme and encourage more self-directed study. Although US students often start out by thinking that this looks easy, many struggle with the responsibility that this puts on them to organize their own work and to make effective use of the opportunities.

- Students from cultures where it is the norm to accept the word of their lecturers, are likely to find it strange where discussion with academics – even challenging their views – is encouraged, as thinking independently and grappling with the topic is valued.

- Academic assessment schemes in the United Kingdom are often different from those in a student's home country. To those students used to getting 'perfect' grades (e.g. GPA 4.0), the UK system can be a shock as it is impossible to do the same under the most commonly used UK grading schemes, where achieving over 70% for a written assignment is exceedingly hard. (Of course, this doesn't mean that they are suddenly doing badly, just that the grading scheme is different!)

- While studying abroad is an opportunity to meet different people and gain new friends, it is not uncommon for international students to find it harder than expected to form real friendships with UK students. This isn't really disinterest, but what is often called 'British reserve' – simply that a national characteristic is that British people tend not to 'wear their hearts on this sleeve' and take a little more time to make friendships. But once a friendship is formed it can last a lifetime. Of course this is a generalization, and there will be exceptions in all directions.

17.5.2 Accessing Support

If a student needs some support while at university or college in the United Kingdom, here are some good starting places:

- Student-run organizations: the Student Union and International student societies are good places to get information and advice from others students who 'know their way around' or are also from the same part of the world.

- University tutors or academic supervisors (titles vary) should be good people to give guidance over academic matters

- There will be counselling and disability services, which are probably found most easily from the institution's web site. (A national web site listing university counselling services is the 'Student Counselling in UK Universities' web site).[15]

- Students will need to register with a local GP practice to get prescription medication.

---

[15] Student Counselling in UK Universities web site: www.student.counselling.co.uk

17.5.3 For Students with Mental Health Problems

Students who have a pre-existing mental health condition would be well advised to take a while to reflect on their reasons for considering studying abroad, perhaps with the support of a counsellor or someone who knows them well. Some will simply relish the chance of the study and cultural opportunities that going abroad offers; they will just need to give some careful thought to what impact their condition is likely to have while abroad, and to check carefully whether the support they will need is available where they are thinking of going. But those who think that going abroad offers an opportunity to escape their problems, to 'start over' or become a 'new person', need to talk this over carefully with someone who can give professional advice, because if their motives for moving are to get away from aspects of themselves that they do not like, then they are almost certain to discover that these come too...

17.5.4 Access to NHS Medical and Mental Health Services

One of the differences that international students tend to underestimate when it comes to health and mental health issues is the role of the NHS in the United Kingdom. Coming from countries where medicine is primarily private and funded either by the patient or medical insurance, the contrast is considerable, so this section gives a brief overview of how NHS services work.

NHS services are paid for from central taxation and all UK citizens have access to the range of services provided. International students are also eligible to use NHS services if they are registered on a course lasting more than 6 months (in Scotland: if registered on a full-time course, no matter how long).[16] Those on a course lasting less than 6 months may still be eligible to access NHS services if they come from a country that has reciprocal healthcare arrangements with the United Kingdom.[17] Those who are not eligible will have to pay the full cost of any treatment, and as this can be expensive it is advisable to have health insurance and to check what it will cover whilst in the United Kingdom. Even those who are able to access NHS services will find that this does not mean that all health care is free of charge, for example:

- Although consulting an NHS doctor is free, there is a standard charge for any medication that is prescribed

- There are charges for eye-tests and glasses, for dental treatments, and for various other types of medical care.

The key to accessing NHS services is for a student to register with a GP. Some universities will have a GP practice on campus, but if not, the institution will be able to advise on the local options. They should do this as soon as they arrive and not wait until they are ill or in need of treatment. Registering will result in the student receiving an NHS card, which they will need to access treatment.

---

[16] Correct as at Feb 2009.

[17] See: www.nhs.uk/Healthcareabroad/Pages/Healthcareabroad.aspx

Not only is the GP the starting point for registering with the NHS, a GP is also the starting point for accessing most NHS services – for example, people cannot normally see an NHS psychiatrist without being referred by their GP. Students from some countries, particularly the United States, may find this strange, but it springs from general principles that underlie the NHS:

- GPs have clinical responsibility for all their patients' medical needs, and whatever level or type of treatment is needed, the GP is aware of this and has usually made the necessary referrals, and it is the GP who keeps patients' medical notes.

- The UK government is keen for as much medical care as possible to be delivered by 'primary care', that is by GP practices. This means that it is increasingly common for GP practices to be staffed by a wide range of medical professionals and for anything from simple prescriptions of medication to minor surgical procedures to be undertaken within the practice.

Although GPs are generalists, when it comes to mental health, it is normal for GPs to be the people who prescribe antidepressants or other common forms of psychotropic medication. Referral to a psychiatrist is only likely to happen when things get more serious (e.g. possible psychosis) or where in-patient treatment is needed ('secondary' or 'tertiary care'). This doesn't mean to say that all GPs are equally expert in matters relating to mental health, and if a student feels that their GP does not adequately understand their situation, it is usually feasible for them to ask to see another GP within their GP practice or suggest that he or she refer them to a psychiatrist or another specialist.

When emergency medical treatment is needed, the student can:

- Telephone their GP practice or NHS Direct[18] for advice (which is accessible 24-hour)

- Go to the nearest Accident and Emergency department at a main hospital

- Phone the emergency services (dial 999 from any landline or cell phone in the United Kingdom) and ask for an ambulance.

Please note that trade names for many commonly used medications are often different in the United Kingdom from those in the United States, and students who are using prescription medication which they will need to get while in the United Kingdom, should make a note of its generic name or take its packet to their GP. Also note that a few medications that are commonly prescribed in the United States are not as easily accessed in the United Kingdom – prescriptions for attention deficit hyperactivity disorder medication being a case in point, as UK doctors and psychiatrists tend to be very cautious about prescribing these.

Private medical care does exist in the United Kingdom, and students who are not eligible for NHS services or prefer to see someone privately, can access these services so long as they have the financial resources. However, where students expect their health insurer to cover this cost, they should look carefully into what criteria apply to their insurance cover, as the differences in qualifications and licensure/accreditation between the United States and

---

[18] NHS Direct: tel: 0845 4647 (within the UK) or www.nhsdirect.nhs.uk

United Kingdom may well mean that the insurer will not pay for them to see the majority of therapists in the United Kingdom.

17.5.5 So, Is It Worth Coming?

International study offers students a wonderful opportunity to study new things, see a different part of the world and its culture and, perhaps just as importantly, to find out more about themselves. There are undoubtedly challenges and demands and there are likely to be some frustrations too if some of their hopes are not fulfilled. Students do need a degree of resilience, to be able to cope with the initial disorientation and be able to handle the inevitable frustrations. Those who are used to fairly intensive support for mental health issues need to think realistically and plan with care, as the loss of familiar support systems combined with the challenges mentioned can exacerbate such problems.

But the rewards can be considerable!

17.6 Conclusion – Where Does This Leave University Counselling?

The educational and developmental roots of university counselling in the United Kingdom are under pressure from several sides. The severity of the mental health problems that students are presenting at counselling services and the historically poor response of NHS mental health services to the student population have pushed university counselling services into a more medical area of work. Moreover, changes in disability legislation, which have encompassed more mental health issues over time, requires institutions to meet their duty of care to students coming within the legislation. Taken together, and over time, university counsellors have developed considerable expertise in responding to this client group, though they are often inadequately funded to do so properly. Yet, the heart of counselling work in universities remains close to the developmental and educational roots of the profession.

The growing influence of NICE on the treatment of common mental health conditions and the current roll-out of the IAPT programme are both promoting CBT as the treatment of choice, while this mode of working currently represents only a small minority of the counsellors working within university counselling services (or, indeed, elsewhere). And the coming registration of counselling and therapy under the HPC may also further push therapists in the United Kingdom working in all settings towards rather prescribed medical-model ways of working with clients.

Although counsellors working in colleges and universities are not employed by the NHS, they will in the main need to be registered professionals. In any case, they will not be able to turn a blind eye to the developments in the therapeutic world outside higher education. The question inevitably comes down to: what are universities employing their counsellors to do?

It seems likely that university counselling in the United Kingdom will soon find itself at a turning point, a moment of choice:

- Will counsellors be able to retain their traditional educational stance and meet the needs of the majority of the students who seek counselling?

  - That is: will universities be interested and able to continue to fund such work?

- Will counsellors continue to see their role extending to work with those students who have more serious mental health problems?

  - That is: will university counsellors be able to do this within the strictures of the NHS, NICE and regulation.

- And, perhaps most crucial of all: will counsellors in universities continue to be able to work right across this range, as they have been doing very ably for some while now?

This last position has much to commend it, but is likely to become much more difficult in the future. Those counselling services in UK universities that have already let go of the 'serious mental health' end of this work – for example where Mental Heath Advisors are located somewhere other than within the counselling service – appear to have already lost this option. But in so doing, they may have jeopardized their future, as university funding will inevitably follow the legal duty of care towards those with the most serious problems.

At this time in particular, we need to be looking to and learning from the experience of university counselling in the United States, where counselling practice has long been heavily influenced by medical insurers and legal constraints. Perhaps we can both learn the lessons and avoid the pitfalls. Time will tell.

References

1. Schwartz, A. (2006) Are college students more disturbed today? Stability in the acuity and qualitative character of psychopathology of college counseling center clients 1992–3 through 2001–2. *Journal of American College Health*, **54**(6).
2. The Children's Society (2009) A good childhood: searching for values in a competitive age. www.childrenssociety.org.uk.
3. Royal College of Psychiatry (2003) Report CR112 *The Mental Health of Students in Higher Education*. www.rcpsych.ac.uk/publications/collegereports/cr/cr112.aspx.

Index

This index was prepared by Neil Manley